"How might psychoanalytic ideas and thinking enhance our understanding and engagement with the creative arts and contemporary life? Based on the work of the longstanding Psychoanalytic Studies Course at the Tavistock, this book provides a surprisingly fresh approach to exploring this question.

Rarely have I read a book that so captured my imagination—exposing me to new and unexpected topics, such as BASE jumping or the inner world of littering, and to such culturally diverse subjects as a moving Palestinian poem or a chart-topping Korean pop video. Drawing on their experience of close observation of infants and psychoanalytic theory, the contributors to this book delve deep, eliciting the reader's engagement.

I loved it! It is relevant and accessible to anyone interested in thinking more deeply about complex states of mind and the world we live in."

—**Dr. Debbie Hindle**, *child and adolescent psychotherapist, Human Development Scotland*

"This book illustrates how psychoanalytic skills developed through the experience of infant observation can be used in many cultural contexts, from poetry and opera to music videos, extreme sports, and social work. The idea that artists and imaginative writers are primary researchers into the mind, exploring psychic change, is held in focus throughout.

The use of material from infant observations is moving and non-judgmental, clearly showing how the inner world of the observer is affected by the experience of observation. The book explores the value and use of these affective responses to further our understanding of human interaction and cultural experience, as well as offering pointers for how individuals and organizations can foster self-reflective practice, consider anti-oppressive approaches, face our own racism, and shift from tracking achievement of competence to understanding the process of learning, with all its uncertainties and anxieties.

This is important reading for those working in public and private sectors."

—**Susanne Lansman**, *PhD, poet, Fellow of the British Psychoanalytical Society*

EXPLORING PSYCHOANALYTIC CONCEPTS THROUGH CULTURE, THE ARTS, AND CONTEMPORARY LIFE

This book explores how psychoanalytic ideas and thinking enhance our understanding and engagement with the creative arts and contemporary life.

Many of us love to read poetry and novels and enjoy the performing arts. All of us take part in contemporary life. But how might a psychoanalytic perspective deepen our understanding or enhance our experience in these areas? What might we discover when we explore the unconscious dimensions of particular cultural artefacts and activities? Based on the work of the longstanding Psychoanalytic Studies course at the Tavistock, contributing authors draw on their experience of infant observation and psychoanalytic theory and apply them to explorations of culturally diverse and wide-ranging topics such as social work, literature, the act of littering, a Palestinian poem, and even a chart-topping Korean pop song.

Blending a deep understanding of clinical work and a broad range of artistic endeavours, this book will be key reading for psychoanalysts, psychotherapists, and anyone interested in understanding how psychoanalysis can inform art and life.

Dr Margaret Lush trained as a child and adolescent psychotherapist at the Tavistock and has worked in clinical and educational settings. She has taught on several Tavistock courses and is currently Joint Course Lead for the Tavistock pre-clinical training course for child psychotherapists. She works in private practice and supervises in Britain and abroad.

Kate Robertson trained as a child and adolescent psychotherapist at the Tavistock and became Head of Child Psychotherapy in Hammersmith and Fulham CAMHS, Course Lead for the Tavistock Psychoanalytic Studies course, and Chair of the Association of Child Psychotherapists. She had to retire early because of health concerns and passed away in October 2023.

Tavistock Clinic Series

Founding Editor: Margot Waddell,
Series Editors: Jocelyn Catty & Kate Stratton

Titles in the Tavistock Clinic Series include:

A for Adoption: An Exploration of the Adoption Experience for Families and Professionals, *by Alison Roy*
Assessment in Child Psychotherapy, *edited by Margaret Rustin & Emanuela Quagliata*
Childhood Depression: A Place for Psychotherapy, *edited by Judith Trowell, with Gillian Miles*
Child Psychoanalytic Psychotherapy in Primary Schools: Tavistock Approaches, *edited by Katie Argent*
Complex Trauma: The Tavistock Model, *edited by Joanne Stubley & Linda Young*
Conjunctions: Social Work, Psychoanalysis, and Society, *by Andrew Cooper*
Couple Dynamics: Psychoanalytic Perspectives in Work with the Individual, the Couple, and the Group, *edited by Aleksandra Novakovic*
Doing Things Differently: The Influence of Donald Meltzer on Psychoanalytic Theory and Practice, *edited by Margaret Cohen & Alberto Hahn*
Group Relations and Other Meditations: Psychoanalytic Explorations on the Uncertainties of Experiential Learning, *by Carlos Sapochnik*
Inside Lives: Psychoanalysis and the Growth of the Personality, *by Margot Waddell*
Internal Landscapes and Foreign Bodies: Eating Disorders and Other Pathologies, *by Gianna Williams*
Melanie Klein Revisited: Pioneer and Revolutionary in the Psychoanalysis of Young Children, *by Susan Sherwin-White*
Mourning and Metabolization: Close Readings in the Psychoanalytic Literature of Loss, *by Rael Meyerowitz*
New Discoveries in Child Psychotherapy: Findings from Qualitative Research, *edited by Margaret Rustin & Michael Rustin*
On Adolescence: Inside Stories, *by Margot Waddell*
Organization in the Mind: Psychoanalysis, Group Relations, and Organizational Consultancy, *by David Armstrong, edited by Robert French*
Perspectives from a Psych-Oncology Team Working with Teenagers and Young Adults with Cancer: Thrown Off Course, *edited by Jane Elfer*
Psychoanalysis and Culture: A Kleinian Perspective, *edited by David Bell*
Researching the Unconscious: Principles of Psychoanalytic Method, *by Michael Rustin*
Sexuality and Gender Now: Moving Beyond Heteronormativity, *edited by Leezah Hertzmann & Juliet Newbigin*
Short-Term Psychoanalytic Psychotherapy for Adolescents with Depression: A Treatment Manual, *edited by Jocelyn Catty*
Surviving Space: Papers on Infant Observation, *edited by Andrew Briggs*
Sustaining Depth and Meaning in School Leadership: Keeping Your Head, *edited by Emil Jackson & Andrea Berkeley*
The Anorexic Mind, *by Marilyn Lawrence*
The Learning Relationship: Psychoanalytic Thinking in Education, *edited by Biddy Youell*
Therapeutic Care for Refugees: No Place Like Home, *edited by Renos Papadopoulos*
Therapeutic Interventions with Babies and Young Children in Care: Observation and Attention, *by Jenifer Wakelyn*
Thinking Space: Promoting Thinking about Race, Culture, and Diversity in Psychotherapy and Beyond, *edited by Frank Lowe*
Turning the Tide: A Psychoanalytic Approach to Mental Illness. The Work of the Fitzjohn's Unit, *edited by Rael Meyerowitz & David Bell*
Understanding Trauma: A Psychoanalytic Approach, *edited by Caroline Garland*
Waiting to Be Found: Papers on Children in Care, *edited by Andrew Briggs*

EXPLORING PSYCHOANALYTIC CONCEPTS THROUGH CULTURE, THE ARTS, AND CONTEMPORARY LIFE

Learning from Observation and Experience

Edited by

Margaret Lush & Kate Robertson

Routledge
Taylor & Francis Group
LONDON AND NEW YORK

Designed cover image: © Courtesy of The Artist and The Modern Institute/
Toby Webster Ltd, Glasgow Photo Cristiano Corte

First published 2025
by Routledge
4 Park Square, Milton Park, Abingdon, Oxon OX14 4RN

and by Routledge
605 Third Avenue, New York, NY 10158

Routledge is an imprint of the Taylor & Francis Group, an informa business

British Library Cataloguing-in-Publication Data
A catalogue record for this book is available from the British Library

Library of Congress Cataloging-in-Publication Data
Names: Lush, Margaret, editor. | Robertson, Kate, –2023, editor.
Title: Exploring psychoanalytic concepts through culture, the arts and contemporary life : learning from observation and experience / edited by Margaret Lush and Kate Robertson.
Description: Abingdon, Oxon ; New York, NY : Routledge, 2025. | Series: Tavistock clinical series | Includes bibliographical references and index.
Identifiers: LCCN 2024036721 (print) | LCCN 2024036722 (ebook) | ISBN 9781032932019 (hardback) | ISBN 9781032932002 (paperback) | ISBN 9781003564867 (ebook)
Subjects: LCSH: Psychoanalysis. | Psychoanalysis and culture. | Psychoanalysis and the arts.
Classification: LCC BF175 .E88 2025 (print) | LCC BF175 (ebook) | DDC 150.19/5—dc23/eng/20241107
LC record available at https://lccn.loc.gov/2024036721
LC ebook record available at https://lccn.loc.gov/2024036722

ISBN: 978-1-032-93201-9 (hbk)
ISBN: 978-1-032-93200-2 (pbk)
ISBN: 978-1-003-56486-7 (ebk)

DOI: 10.4324/9781003564867

Typeset in Palatino
by Apex CoVantage, LLC

In memory of my co-editor and friend Kate Robertson,
17th January 1958—11th October 2023

CONTENTS

SERIES EDITORS' PREFACE

Since it was founded in 1920, the Tavistock Clinic—now the Tavistock and Portman NHS Foundation Trust—has developed a wide range of developmental approaches to mental health which have been strongly influenced by the ideas of psychoanalysis. It has also adopted systemic family therapy as a theoretical model and a clinical approach to family problems. The Tavistock is now one of the largest mental health training institutions in Britain. It teaches up to 600 students a year on postgraduate, doctoral, and qualifying courses in social work, systemic psychotherapy, psychology, psychiatry, nursing, and child, adolescent, and adult psychotherapy, along with 2,000 multidisciplinary clinicians, social workers, and teachers attending Continuing Professional Development courses and conferences on psychoanalytic observation, psychoanalytic thinking, and management and leadership in a range of clinical and community settings.

The Tavistock's philosophy aims at promoting therapeutic methods in mental health. Its work is based on the clinical expertise that is also the basis of its consultancy and research activities. The aim of this Series is to make available to the reading public the clinical, theoretical, and research work that is most influential at the Tavistock. The Series sets out new approaches in the understanding and treatment of psychological disturbance in children, adolescents, and adults, both as individuals and in families.

In *Exploring Psychoanalytic Concepts through Culture, the Arts, and Contemporary Life: Learning from Observation and Experience*, Margaret Lush and Kate Robertson draw on the work of a longstanding Tavistock master's degree course in order to explore the different ways in which psychoanalysis can "illuminate aspects of cultural and contemporary life beyond the consulting room". The Psychoanalytic Studies course, which Robertson led for many years and on which Lush herself taught, has been influential in introducing psychoanalysis to generations of students from a range of professional backgrounds, many of whom have gone on to clinical training themselves. As Lush and Robertson make clear in this edited collection, the course is a rich opportunity for students and teachers alike to explore the interrelationship between psychoanalysis and culture in its many forms. Some of the teachers on the course contributed chapters to describe the pedagogical endeavour involved here: helping students to explore the ways in which psychoanalytic thinking may open up areas of understanding of cultural life, and vice versa. The remainder of the chapters, written by former students, some returning to earlier work after many years' experience, bring into vivid colour the diverse ways in which they have applied this learning, both on the course itself and since. Some contributors are returning to their work after as much as 20 years' professional experience, illustrating the far-reaching influence of the course, and the Tavistock, in the minds of its former students.

The book is divided into four parts reflecting different areas of cultural experience, each introduced by Margaret Lush. The first part, "Learning through Infant Observation", begins with a chapter by Barbara Segal on teaching infant observation in a way that may enable students to internalize the observational stance and take it into other areas of enquiry. The chapters that follow range from accounts of an infant observation (by the late Jenny Abbott), to readings of a nursery rhyme (Tsutomu Ichige) and of an art installation (Deirdre Ingham), to reflections on the nature of observation itself and how it can inform a career (Olivia Sagan). Part II, on poetry, begins with a contribution by Judith Edwards on the ways in which the two disciplines may be experienced as "in orbit". Anne Kane and Elina Matter then contribute chapters on Jo Shapcott and the Palestinian poet Mahmoud Darwish, respectively. The third part, "Literature and the Performing Arts", starts with Michael Rustin's account of the seminar series he ran for many years on psychoanalysis, drama, and society. This is followed by chapters on Beckett's *Rockaby* (Maryam Ghasemi), Puccini's *Turandot* (Tomaso Quaini), and the novels of Kazuo Ishiguro (by the late Diana Webster Thomas). The final part, "Contemporary Life", picks up on the diverse ways in which former students of the course have used its learning in the service of understanding contemporary culture, from a pop song (in an analysis by Yong Suk Lee), to BASE jumping (Gabrielle Smith), to littering (Leila Taheri). This part closes with an account by Clare Parkinson, until her recent retirement a Senior Social Worker and lecturer at the Tavistock, of the ways in which the social work profession, and the learning endeavour within it, may be illuminated by psychoanalytic theory and practice.

Exploring Psychoanalytic Concepts thus captures something essential about the Tavistock's endeavour. It follows a tradition of psychoanalytic writing about cultural life that has been a central feature of the Series,[1] and indeed also of the work of its founder, Margot Waddell. Waddell (who presided over the Series from its inception and is now named as its Founding Editor) has done a great deal to integrate a literary sensibility with psychoanalytic understanding in her books[2] and numerous papers. Waddell writes about "the triumph of the human spirit . . . founded in some of the kinds of thinking that lie at the heart of creative expression, whether in painting, literature, music, sculpture or . . . in the psychoanalytic process itself".[3] Something of this triumph is evident in *Exploring Psychoanalytic Concepts*, in the ways in which its contributors' close attention to different cultural artefacts and practices have brought them to life in such vivid ways, producing an "expansion of meaning, the expansion of the understanding of oneself and of others, of one's being in the world".[4]

The book's engagement with cultural experience sits alongside some significant losses. Two of the contributors, Jenny Abbott and Diana Webster Thomas, died before the book went to press. And Kate Robertson, who conceived of the book along with Margaret Lush and did so much to inspire both the Psychoanalytic Studies students and the contributors to this book, died in 2023. Margaret Lush pays testament to Kate Robertson's role in the genesis and development of *Exploring Psychoanalytic Concepts* in her Afterword, as well as dedicating the book to her.

Notes

1 D. Bell (Ed.), *Psychoanalysis and Culture: A Kleinian Perspective* (London: Karnac, 1999). M. Rustin & M. Rustin, *Mirror to Nature: Drama, Psychoanalysis and Society* (London: Karnac, 2002). H. Canham & C. Satyamurti (Eds.), *Acquainted with the Night: Psychoanalysis and the Poetic Imagination* (London: Karnac, 2003).

2 M. Waddell, *Inside Lives: Psychoanalysis and the Growth of the Personality* (London: Routledge, 2002). M. Harris Williams & M. Waddell, *The Chamber of Maiden Thought: Literary Origins of the Psychoanalytic Model of the Mind*

(London: Routledge, 2013). M. Waddell, *On Adolescence: Inside Stories* (London: Routledge, 2018).

3 M. Waddell, "All the light we cannot see": Psychoanalytic and poetic reflections on the nature of hope. *International Journal of Psychoanalysis, 100* (2019, No. 6), p. 1408.

4 Waddell, "All the light we cannot see", p. 1410.

ACKNOWLEDGEMENTS

I am grateful to have been involved in the Tavistock Psychoanalytic Studies course over a number of years, from 2013 on. I can confidently express similar gratitude on behalf of my co-editor, Kate Robertson, as the many conversations we had during her lifetime confirmed that we shared a love of the course and found working with the students and staff intellectually stimulating and emotionally rewarding.

I would like to thank the parents of the observed infants, who have generously allowed us to include observational material and, in the case of "Sam" (Chapter 2), have agreed to us including the observer's paper, written as her regular visits to the family drew to an end.

Special thanks are owed to the contributors—the former students and staff who worked hard to write new material or to develop and adapt their original work to create the chapters. They have all been endlessly patient and responsive to the many small queries that inevitably arose during the process of compiling and editing the book.

Michael and Margaret Rustin have been deeply involved in the Psychoanalytic Studies course from its beginning, and, in addition to acknowledging that work, I would also like to highlight their exceptional contribution to the psychoanalytic thinking at the Tavistock more broadly over such a long period. Many, including the editors of this book, have learnt, and continue to learn, so much from them.

Many thanks are due to the dedicated editorial team, Aakriti Aggarwal and Kate Hawes, as well as Eric and Klara King who brought their long experience and meticulous attention to detail to the process.

The editors of the Tavistock Clinic Series, Jocelyn Catty and Kate Stratton, have been hugely encouraging, particularly when the task of completing the book fell solely to me, and I am grateful for their astute feedback. I am proud that this is the first book in the Series where Margot Waddell's role is honoured with the title "Founding Editor". Hers is indeed a valuable legacy.

Margaret Lush

ABOUT THE EDITORS AND CONTRIBUTORS

Jenny Abbott was a BAFTA-nominated documentary maker at the BBC, responsible for series such as *Reputations*, *Great Britons*, *Nurses*, and *Living with Cancer*. Having completed her Masters in Psychoanalytic Studies at the Tavistock, she was in training at the Institute to become a psychoanalyst when she was diagnosed with Stage 4 lung cancer. She died in 2021, having founded a charity, EGFR Positive UK, to provide support to patients with her lung cancer mutation.

Judith Edwards is a retired consultant child and adolescent psychotherapist who has taught and supervised on various courses at the Tavistock since the 1980s. She was course lead for the Tavistock's Psychoanalytic Studies course for ten years, until July 2011; since retirement, she has worked there as a visiting lecturer and also at Roehampton University. A past editor of the *Journal of Child Psychotherapy,* she has edited and published several academic books internationally, including *Being Alive: Building on the Work of Anne Alvarez* (2001), *Psychoanalysis and Other Matters* (2019), and *Grandmotherland* (2023). Apart from her clinical experience over the years, one of her principal interests has been in the links between psychoanalysis, culture, and the arts, and in 2010 she was awarded the Jan Lee memorial prize for the best paper linking psychoanalysis and the arts during that year.

Maryam Ghasemi has a background in sociology and social research and has studied and worked within the field in Iran, Sweden, and the UK. She then embarked on a training in the British Object Relations tradition of psychoanalysis in London and has worked as a psychoanalytic psychotherapist in the NHS, in third-sector organizations, and in private practice. She currently lives in London and works at the Fitzjohn's Unit at the Tavistock and Portman NHS Foundation Trust. She is also in the process of completing a training in Lacanian psychoanalysis.

Tsutomu Ichige is a Japanese clinical psychologist. After postgraduate training in child psychotherapy, he worked as a child and adult psychotherapist in a psychiatric clinic, psychological assessment, and psychiatric rehabilitation. He then moved to the UK, where he studied on the Psychoanalytic Studies course at the Tavistock. Since returning to Japan, he has been engaged in clinical practice in a child psychiatry clinic.

Deirdre Ingham is an IPCAPA-qualified child and adolescent psychoanalytic psychotherapist. In her earlier career, she studied art at Nottingham Trent University and trained as an art psychotherapist at the University of Sheffield. She currently works as a parent–infant psychotherapist in a perinatal mental health team in London. Alongside her clinical work, she teaches on the doctorate course in Child Psychotherapy at IPCAPA, and on the MSc Psychodynamics of Human Development at the British Psychotherapy Foundation. She has an ongoing interest in the relationship between psychoanalysis, art, and early infancy.

Anne Kane is a psychoanalytic psychotherapist who trained at the Association for Group and Individual Psychotherapy (AGIP) after completing the Psychoanalytic Studies Masters course at the Tavistock. She also teaches and provides supervision. Before formally pursuing an interest in psychoanalysis, she worked for many years in social justice and equality policy, research, and campaigns. She has a particular interest in disability discrimination and disablement as part of a wider interest in how psychoanalysis can help understand and combat the dynamics of prejudice and the resilience of structural discrimination.

Yong Suk Lee is a psychiatrist in South Korea who studied medicine and psychiatry at the Ajou University School of Medicine. He worked as a psychiatrist in Yongin Mental Hospital and as a director in the Community Mental Health Centre in Yongin-Si. After gaining his Masters in Psychoanalytic Studies at the Tavistock, he now works in private practice and teaches as an advisory professor for psychiatric residents at Ajou University Hospital. He is a Member of the Korean Association of Psychoanalytic Treatment and the Korean Neuropsychiatric Association.

Margaret Lush is a Tavistock-trained child and adolescent psychotherapist with a background in music and a strong interest in the arts. She has worked in various clinical and educational settings, including, over a long period, at Gloucester House, the Tavistock Children's Day Unit. She was Book Reviews Editor of the *Journal of Child Psychotherapy* for many years. She has taught on several of the Tavistock courses and is currently Joint Course Lead for Perinatal, Child, Adolescent and Family Work: A Psychoanalytic Observational Approach, an applied course that also forms the pre-clinical training for child psychotherapists. She works in private practice and supervises trainees and clinicians in Britain and abroad.

Elina Matter is a Research Associate with a multidisciplinary background, including a Bachelor's of Liberal Arts from King's College London, an MSc in Psychology, and an MSc in Mental Health Research from the University of Nottingham. Elina has extensive mental health research experience having worked on National Institute for Health and Care Research–funded projects focused on the experiences of parents of young people with self-harm and suicidal behaviour. She was a student on the Psychoanalytic Studies course at the Tavistock in 2017, where she is now also a visiting lecturer teaching the Poetry Applications unit.

Clare Parkinson is a social worker and social work academic. Over two decades she has taught social work students from qualifying to doctoral level at the University of East London and the Tavistock. She is proud to be in the class of '95, which is the first cohort to have completed the Tavistock Masters in Psychoanalytic Studies.

Tomaso Quaini is an Italian psychologist with a passion for art in its different forms. Following his professional qualification, he moved to London, where he pursued his interest in psychoanalysis. He was a student on the Psychoanalytic Studies course at the Tavistock and Portman NHS Foundation Trust and was awarded his Masters in 2015. He is currently training as child and adolescent psychotherapist at the Tavistock.

Kate Robertson trained as a child and adolescent psychotherapist at the Tavistock and was deeply committed to working with troubled young people in the public sector. After working in various clinical and education settings, she become Head of the Child Psychotherapy Discipline in the Child and Adolescent Mental Health Service in Hammersmith and Fulham in 2012. She took over from Judith Edwards as course lead for the Tavistock Psychoanalytic Studies course in 2011, remaining in that role until 2018. From 2020 on she was Chair of the Association of Child Psychotherapists, where she had a particular interest in promoting diversity within the profession. She left that role at the beginning of 2023 because of ill health, and she died in October 2023.

Michael Rustin is a Professor of Sociology at the University of East London, a Visiting Professor at the Tavistock and Portman NHS Foundation Trust, and an Associate of the British Psychoanalytical Society. He has taught on the Tavistock's Psychoanalytic Studies course since it began. He has written widely about psychoanalysis and its social, political, and cultural applications. His books include *The Good Society and the Inner World* (1991); *Researching the Unconscious* (2019); *The Inner World of Doctor Who,* with Iain MacRury (2014); and, with Margaret Rustin, *Narratives of Love and Loss: Studies in Modern Children's Fiction* (1987/2002), *Mirror to Nature: Drama, Psychoanalysis and Society* (2002), and *Reading Klein* (2017).

Olivia Sagan is Head of Division of Psychology, Sociology and Education and is also currently Director of the Centre for Applied Social Sciences at Queen Margaret University Edinburgh. Her area of research expertise lies in phenomenological qualitative research, exploring first-person narrative of mental distress and its interface with creative expression and autonomous strategies for wellbeing. Her most recent work has been focused on exploring the experience of loneliness within mental illness and how individuals arrive at a range of strategies to work with this phenomenon and derive meaning and insight from it.

Barbara Segal is a consultant child and adolescent psychotherapist who trained at the Tavistock. Her background is in English Literature and Drama, which she studied at the University of Cape Town, South Africa. She worked at Great Ormond Street Hospital and then University College Hospital, London, where she worked on the Teenage Cancer Trust Unit. She became Head of Child Psychotherapy Services, continuing to develop the tradition of paediatric liaison work at UCLH until her retirement from the NHS in 2010. She continues to see patients privately and to teach and supervise in London and abroad.

Gabrielle Smith is an Australian-born, London-based assistant editor working in film and television. Her film credits include *The Full Monty, Atonement, Slow West,* and *Three Billboards Outside Ebbing Missouri.* She completed the Foundation Course at the Institute of Psychoanalysis in 2011 and an MA in Psychoanalytic Studies at the Tavistock and Portman NHS Foundation Trust in 2013. She volunteered for several years for MIND in Camden. She is currently a story editor for the podcast *No Laughing Matter.*

Leila Taheri is a creative director working in advertising. In parallel, she leads Friends of the Welsh Harp, a grassroots group caring for the Welsh Harp (Brent Reservoir) in North West London. She has a Masters in Psychoanalytic Studies, focusing her dissertation on the hidden inner world of littering. She has been featured on BBC News, BBC World Service, ITV, in *The Guardian,* and local media outlets for her work. She is a founding member of Edgy Collective, a storytelling and design collective reimagining public spaces. Leila also runs nature workshops for children, with the aim of creating deep and lasting imaginative connections.

Diana Webster Thomas was a student on the Psychoanalytic Studies course at the Tavistock and the University of East London. Her professional work, before her retirement, was as a teacher of English. After completing her Master's degree she undertook a PhD at the University of East London, which she was awarded in 2013. Her thesis is an original application of post-Kleinian psychoanalytic thinking to understand the novels of Kazuo Ishiguro. It contains a substantial discussion of the literary context of Ishiguro's work, the psychoanalytic theory that underpins her analysis of it, and a detailed analysis of the six of Ishiguro's novels that were in publication at the time of her research. Her contribution to this book is an abridged version of her Introduction to her thesis and its chapter on *The Remains of the Day,* which has been chosen as one of the best known of Ishiguro's novels.

Introduction

For many people, their image of psychoanalysis is of a patient lying on a couch watched over by a psychoanalyst, possibly Freud himself, sitting behind the patient's head and listening attentively. That could be described as the classic picture of clinical psychoanalysis in the popular imagination, and it does indeed represent the traditional psychoanalytic setting that remains the cornerstone of psychoanalytic practice today. The image shows clinical psychoanalysis as predominantly a two-person endeavour, taking place within the quiet and privacy of the consulting room.

Although psychoanalytic theory, including the many theoretical advances that have come about through psychoanalysts' experience with their patients, provides the underlying framework of the chapters in this book, our focus is not on the practice and method of clinical psychoanalysis. Rather, the volume is concerned with a different but related area, which we would describe as making use of psychoanalysis to illuminate aspects of cultural and contemporary life beyond the consulting room. Embedded in the ethos of the book, and the Tavistock Psychoanalytic Studies course it grew out of, is the recognition that drawing on psychoanalytic thinking in this way is a valuable pursuit in its own right.

The Psychoanalytic Studies course (known within the Tavistock's portfolio of courses as M16) is a non-clinical Masters course where the emphasis is on learning from experience and on giving students the

DOI: 10.4324/9781003564867-1

opportunity to bring their developing psychoanalytic thinking to the arts, poetry, literature, society, and, more widely, any activity that humans are involved in. In contrast to the dyadic nature of clinical psychoanalysis, within the course ideas are generated and considered predominantly in small seminar groups, where the seminar leader and the student group think together to make sense of their object of study.

Linked with the particular sort of learning the course encourages is the distinctive approach to teaching it necessitates, and, in addition to the focus on psychoanalytic thinking in relation to the arts and contemporary life, this volume is also concerned with exploring the nature and quality of learning and teaching on the course. In other words, we are also interested in how students are taught the value of psychoanalysis in illuminating aspects of cultural life.

The idea of compiling the book was born during the time that Kate Robertson was the Psychoanalytic Studies Course Lead, and Margaret Lush was a tutor and dissertation supervisor. We were consistently impressed by the quality of much of the work done by the students, which was original and creative and offered a fresh perspective on a wide range of topics. The way the course is structured means that there is considerable scope for students to follow their own interests and to choose where to direct their developing psychoanalytic gaze, and this contributes to the range of subjects explored in their written work. We believe that the resulting work deserves a wider readership and will be of interest to many outside the course. Although students' and former students' work is rarely showcased in this way, we wanted their work to form the main content of the book, framed and set in context by three chapters by course staff.

We envisage that the book will appeal to students of psychoanalysis, anyone interested in thinking about the arts from a psychoanalytic perspective, and students of infant observation, interested in the process of observation itself and how skills developed through infant observation become embedded and available for use by the student in other contexts. As some readers may be unfamiliar with psychoanalytic ideas, we have included an Appendix, which gives a brief explanation of some fundamental psychoanalytic concepts referred to in the chapters.

It is important to note that, unlike many of the Tavistock courses, Psychoanalytic Studies is a non-clinical course, which means that students are not training to be psychoanalysts or psychotherapists at this point, although some may subsequently go on to a clinical training. The course offers an introduction to psychoanalytic ideas and psychoanalytic thinking and is open to applicants from any professional background. Students come from diverse backgrounds and professional fields, are at different stages in their careers, and cover the age range from the early twenties to after retirement. In recent years there have been increasing numbers of international students, and this diversity has added to the rich inter-disciplinary mix.

Some students come to the course with a basic knowledge of psychoanalytic ideas, some have an interest but little knowledge, others might have become interested in psychoanalytic theory as a result of being in analysis themselves. Many are highly accomplished within their subject or professional field—for example, English Literature—and are interested to find out how psychoanalytic thinking might add another dimension to their work. The cohort often includes psychotherapists or counsellors who want to learn more about a psychoanalytic approach. It is a reasonably short course—only one year of full-time study or two years part-time—and we have found it remarkable that students are often able to make sophisticated use of complex psychoanalytic thinking within such a short time.

Any course working with non-clinical psychoanalytic students faces the challenge of how to teach them effectively, as the traditional home of psychoanalysis is, as we noted at the outset, the clinical setting of the consulting room. This has been called "the laboratory" (M. J. Rustin, 2001, 2019a), where psychoanalytic understanding has been developed and psychoanalytic concepts have been refined over time through close attention to patients' presentations and the material they bring into the session. In a clinical training the students learn psychoanalytic theory, and this gives a vital theoretical framework, but much of their learning takes place through working with carefully selected patients and the close supervision that goes alongside. Clinical students learn about their own unconscious processes through experience of personal analysis. Michael Rustin likens the training of psychoanalytic child and adolescent psychotherapists to a craft apprenticeship (M. J. Rustin, 2007): the trainee is learning through doing and, in this way, learning from experience. However, students on a non-clinical course don't see patients, nor do they have to be in analysis.

This situation brings a certain set of challenges for teachers, and our experience is that the course has been a fertile ground for staff to develop their thinking and their skills in teaching students about the relationship between psychoanalysis and different aspects of cultural and contemporary life. We see this as fundamental to the students' engagement with the task, and we believe that the distinctive approach and quality of the teaching play a large part in the production of the wide range and high standard of the student work.

Although in the early days of psychoanalysis its method was to delve into the patient's past to uncover the origins of conflicts and neuroses, it is, as it is practised today, concerned more with the activity of the unconscious mind and emotional experience in the "here and now". The patient's internal world (see Appendix, "1. The inner world and the good object") and states of mind are explored as they reveal themselves in the analytic session and, particularly, within the patient's relationship to the analyst.

The course name, "Psychoanalytic Studies", might suggest something purely theoretical and academic. The students could learn *about* psychoanalytic theory by studying the works of Freud, Klein, and later theorists, as they do in the theoretical strand, and that would be interesting and intellectually stimulating. However, if that made up the entire content of the course, the students would be engaged in a primarily cognitive rather than experiential and emotional process, and, importantly, their learning would not encompass the essence of psychoanalysis. The psychoanalyst Wilfred Bion emphasized the importance of learning from experience as a genuine form of learning that takes root securely in the mind, and he conceptualized the process that needs to take place between a mother (or primary caregiver) and the infant in order for the infant to develop the capacity to really learn from experience (Bion, 1962a) (see Appendix, "4. Containment"). This genuine learning has a very different quality from rote learning or acquiring and remembering facts.

The course started as a collaboration between the Tavistock Clinic and the University of East London, with the aim of creating a psychoanalytic course that was also interdisciplinary. This relationship enabled the course to draw on staff from a range of professional and academic backgrounds: the Tavistock provided psychoanalytic clinicians who had a strong interest in literature or the arts, and they were joined by academics from the university who combined expertise in a particular subject area with an interest in and knowledge of psychoanalysis. The course was set up as a structure with three main strands—Infant Observation, Applications, and Psychoanalytic Theory—and it is in the Applications strand where the interdisciplinary approach is most embedded. Although subsequent course leads have developed the course in their own ways, this tripartite structure continues, and we believe that it is the combination of these three elements that creates the conditions for such creative and original work to be produced.

Learning from experience is central in the infant observational process, where students learn, through spending one hour a week in the family home over an extended period, how mothers and babies relate within their nuclear and extended families. Student observers develop an increased understanding of what goes on underneath the surface, and they see how the baby's personality is shaped by the individual and unique relational experiences he has. As is described in Chapter 1, the small infant observation seminar groups are run by child and adolescent psychotherapists, and students are encouraged to observe closely and record what they notice in increasing detail, but also to be alert to their own emotional experience. The process helps students develop those capacities over time, and, with the aid of the seminar group, they become more adept at using their emotional experience to help make sense of unconscious processes. Unconscious processes will be at play in the infant's mind, within the infant–mother relationship, within the dynamics of other family relationships, and, importantly, also between the observer and the observed. The observer has the experience of being in the presence of early and primitive states of mind, and much of the communication is nonverbal. The student observes within the same family for one academic year and over this period comes to understand how a personality is formed through complex interactions between the infant's innate constitution, experiences within his earliest relationships in a changing societal context, and his capacity to make use of what's available to him. The student comes out of the course understanding that there is not a single self, but that the self is multifaceted and states of mind are fluid.

Traditionally there has been a marked divide between "clinical psychoanalysis", which, as described, refers to analysis that takes place inside the consulting room, and "applied psychoanalysis", the term given to psychoanalytic thinking outside the consulting room. In their introduction to *The Culture-Breast in Psychoanalysis* (Giffney, 2021), Bainbridge and Yates (both of whom have taught on the Psychoanalytic Studies course) draw attention to "the complex debate that has been long been raging between psychoanalysis as a 'pure' form of clinical practice and the application of psychoanalytic concepts, theories and strategies to the experience of the cultural and social environment" (Bainbridge & Yates, 2021, p. xvi).

The idea of the "application" of psychoanalytic ideas gives rise to two questions. First, what is the nature of the model being applied, and, second, what is the nature of the application?

The model is the British Object Relations school of psychoanalysis, the main proponents of which were Melanie Klein, followed by post-Kleinians, notably Bion, Segal, Rosenfeld, Britton, and Steiner. This Kleinian tradition also forms the bedrock of the Tavistock clinical psychoanalytic courses. The theory strand forms a third of the course, and the first year is spent studying Freud, with the opportunity to learn about the beginning of the psychoanalytic approach and to follow the development of Freud's thinking. The course starts by considering Freud's position and the particular standpoint that shaped his worldview; the birth of psychoanalysis is placed within Freud's cultural context as a Jewish man in "*fin de siècle*" Vienna. As the development of Freud's thinking is followed closely in this way, what becomes clear is how open he was to his experience.

Freud, Klein, and the post-Kleinians are taught in the theory module and provide the main theoretical framework underlying the essays here. (Brief explanations of some of the main Kleinian concepts and post-Kleinian developments drawn on in these essays are given in the Appendix.) Students are also introduced to Winnicott's work, and there is some inclusion of Lacan and Anna Freud in the theory syllabus.

The word "application" could evoke particular and perhaps misleading associations—the application of paint to a wall might come to mind. One might wonder whether the approach is to "put psychoanalytic concepts onto" the subject being explored.

However, the relationship between the psychoanalytic perspective and the object or area being studied is considerably more nuanced than that, and the complexity of this relationship has particularly interested some course staff. Many writers point to early examples of the application of psychoanalytic thinking—the well-known studies by Freud of Leonardo (1910c) and Michelangelo (1914b)—that "focus on the artist's personality, what is known about his life and what can be inferred from his work" (M. J. Rustin, 2019a, p. 270). Since Freud's time, psychoanalytic writers have considered a variety of approaches to literary or artistic works, and methods continue to develop.

Baudry (1984) classified four main psychoanalytic approaches to a literary text,

1. The analyst interprets a literary work as a case history.
2. He associates it with the mind of the author.
3. He deals with the text in its own right. It is related to some mental phenomena—for example, the primal scene.
4. He focuses on the aesthetic response of the reader.

There are a number of units within the Applications strand, including drama, poetry, literature, art, music, and film. There is also a social and political unit that tackles subjects such as climate change and racism. Partly through his involvement with the course over many years, Michael Rustin has developed his view of how we can understand the relationship between psychoanalysts and the cultural artefacts they are studying. He has explored this relationship in depth in his chapter, "Psychoanalytic Cultural Methods", in *Researching the Unconscious* (M. J. Rustin, 2019a). He notes that the psychoanalyst in the consulting room is concerned with unconscious phenomena, and he wonders whether cultural artefacts or their creators "have an 'unconscious' dimension that psychoanalysts are in a privileged position to understand" (p. 270). However, he believes that the relationship between psychoanalysts and their patients is different from the relationship between psychoanalysts and cultural objects they study; he describes this difference: "[A]rtists are themselves creators of understanding with the ability to understand and describe the phenomena of unconscious mental life as great and often greater than psychoanalysts" (p. 270).

Rustin draws attention to the well-known exchange between Freud and a speaker at his 70th birthday, who said that the founder of psychoanalysis was "discoverer of the unconscious". Freud immediately corrected this view, and responded: "The poets and philosophers before me discovered the unconscious . . . what I discovered was the scientific method by which the unconscious could be studied" (p. 270). Rustin points out, therefore, that artists and imaginative writers should be seen as primary researchers into the mind, as psychoanalysts are themselves, and he sees no hierarchy whereby psychoanalysts could be justified in believing that they have superior or greater in-depth knowledge of the human mind, as has been implied by some writers.

Although most of the chapters here are written by students or former students, we have included three by staff, one at the beginning of each of the first three parts. Of these, two are concerned, among other things, with the relationship between psychoanalysis and a particular genre—in one case, poetry (Edwards), and in the other, drama (Rustin). In other words, both authors examine the nature of the application of psychoanalytic thinking in those areas. Each author incorporates reference to their teaching on the course in a different way. Rustin examines how the study of drama is illuminated by psychoanalytic concepts and vice versa, and he does this through giving an account of how this was done on the course, as he developed the "Psychoanalysis, Drama and Society" Applications strand over many years. Both authors are clear about what the relationship between the genre and psychoanalysis is not—they do not ascribe superiority to psychoanalytic understanding, and they concur that the relationship in each case is a complementary and mutually illuminating one. Poets and playwrights have a deep understanding of states of mind and psychic processes within and between people and have been able to give expression to these in ways that audiences find compelling. Psychoanalysis is also interested in those areas. The two chapters show how students are taught about the value of psychoanalysis in illuminating aspects of cultural life and how, in relation to each of the disciplines, maintaining a focus on their emotional experience of a poem or a dramatic scene is a central part of the learning process. The other staff chapter by infant observation seminar leader, Barbara Segal, enables us to see how a similar focus on the students' emotional experience underpins their learning in infant observation.

As discussed previously, infant observation is a process in which the student is immersed in learning from experience. The development of the students' sensitivity to feelings, including those that are painful and difficult to bear, is an important element. This emotional experience is drawn on in the reflective seminar, and the different feelings evoked in the observer during the observation hour are considered to help make sense of unconscious dynamics. The student also needs to find and maintain an observational stance whereby they are not actively involved in the family's activities, but nor are they detached and unresponsive. The task for the observer is to find a state in which they can be as open and receptive as possible, using all their senses so they notice and take in the details of the interaction between the infant and caregiver and the changing dynamics that they, too, are part of. In this observational role and through their increasing alertness to their feelings, students develop a particular way of "being with" and a particular sensibility.

We wonder to what extent the students' experience of infant observation and this particular way of being with informs and suffuses how they engage with the poetry, literature, and performing arts explored in the Applications strand. The tripartite structure of the course as a whole aims to develop a triad of skills—"Looking, feeling and thinking" (Edwards et al., 2006)—and we believe the experience of being an infant observer develops and enriches the way students look at an artwork and experience it emotionally. This particular type of engagement underpins Ingham's exploration of the art installation, *Untitled (Possil at last)*, and the experiential aspects of being an audience member are highlighted in Quaini's chapter on the opera *Turandot*. Students are using their developed observational skills and openness to emotional experience to deepen their understanding of an artwork, theatre performance or poem. As Taheri's chapter in Part IV shows, this openness to learning from experience can also aid students' efforts to understand dynamics within social or societal situations.

The defining feature of clinical psychoanalysis is the presence of a live patient, and it is in the relationship between the analyst and the patient that the analytic work takes place. There is no patient in the sort of applications we are describing. However, if emotional experience is central in applied work in the way described above, it is arguable whether the divide between the two is as stark as has traditionally been thought; perhaps the applied approach and the sensibility it promotes might even be fruitful in the training of clinical students. Giffney (2021) advocates a development of this way of engaging with cultural artefacts as a component in clinical trainings, and a similar way of working is being introduced into the pre-clinical training of child psychotherapists at the Tavistock.

The approach described so far is one way of bringing psychoanalytic thinking to a work of art or literature, but some of the chapters here demonstrate another approach, which is different again from the four methods listed by Baudry. As described in the Appendix, a cornerstone of Kleinian theory is the concept of the inner or internal world. Bringing a psychoanalytic perspective to literary texts, writers in the post-Kleinian tradition, such as Waddell, have explored the inner worlds of fictional characters as they mature and go through processes of psychic change. Waddell's exploration of Dorothea in George Eliot's *Middlemarch* (Waddell, 1998b) and Emma Woodhouse in Jane Austen's *Emma* (Waddell, 1998b, 2018) are two accessible examples.

A focus on the inner world is what Thomas brings to her chapter, in which she explores the states of mind of Stevens, the butler, in Ishiguro's novel *The Remains of the Day*. Although this approach is less experiential, there are, again, links with the process of infant observation, where interest is in the formation of the infant's inner world that takes place in interaction with the inner worlds of the mother and other family members. Exploration of the characters' inner worlds also features in Ghasemi's essay about Beckett's play, *Rockaby,* and in Quaini's *Turandot* there is a vivid description of a coming together of the internal worlds of two of the main protagonists, as well as an in-depth exploration of the inner world of Turandot herself.

As this volume is titled *Exploring Psychoanalytic Concepts through Culture, the Arts, and Contemporary Life,* it is important to clarify what we mean by "culture" here. We are all embedded in the cultures we grow up in, and we inevitably bring conscious and unconscious assumptions, influenced by our culture, to any object of study. There has been increasing awareness of this in recent years and greater integration of spaces for reflection on the self, and on the impact of individuals' cultural backgrounds on their observational vertex, into non-clinical and training courses. It is now widely accepted that any interpretation is a culturally informed one. Increasing research in other cultures—for example, in the field of child development—has forced European and American researchers to question previously held assumptions about the universality of some earlier findings. The importance for the infant's development that psychoanalysis traditionally places on the psychic capacities of the mother has also been questioned, as in some sociocentric rather than egocentric societies infants spend little time with their mothers and are, instead, looked after by a range of members of their extended families. Freud's view of a universal model of human development has also been, and continues to be, challenged.

When students from abroad apply for the course, what some of them are interested in is whether the psychoanalytic theoretical concepts they have read about, such as the Oedipus complex, have as much relevance in their culture as in Western culture. As becomes clear in the chapters by Judith Edwards and Barbara Segal, the involvement of students from other cultures has always enriched work in the seminars and has brought the opportunity for students to share artefacts from their cultures, which reveal similarities and differences when their unconscious themes are explored. Perhaps not dissimilar to other psychoanalytic courses, particularly clinical courses, Psychoanalytic Studies has not attracted a diversity of UK students, and this is being taken up more robustly now under more recent course lead, Dexter Benjamin and Felicity Tyson. Questions of cultural influence, specificity, and universality are being discussed more on the course now than they were at the time when many of these essays were written.

For the purposes of this book, the editors and authors are predominantly thinking about "exploring psychoanalytic concepts through culture" in the sense of engagement with what Michael Rustin calls "artefacts of cultural production" (M. J. Rustin, 2019b), meaning artworks, poems, plays, films, literature, and so on.

Some of the authors have chosen to engage with artefacts from within their own cultures. Yong Suk, who is Korean, explores a Korean pop song; Japanese student Tsutomu Ichige focuses on the function for a mother and baby of a Japanese nursery rhyme; Elina Matter, Palestinian herself, discusses the Palestinian poet Darwish, and Italian Tomaso Quaini's subject is an opera by the Italian composer Puccini. These essays explore themes such as oedipal dynamics, processes of psychic integration and disintegration, loss and mourning, and narcissistic states (see Appendix, "5. Oedipus complex"; "6. Narcissism"; "8. Mourning"). What is striking is that the states of mind and the processes of movement between states suggested in these works created within varied cultures do, in these cases, appear cross-culturally. As Yong Suk concludes, perhaps it is the universality of these states of mind, which strike a chord of recognition in the minds of a wide audience across the world, that led to the song becoming a worldwide hit.

There are various ways we could have structured the book, and one might have been to reflect the tripartite nature of the course and include three parts, based on the Infant Observation, Applications, and Psychoanalytic Theory strands. Another three-part structure could have been built around the areas of student learning highlighted by Edwards: looking, feeling, and thinking. However, although each of these strands contributes a valuable and distinctive perspective and the three areas of learning are equally important, the aim of the course is to create the opportunity for students to bring together the learning done within each of the strands, so the different perspectives and skills they are developing become integrated into a multidimensional view of their object of study from experiential and theoretical viewpoints. Cross-fertilization between strands and between disciplines is embedded in the design of the course.

Our aim throughout has been to group the material into sections that have a focus while keeping that focus broad enough to encompass the wide range of subject matter students have chosen to engage with and the multiple ways they have made use of theoretical psychoanalytic ideas. We therefore decided to structure the volume in four sections: Part I: "Learning through infant observation"; Part II: "Poetry"; Part III: "Literature and the performing arts", and Part IV: "Contemporary life". Each part is preceded by a brief introduction that draws out overarching themes. However, the nature of the course and the understanding that infant observational skills and psychoanalytic thinking have wide applications leads to interesting areas of overlap, and several chapters could equally well have been placed in different sections. The infant observation part includes chapters on music and art, and the chapter on Psy's "Gentleman", in Part IV on contemporary life, could have been grouped with chapters on literature and the performing arts. Readers will notice that themes reappear in different guises and reverberate throughout the book in interesting ways.

The Psychoanalytic Studies course has run over a long period and continues to develop, enriching the NHS organization it is part of with its focus on psychoanalysis, the arts, and society. Most of the chapters here were written by students as part of their ordinary studies and are derived from their original essays or dissertations adapted to a suitable length. Two are written by former students who, many years later, revisit a theme that particularly interested them, and in each case they demonstrate how their learning on the course provided a foundational framework in their later working lives. One of these is the final chapter, written by Clare Parkinson, who was a student when the course first started, going on to become a senior staff member at the Tavistock, teaching social workers. She revisits her Masters dissertation after 25 years, reflecting on the continuing importance of learning from experience but describing the difficulty in maintaining a reflective and thoughtful holistic approach where the emphasis in National training standards is on achieving competencies in individual and specific skills.

With the exception of the contributions by staff members, the chapters are written not by psychoanalysts or clinicians with many years of clinical experience, but by non-clinical students or former students at different stages in their process of learning from experience. The editors believe that this collection of essays vividly captures the essence of the course and the traditional Tavistock ethos with its emphasis on experiential learning, and the book demonstrates the quality of that learning (and teaching) on the Psychoanalytic Studies course.

PART I

LEARNING THROUGH INFANT OBSERVATION

Part I focuses on the practice of infant observation and the development and use of infant observational skills in broader contexts. Chapter 1 is by staff member and highly experienced infant observation seminar leader, Barbara Segal. For readers unfamiliar with the infant observational method, it gives an excellent introduction; readers who already understand the approach will find much to enjoy in the thought-provoking discussion of substantial and poignant observational material. Cultural considerations are touched on as the implications of coming to an observation from a culturally different viewpoint are explored briefly in relation to each of the two central observations. Several themes inherent in the infant observation process emerge in Segal's chapter and come to the fore explicitly or implicitly in each of the subsequent chapters: these interrelated themes could be broadly delineated as multilayered complexity, non-verbal communication, reflection, and psychological digestion.

Part of the multilayered complexity relates to the concept of containment (see Appendix, "4. Containment") and the layers of containment that are both needed and provided within the infant observational structure. As Segal describes, there are two parts to the infant observation process: the observation itself and the observation seminar, where one student's observation is discussed in detail in each seminar. There is an element of containment for the observed family in the regular and attentive presence

DOI: 10.4324/9781003564867-2

of the observer, who, in turn, needs to feel contained by the observation seminar. Because of the intensity and power of the infant's primitive emotional states, anxieties, and projections, students and staff also need to be contained by surrounding course and organizational structures. As Margaret Rustin (2011) describes: "Containment is an onion-like phenomenon in structure—many layers are required when the task is the growth of the mind" (p. 2).

Communication within observations is also multilayered, and observers and their seminar groups work to make sense of different levels of conscious and unconscious verbal and nonverbal communication. Segal draws attention to the containment and thinking in the groups and notes how the seminar can facilitate the opening up of the development and emotional experience of the students. In relation to one observer, she says: "It is important to notice here how the seminar facilitates the opening up of these themes; that the trust that develops in the seminar enables this observer to bring his more personal responses to the observations, and the strength of these responses elicits a deeper understanding of the meaning of what has been observed and described." Thus, the multiple layers inherent in the process support increasingly in-depth understanding.

Towards the end of the academic year, each student writes a paper telling the story of their observation and the baby's development during the period of observation. Their focus is on the baby's psychological development within its family relationships and their understanding of conscious and unconscious factors that have come to the fore over time. The process of writing gives students a further opportunity to reflect on specific aspects of the observation and the experience as a whole, and the paper is grounded within a psychoanalytic framework through references to relevant psychoanalytic theories that illuminate and support inferences. Students are also encouraged to draw on concepts from the child development research literature, where relevant.

Chapter 2, which tells the story of the first 18 months of baby Sam's life, is based on the infant observation paper written by Jenny Abbott, who sets her experience of psychoanalytic observation in the context of her background as a documentary-maker. She describes how she came to the course experienced in one sort of observation but quickly came to understand that psychoanalytic infant observation was something very different, which meant that she needed to "unlearn" many of her previous ways of seeing and gathering information. As Abbott describes, the infant observation process involves an unfolding over time, and as an observer she was "required to watch, listen, and wait until the emotional meaning of what I had observed made itself known through reflection and time". She uses an evocative phrase to describe the place of nonverbal communication, writing, "I had to learn to be sensitive to pre-linguistic communication, *the tiny shifts and gestures that told a story beyond language*." The idea of a "story beyond language" underlies all the chapters in this part.

Chapters 3, 4, and 5 each demonstrate students, or former students, making use of the skills they develop through infant observation in wide-ranging ways. Tsutomu Ichige's chapter, "An Exploration of a Nursery Song, 'The Police Dog', as a Container", and Deirdre Ingham's chapter, "Mother-less: A Psychoanalytic Observation of an Installation by Cathy Wilkes", are based on original essays done within the Applications strand, but it is clear how in each case the student's observational experience underlies and informs their approach. Ichige's chapter explores the place of a traditional Japanese nursery rhyme within the mother–infant interaction he observed. The sung nursery rhyme draws the reader's attention to the place of music in infancy, but the broader musicality of the fluid reciprocal interaction between the mother and baby and their responsiveness to each other also comes through strongly. Ichige makes use of observational material to stimulate his thinking about the subtleties of unconscious processes within the mother–infant container–contained relationship, which comes under great pressure in the face of infantile annihilation anxiety. He highlights that it is not only receptivity and reflection that is needed for containment, but another vital aspect: psychological digestion. He says, "if only offering empathy, the container could just stay in sympathetic vibration with the infant's painful emotion, leading not only to the container being emotionally overwhelmed but also reinforcing the infant's pain. The process of psychological digestion is also an essential aspect of the containing function."

The original thinking Ichige brings to the interrelated states of mind of the infant and the mother when they are under the sway of intense and primitive anxieties reminds us that it is not only the clinical consulting room that is the psychoanalytic laboratory—the infant observational setting has that potential too.

Ingham's exploration of the art installation by Cathy Wilkes, *Untitled (Possil, at last)*, demonstrates the approach we describe in the Introduction. As she says, the essay is not an analysis of the artist, but a reflection on what Wilkes' work communicated to her. Ingham draws on her background as an art psychotherapist, enriched by the sensibility she developed through infant observation, to reflect on the work as a whole and its individual elements. She brings in the idea of zooming in and moving out, using her eyes and her "emotional lens", at times taking in the whole, at other times focusing on small fragments and details. In this way she draws a parallel with the infant observation process, where, as she says, "At times the whole scene is taken in, and at other times small fragments, gestures, and words might capture the observer's attention." Another parallel with the clinical analytic situation is suggested here as the analyst also pays attention to both the overall emotional atmosphere and the detail of the patient's material. Different layers are attended to, taken in, reflected on, and digested.

The part ends with Olivia Sagan's chapter, "The Is-ness of Things: Reflections on Observation in Contexts Where Words Are Hard to Find". It has been a long time since Sagan completed the Psychoanalytic Studies course—almost 20 years at the time of writing—and she reflects here on how, in the intervening years, she has digested her observation experience and incorporated the approach into her work as a researcher, teacher, counsellor, and psychologist working with deprived populations in a range of settings. The theme of nonverbal communication runs through the essay as she notices how, particularly for deprived, traumatized, and oppressed populations, language is just not available to them as a way to tell their story; they are far from being able to make use of the "talking cure" as it has traditionally been understood.

Sagan repeatedly emphasizes the value of being able to observe in detail and, echoing Abbott's words, watch, wait, and listen to what is communicated through other means. She describes how, in her work with psychiatric patients, something of their unbearable experience was communicated to her as she could find herself feeling "wasted, unheard, impotent". Their feelings were communicated by means of "the ebb and flow of projective identification".

When discussing her recent training as a counsellor, where the skills taught presuppose some capacity in the client for verbal communication, Sagan states that it was the single skill of *being* that allowed her to be human. Perhaps it is not only the "being" but the repeated "being *with*"—a skill honed through infant observation—that allows these very deprived people to begin to feel that there might possibly be someone who could be interested, could listen, take in, and provide some sort of a container for experiences that are beyond words.

The chapters in this part illustrate not only how infant observation can be a hugely enriching activity in itself, but also the way in which the observational attitude and skills developed become part of the observer and available in their work and life, deepening their interactions with individuals and their encounters with works of art.

CHAPTER ONE

Teaching infant observation

Barbara Segal

Child psychotherapists and psychoanalysts feel passionate about infant observation. The method of observation of an infant in the training of child psychotherapists was pioneered by Esther Bick, at the Tavistock Clinic, in 1948. This naturalistic observation method is now widely undertaken, not only as a prerequisite for psychoanalytic training, but also in other non-clinical courses at the Tavistock, such as the course at the centre of this book, Psychoanalytic Studies, and also for the enrichment of the work of other professionals, such as teachers, doctors, social workers, and others. Today the international body of students from a wide range of professional backgrounds is engaged in infant and young child observation, and many talk of the experience as having been life-changing. It has been striking to see the emergence of the multifaceted impact of the observation experience on the students, on their learning and on their professional role. On the Psychoanalytic Studies course the impact has been influential in the study of literature, art, film, and theatre, which is addressed elsewhere in the book.

There is much to learn as a teacher in this field, even with many years of experience in teaching observation. One listens to and tries to learn from what the multinational students bring to the course and from how "meaning is attributed to difference" (Ellis, 1997), the issues of inclusion, diversity in culture, language, the ethos of both the observer and the observed family, and the challenges for students arriving at the Tavistock, with its

DOI: 10.4324/9781003564867-3

reputation, only to learn that the Tavistock does not help you to find a baby to observe. At the time of writing, students are being taught online due to the international pandemic and are having to introduce themselves to possible families by remote means and to begin their observations by video. It has been uplifting to note that their keenness to find a baby or toddler to observe has not been dampened, and the usual atmosphere of excitement, as well as trepidation, which is so marked at the beginning of the academic year, is clear to see.

Over time one can observe a slow dawning in the student of hitherto unknown aspects of the self and changes or personal transformations that can occur. This kind of opening up and experiencing new insights is illustrated a little further on. Linked to this unfolding is the crucial containing experience of the small seminar group where observations are discussed.

Method

Students are asked to make appropriate contact with a mother (and father or mother's partner) about to give birth, or with one with a very new baby, in order to set up a series of hour-long observations on a weekly basis. Students are told that these take place in the baby's home (most usually) in order that the student may watch and learn about the baby's development within his or her own setting. The learning objectives for the student are complex and subtle—i.e., to try to observe and experience in as open and non-judgmental a way as possible the burgeoning development and expression of the infant's capacities to relate to the main carer (usually the mother) and the other important figures in his world, including the observer, as well as to help the student to make sense of the communications of the baby's needs and feelings and to try to understand how and to what extent those communications are received. The overall aim is to attempt to understand the unconscious aspects of behaviour and patterns of communication. Sue Reid writes,

> The emphasis in this method of observation is on what is seen and *felt* during the observation, and premature attempts to explain and make formulations are actively discouraged. . . . The student is encouraged and supported to see *what is there to be seen* and not to look for what they think should be there . . . the observer has no idea what he or she will see and therefore is exposed to a whole new level of perception of human relationships. This is both disturbing and exciting.
>
> [Reid, 1997, p. 1]

In a paper on teaching observational skills on the Psychoanalytic Studies course, Judith Edwards (2006) writes that "the skills of watching, waiting, and wondering are developed and increasingly seen as valuable tools for insight" (Edwards et al., 2006, p. 222). She cites the idea of "accumulated actions, involving, in the developing mother–baby dyad, often repeated sequences of holding, of feeding, of cleaning and of conversing, building a force field of reciprocal meaning, a getting-to-know about the world, which evolves over time" (p. 222). She believes this cultivation of the knowledge process on the course, and the space for reflective self-development that evolves in the observation module, "will enable the student to link insights with other elements in the course, and move towards understanding from a psychoanalytic perspective" (p. 222).

Janine Sternberg (2005) lists the different layers of the task the student will be engaged in as she undertakes the observation: "to look, notice, feel, be aware of how what she sees impacts on her, reflect, remember, process, think, and then write about it all" (p. 6).

Given the provenance of psychoanalysis, our teaching objectives are rooted in a European framework of psychoanalytic theory, especially that of Melanie Klein, as well as Winnicott, Bick, and Bion. However, the aim is not to teach students psychoanalytic theory but, rather, to use the theoretical concepts to inform and focus the observations.

The importance of reliability and boundary keeping is emphasized. Over time, students learn about the interference that cancelled visits and changes of time can create. Observers are advised to be friendly, non-intrusive, and interested, but not to be too open with personal information about themselves. The reasons for this way of conducting oneself are explained but really become fully appreciated only when something is played out in the observation experience and the student begins to understand the unconscious and transference factors at play (for example, the cancellation of a session by the mother after a holiday taken by the observer). Kate Robertson calls this understanding of the nature of the observer/family relationship "the internalisation of the setting" (K. Robertson, personal communication, November 2020).

"Infant Observation training is essentially an experiential form of learning with two major components: the observation itself and the observation seminar" (Davids, Miles, Paton, & Trowell, 1999, p. 17). While the task of observation itself seems straightforward enough, the emotional proximity of the observer to the rawness of infantile anxieties, without the option of intervention, makes the task far more complex. To quote again from Davids et al., "The observation seminar is the place where some of this complexity can be disentangled to facilitate the process of observation. The containing function of the seminar assists the observer in the extraordinarily difficult task of refraining from active intervention" (p. 17). This containment is described by various writers as being comparable with Bion's (1962a) notion of the mother's modification, and handing back in an acceptable form, of the infant's raw, unprocessed projections. Examples of this idea of containment by the seminar are presented in further on.

Can students be prepared for the emotional impact?

Some attempt is made to prepare students for the emotional impact of being observers of a new mother and her infant. Emotion will assume a very prominent place in this exercise and will need to be observed and recorded. It should be seen not as a distraction, but as the most useful tool in achieving further understanding. One never does know exactly what emotional impact a particular observation might have on a particular observer. Clearly, such close contact with strong infantile feelings will awaken such feelings in an onlooker. An observer's own infantile self may be painfully evoked if there have been deprivations and unmet longings in their own infantile experience; memories of one's own failed attempts to pacify or contain one's own infant may be invoked; one may look with longing at the support the observed young mother is receiving from her partner or from her mother; one might feel like an unwanted outsider. I have been asked in tutorials or seminars, "Why were we not told this could be so painful and difficult?"

This exposure to the emotional impact of the observations in learning about early emotional development through such close contact with an infant and his mother, as well as one's own response to the observed couple, is what requires a containing and supportive network. This applies not only in the observation seminar but in the training institution too.

The early weeks with a new group of students can be very disheartening, and the teacher may feel they haven't addressed the objectives or the instructions adequately. The poor quality of the descriptions and the paucity of detailed information are very likely to be linked with the trepidation experienced by the student within the observation hour. Worries about remembering sequences of the observations, due in part of course to the acquisition of this new skill in disciplined observation, taking in and remembering, point to the possible agitation experienced about the awakening of primitive anxieties, discussed above. There is also the element of scepticism about whether what they are watching makes any sense at all, whether it is relevant to note, remember, and record movements the infant makes, such as apparently random leg or arm movements or tiny changes in facial expression, or a sudden vocal sound. It is hard to believe these activities can be meaningful. Somebody asked in a seminar one day early on the course: "What IS the Tavistock? I know it's famous and everyone knows about it, but what is it?" I understood this as an expression of utter bewilderment about an unfathomable exercise, this new way of looking at an infant's experience, which was very far away from this student's professional life hitherto.

One of the complex issues that may arise is that of the impact of diverse cultural codes on the observed baby and his family, and also on the observer. This raises questions about how to understand the observed baby's internal world (his very own experience) as well as how to comprehend the cultural realities of the observed family and of the observer. Lynda Ellis (1997) refers to "the potential for prejudice, value conflict and moralizing" (p. 57).

Such complexity is expanded on the details of the observations discussed below. Differences in culture and customs, as well as in social consciousness, appear as important factors in the experience of the observed family, the observer, and, indeed, in the group of the students in the seminar.

I am grateful to the students who have allowed me to use their observation material.

"Kelly"

The description that follows recognizes some of these dilemmas and was voiced in one of my seminars as we were entering the second term in the second year, showing how these themes may arise well into the two years of observation. It was the turn of one observer, whom I shall call Kelly, to present her first observation after a three-week Christmas break, during which she had returned to her home abroad.

The task of setting up the observation for Kelly had been very difficult, as she felt unable to telephone the mother, a complete stranger, to request a first meeting. It transpired through discussion in the seminars that Kelly considered this presumptuous. It emerged that Kelly's own culture has an established code of conduct around social mores that amplify politeness and avoid causing potential offence or intrusion.

Over the first year of the observation, the seminar had been experiencing rather serious concerns about baby Nina's failure to engage her mother's focused attention to her needs. We had been distressed at times by mother's attempts to "force feed" Nina with a spoon despite her resolute shutting of her mouth and turning her face away from mother. We felt that mother was driven by her own needs. The observer had been saddened by

Nina's depressed demeanour and apparent experience of what she called "loneliness" when Nina's mother ignored her, frequently left the room, or simply neglected to pick up on her cues. On exploration we learned that the word "lonely" was used to describe a flat, blank, affectless expression and lack of response in Nina.

In Kelly's previous presentation we had spent some time discussing her responses, both internal and external, to these happenings and asking her about them. The seminar's interest in the observer's responses was prompted, I am sure, by our experience of her as, at times, somewhat impassive, which led to a concern that Nina might be exposed to an expressionless observer at these painful times, so exacerbating her "loneliness".

Before commencing her current observation visit, when Nina was just one year old, Kelly read us a brief paragraph, summarising a visit before Christmas, when mother had been asleep, and she had observed Nina with her father. She had been delighted to observe that father was totally engaged with Nina, played and laughed with her, and that the atmosphere was relaxed and happy.

She then presented her more recent observation. I quote a section from the start:

> Mother opened the front door, and I saw Nina walking into the hall. She looked very different since my last visit nearly one month ago. Her hair had grown longer, more wavy, and soft. She was wearing a pink dress and pink tights and looked lovely. I sat on the sofa in the living room, and mother sat on the other sofa. Nina came near me and looked at me curiously but went towards mother quickly shortly after I had spoken to her. She sat between mother's legs and looked back at me shyly but intensely. She went to the corner of the room, picked up a toy mobile phone and was walking around holding it with her left hand on her left shoulder. Mother asked, "who are you talking to?" Nina came near me, gave it to me, and moved away. She soon came back, took it from my hand gently and went to mother. Mother looked out of the window and stood up suddenly, saying "the postman has come", and went to the hall. Nina looked surprised and stood shouting "Ma!" and ran into the hall. They returned; mother sat next to me, opening letters. I told mother I was surprised to hear Nina speaking for the first time. Mother said, "She says mamma and dada" and called Nina and said "say mamma". But Nina stood in front of mother and smiled delightedly at her. Mother asked her again, Nina opened her arms wide and put her head and arms on mother's lap. Mother looked embarrassed but hugged her and kissed her face. Nina picked up a letter, stood up, holding the letter up and turning round and

round, looking up at the flapping letter in her right arm. Mother told me that Nina had woken up at two o' clock that night and scratched herself all over her body, because she was itchy. Mother had played with her and bounced her in the air. I asked mother to tell me whether Nina had tried to attract her attention or wanted to play with her. Mother murmured "she wanted my attention . . ."; suddenly mother sat on the floor to play with Nina. Mother's reaction was as if I had urged her to do that.

As the observation progressed, the detail became clearer and finer, and a very lively visit was presented. We heard that mother hardly left the room during the observation; Nina became drawn to the observer as the visit went on, bringing her toys, playing with much concentration with her handbag, climbing repeatedly onto mother's lap for a breast-feed, then returning to the observer. At the point where mother kept her out of the kitchen while she prepared her lunch, Nina "looked lonely and came towards me, opening her arms. I was squatting and ready to hug her."

The whole atmosphere of the observation was very different from what we had become accustomed to, and the seminar felt excited. The observer, usually struggling for words, was inspired and interjected with more remembered detail, with her ideas about the meaning of what she had observed and experienced and her wonderment at Nina's apparent attachment to her. She said two things had brought her much relief: one was observing father with Nina, and their lovely interaction; the other was my having said, when she had last presented, that she did not have to sit immobile and expressionless if Nina was distressed and looked to her for comfort.

We were struck by mother's attempts at engagement and the observer's livelier presence. Clearly, when she had observed father's interactions, Kelly had felt great relief from her distress about Nina's situation. She also seemed enabled to let go of the institution's (my) restraints on her and feel "permission" to become engaged. It seems to me very likely, too, that the observer's recent visit to her home and family abroad had also had an impact on her experience in the first observation visit after her return. I suspect that the parting from her family put her in touch with the isolation and sense of separateness of Nina and her mother—their "loneliness". She, too, had a need to be in emotional contact. It seems she might have brought with her a new confidence provided by the affection of her family and her sense of belonging in her own country. Instead of remaining apparently detached, yet noticing the sadness engendered in her (as she had described to the seminar previously), she intervened, commenting on Nina's speech and revealing her curiosity about mother's activities with Nina during the night. This resulted in an altered perception in all three of them about their relationships to each other, including the observer. Nina seemed to "re-find" the observer after the break and her cautious greeting; she seemed to associate the mobile phone and the lovely, fluttering, newly arrived letter with the comings and goings of the observer. Nina's interest in what the observer brought with her, in the shape of her handbag, standing for Kelly's new willingness to be open to mother and Nina's developing engagement, is evident, I suspect. I also wonder whether mother's interest and curiosity in the observer's comments and questions about Nina revealed to mother the observer's sustained holding of Nina and the family in her mind over the holidays.

It would seem that the observer's capacity to make these interventions arose out of her experience during her previous presentation, when the seminar had taken very seriously her discomfort and upset about Nina's state of mind and had explored with her own reactions and her ostensible non-involvement in the observation hour. I think she experienced the sense of containment by the seminar, to which I referred earlier, which can be likened to the mother's striving to make sense of feelings that are too raw for the infant to process itself.

The impact was felt by the seminar group, who, interestingly, expressed a more empathic warmth towards mother's (and not only Nina's) struggle with weaning (the to-ing and fro-ing from the breast), and the seminar was touched by mother's taking a cue from the observer's question to mother about why Nina had woken in the night and what might have caused her restlessness. The seminar was thoughtful about the change in Kelly, and the students began to talk about their own changing experience of their observations. Someone said, "I'm beginning to get it. . . . I think we are only just getting to understand what being an observer is all about, and how to let ourselves really be there; but what a long time it takes, and how complex it is!"

I have tried to convey the richness of this observation, in terms of Nina's eagerness for exploration and engagement, mother's later repeated attempts to try to follow Nina, and the observer's increasing involvement in the process of observing and allowing herself to become a part of the experience, without grossly overstepping any boundaries. What was also of interest was to notice the change in the quality of the written description as the observation progressed, as the observer shed some of her inhibitions in allowing herself to experience the impact of close proximity.

As time has passed since this observation, I believe we have become more aware of the challenges for some students when observing an infant in a family, especially when coming from overseas and needing to develop their own understanding of different cultural customs. We have perhaps been slow, too, to think about what we can learn from cultural differences.

What, for example, is the appropriate distance to keep within an observation. and what informs the distance that a student takes? Kelly's experience exemplifies the layers of potential obstacles our students may face. Kelly found herself a long way from home, embarking on a new course with the unfamiliar discipline of observation, while she was isolated and perhaps lonely. She was not fluent in English when she arrived and might have missed out on some of the early seminar discussions. Perhaps there was a mirroring of experience in the difficulty of close attunement—for a mother with her first baby, and for the observer in her new identity. The picture of Nina's father enjoying his baby girl with much warmth seemed to act as a catalyst for a more lively contact and seemed to offer a much needed different perspective, which also touched Kelly in a new way.

What follows is a final example of observational material from Martin, which draws together some of the themes raised above. The ongoing development and emotional experience of the students undertaking this complex task, engaged in the process of their own learning from experience, is at the very heart of the study of infant and young child observation. It is important to note here how the seminar facilitates the opening up of these themes; the trust that develops in the seminar enables this observer to bring his more personal responses to the observations, and the strength of these responses elicits a deeper understanding of the meaning of what has been observed and described. One might say that the observer has himself experienced something of what the child is feeling. (One of the tasks of the seminar group is to explore this in relation to who an observer is drawn to identify with. Is it the baby, the mother, or the father?) In addition, and most importantly, in this example the observed child is seen to have developed a capacity for self-reflection. To what extent might this be linked with his experience of the observer's unflinching, regular attentiveness towards him for an hour a week over an extended period?

Martin

Martin started his observation when Simon was 3 weeks old. He described the family home and atmosphere as "a male place", having been struck by accounts of infant observations as mostly female-dominated. Simon had one sibling, an older brother. Father was out of the house at work all day. His impression of mother, who was welcoming and friendly, was that she was a very energetic woman who demanded quite a lot of herself and others, believing that people should "pull themselves together". During her maternity leave mother was still very active in her career. Martin described what he felt was a tension between mother's busy-ness and her dedicated devotion to Simon. He talked about her apparent incapacity for reverie, as he felt he had not seen much of this state of mind in Simon's mother during the observations. Martin was referring to Bion's (1962a) term, "reverie", which describes "a state of calm receptiveness to take in the infant's own feelings and give them meaning" (Hinshelwood, 1989, p. 420), and Simon's repeated attempts at engagement to be answered by his mother's gaze. Martin writes about an observation at 4 months, when mother was exhausted after a journey. She had fed Simon from one breast and abruptly stopped. He looked up at her questioningly, then protested.

> She stands him in front of her. His face is inches from hers. He is leaning forward slightly and looking at her eyes. He starts crying. In seconds his face and head become pink, then red. He closes his eyes. His eyebrows become dimpled. His hands are fists, and he moves his arms back and forward determinedly. His legs are bent at the knee. His cries are angry, hopeless protests. Mother stares blankly at Simon. Her face is empty and tired. He finds nothing in her face.

The pain felt by the observer is palpable.

However, there is another observation during which Simon succeeded in engaging his mother after loudly making known his need to be held and fed. At the end of the feed:

> He opens his eyes and looks up. Mother is talking to his brother. It seems to me that Simon is looking intently and lovingly at his mother. I really want mother to look at him. After a while she looks down and sees Simon looking up at her. She perhaps sees the same thing as I have, because she bends further over him, shoulders hunched, and looks back at him. Simon's gaze is constant and serene, his eyes are large and clear. Mother's expression is troubled, until gradually her face clears. To me it feels vital that Simon should secure his mother's gaze. I feel relief and elation.

The observer worried that although mother was loving and caring, there were only fleeting moments in the observation hour when this kind of experience of reverie was seen. The observer felt that he didn't see much evidence of a sensitive, responsive mother able to receive her child's quest or fear and find a way to modify it to something bearable. We wondered why Simon's mother needed to keep so busy, about her own experience of being mothered, and what feelings she might need to keep at bay.

It seems clear that the observer is straining to watch whether mother will answer her baby's search for a loving response. He is closely identified with Simon and feels helpless, then joyful. In discussions we had thought about the ways in which Simon sometimes protected himself from being dropped or unnoticed and his psychic pain by adopting a muscular kind of brittle independence (Bick, 1968).

As time passed, the observer noticed the ways in which Simon communicated something of the developing relationship between himself and the observer and notably his appreciation of the idea of containment. We had noticed the way Simon was able to reach out and how much he protested when what he was seeking was not there—a strong lively force, able to seek what he needed. In a similar way, he sought out Martin and started to give him something on greeting him. At 15 months he gave Martin, and then took back, a little plastic toy:

> . . . and then, while shouting "Ook! Ook!" (Look! Look!), he stands against the toy kitchen unit and with both hands pulls the washing-up bowl out of the sink and drops it on the floor. Mother, incredulous, asks, "What on earth are you doing?" Simon puts his right hand, holding the horse, in the hole where the bowl was. He turns his head towards me, again saying "Ook! Ook!" There is an intensity to his actions. He is breathing hard, and his eyes are bright."

We thought in the seminar that Simon was a baby who could reach out and was therefore expressing a realization of Martin's availability for and interest in him every week, in the handing over and taking back the little horse (the coming and going, the presence and absence?) and that Martin noticed and responded to the emotions within his play and would feel for (or with) him. In place of the empty bowl, Simon clutched a meaningful small creature within a newly created space and held it there, excitedly showing Martin. He was identifying or indicating an experience of containment. He could do this because he was a baby who had made the most of what his mother had to offer him.

In the same way, two months later, Martin arrived to see him playing with a plastic sorter toy.

> He sits upright, his legs flat in front of him. He is concentrating hard and breathing heavily. He tries to put a counter in the wrong slot. He tries another counter, and it works. He picks up a third counter and puts it carefully into a white cup. Holding the cup, he stands up and walks towards me, stands in

> front of me, looks up, and makes little cooing noises as he holds out the cup. I say thank you and take the cup. He pauses, looking at me in a serious way, then walks off quickly, babbling happily.

In a more sombre observation Martin presented a visit when Simon's mother, older brother, Simon, and Martin had gone into the garden to look at the chickens.

> Simon holds his mother's hand. He is silent and looks down . . . at the stockade Simon watches anxiously as his mother and brother collect some feed. . . . He follows them to the coop, walks in front of his mother, and reaches up his arms for her to lift him over the fence. He looks desperately at her. "It's too muddy," she says, He stands silently as he watches his mother lift his brother over the fence. Simon raises his arms towards me, his face imploring. He makes sharp little grunting noises. "I'm sorry", I say, feeling guilty. He drops his arms and turns away from me . . . the feeding done, mother carries an excited older brother back over the fence. Simon goes to his mother, his head down. She holds his hand. His head stays down. We walk back to the house, Simon quiet and downcast.

After this presentation the seminar felt protective and empathic towards the observer and his discomfort and even pain at denying Simon what he longed for. The observer described his real upset at witnessing this rebuff, and we began to understand how Martin had been open to receiving Simon's distress and had taken the acuteness of the situation into himself. We wondered what part this played in enabling Simon to go inside with his mother. As well as his hand being firmly held by his mother, having his grief "held" by a sensitive observer, someone who had witnessed and shared the moment and made it bearable by so doing perhaps contributed to him managing the experience.

However, we also thought that Martin was describing how Simon was resorting to using a "second skin" protection to move forward: he dropped his head and stoically accompanied his mother indoors, without a backward look at the chickens or any florid show of fury and upset.

The seminar also heard that some weeks earlier mother had told Martin that she intended to send both boys to boarding school, because it "made boys into leaders". Martin had been holding on to this information for weeks. There was a "collective groan" (Martin's words) from the seminar group, who were strongly identified with Simon. There was concern about whether this way of thinking in the family and Simon's tendency to resort to the defence of a second skin would overtake his own developing emotionality and his touching capacity to recognize and respond to something gentler and more reflective as a way of interacting with his world?

There was a sad atmosphere in the seminar, and the students were concerned that the parents were acting without thinking. Another male student texted Martin after the group, to say how much he felt for Martin. The question in our minds was whether Simon, who had often had his early communications rejected, would introject "something which is unresponsive to the communication of feeling" (Waddell, 1998a, p. 14). Our hope that Simon's own strengths in trying to capture his mother's responsiveness, and the experience of having some of his painful feelings understood and held, would allow him to develop into someone sensitive and responsive.

On reflection, it is interesting to consider whether covert judgements were influencing our views about Simon and his family. The need for Simon to show a stiff upper lip and to stand on his own, demanded by the busyness of his mother and the boarding school culture of the family, was considered as a defence against being dropped and a lack of feeling. This resonated with our view of psychoanalytic understanding about how to manage painful feelings. Perhaps, the observer's strong identification with Simon, and the seminar group's connection with the observer, may have left the seminar less able to think about the strengths that were being propounded by the family in relation to independence—something that may have been needed by Simon to prosper in this particular cultural context, hopefully taking with him the capacity for sensitivity of feeling. Regardless of this, the slow unfolding of the experience is what both the observer and the seminar group are concerned with.

Conclusion

I read something by Fintan O'Toole, drama critic with the *Irish Times*, that encapsulated some of the ideas I have been preoccupied with here. In the 1960s Brian Friel, the Irish playwright, went, at the invitation of the great theatre director, Tyrone Guthrie, to Minneapolis in Minnesota, where Guthrie was founding his new theatre.

> For six months [Friel] spent his days and evenings in the theatre, "literally skulking about in the gloom of the back seats", until a doorman challenged him. As he was trying to explain his function one of the actors stepped in to rescue him with the words, "He's okay . . . he's an observer". As Friel later recalled, "that fortuitous christening gave me not only an identity but a dignity: an observer, part of the great communal effort—pass friend".
>
> [O'Toole, 2015]

Postscript

As I was finishing writing the chapter and wondering whether I had sufficiently embraced the idea of observation, I watched the documentary film, *My Octopus Teacher*. Craig Foster, a naturalist, free diver, and wildlife film-maker, described a relationship that developed between an alien animal, a cephalopod or octopus, and himself, in the icy depths of the kelp forests in the ocean off the Western Cape in South Africa. After a spell of debilitating burn-out and feelings of emptiness and apathy, he was looking to re-connect with the natural world. Every day over many months he observed her, visited her in her den, and tracked her movements, eventually winning her trust. The film gradually revealed how the octopus shared the mysteries of her world. A close bond developed. His immersion in her extraordinary mind and life captivated him, profoundly affecting his state of mind. It seems she was equally enchanted by his sustained and relentless discipline in diving and watching her each day.

I was forcibly struck by the link with my preoccupation with writing about infant observation. It was the consistent, detailed observation and interest in every small thing (and huge momentous happenings too), and the animal's trusting of this, that created a significant emotional contact . . . a relationship.

Reflecting on the depth of the impact on him, Craig Foster expressed his thoughts on how the octopus had taught him to feel that humans can be part of the natural world too. There can be a friendship between species. We are all part of humanity.

CHAPTER TWO

Sam: observations and reflections on the first eighteen months of life

Jenny Abbott

When I applied to study on the Psychoanalytic Studies course, I was particularly drawn to a part of the course called Infant Observation. At the time, I had no real idea of what this would involve, but I had spent nearly twenty years at the BBC making documentaries, and I thought that observation could be something I was good at. As part of my job, I was used to standing with a camera crew and observing, often filming people at their most vulnerable. I had filmed births, weddings, deaths, I had spent days in A&E departments, on psychiatric wards, and in homes for people with dementia. When I was researching a project, I would follow people around for weeks, watching them do their jobs or interact with their families, getting to know them and something of their lives. I was propelled in my job by a deep curiosity about how people lived, their motivations and challenges, and I tried to honour their stories as best I could. I thought I was good at seeing and understanding. As it turned out, infant observation would require a whole new way of seeing, and I had to "unlearn" many of the old ways.

Observing for a documentary requires an active participation, an interpretation on the part of the film-maker, or, as Grierson put it, "the creative treatment of actuality". Often these interpretations, though rooted in observation, are made quickly (there is a budget and a product required after all), influenced by pre-conceptions, the work of other documentary makers, and one's own feelings or desires (conscious or not), all of which

DOI: 10.4324/9781003564867-4

can remain largely unexamined, despite the emotional intensity of what is being observed and filmed. In the two years in which I made weekly visits to baby Sam and his mother, I had to learn to make a new space in my mind in which my thoughts and emotional responses could be held until meaning became clearer, to tolerate the anxiety, discomfort, and uncertainty, which is part of this process. I had to learn to be sensitive to pre-linguistic communication, the tiny shifts and gestures that told a story beyond language. I had to learn to observe with close attention, alive to the importance of the regularity of my visits and of consistency in my position and reactions. It was having to tolerate "unknowing"; however, that seemed most in contrast to my observational position as a documentary maker—I was required to watch, listen, and wait until the emotional meaning of what I had observed made itself known through reflection and time. I could not edit this story in the way I was accustomed to; there would be no splicing and sticking together bits of film in a new order to suit my version of the story I hoped to tell. I had to allow this story to tell itself.

Observing in this way was challenging but immensely rewarding; and my weekly infant observation seminars led by Angelina Trellis-Fishman soon became a highlight of the course. I am deeply grateful to the mother who allowed me to visit for two years; the experience she and Sam gave me was hugely influential in developing my own desire to train as a psychoanalyst.

What follows is the essay I wrote at the end of my infant observation, based on observations and reflections on Sam's first 18 months of life. It is primarily rooted in the words recorded after my weekly hour long observation visits. As Esther Bick wrote, "here, in the house of parents with a new-born baby, the observer . . . is confronted with a situation of intense emotional impact" (1964, p. 559). The thoughts presented here began to emerge through reading and discussing what I wrote about the emotional experience of being with Sam and his mother.

* * *

At the age of 18 months, Sam appeared to be a healthy, engaged, and delightful infant, who was advanced verbally and physically and displayed an intense curiosity about the world around him. He was accommodating, loving, and playful in his relationship with his mother and showed himself to be loving and generous with his grandparents, his sibling, and with me, his special weekly visitor. Sam was also able to express his own needs and desires, as well as being able to tolerate some frustration when things did not go according to plan. I was in the family's home to learn about the development of this unique baby in this particular family, and I was present during the ordinary ups and downs of the first 18 months of Sam's life. His mother was attentive and obviously loved her son dearly, but having a new baby inevitably brings intense anxieties, and it seemed at times that she worried a lot about his ability to survive the precarious first year or so of life.

This is the story of how Sam and his mother negotiated their way through these tricky early months together; how Sam helped his mother relax into being a mother for the second time; and how she, in turn, found a way to allow and encourage Sam's own personality and identity to develop.

"Ghosts in the nursery"

I met Sam and his mother, Louise, when he was just 3 weeks old. He had an older sister, Rebecca, who celebrated her birthday the week of my introduction to the family. Sam's parents are both in their mid- to late thirties (I only met Jonathan, his father, once). Both parents are professionals. Louise worked had part time up until Sam's birth, but, during the period of the observation, decided not to return to work when her maternity leave ended. Louise is slight, with an open and intelligent face, and she has a wry sense of humour. She is energetic and competent, with a preference for everything to be in order. Sam, at the age of 3 weeks, was a fine-featured baby with a shock of blonde hair and deep-blue eyes.

Louise was very willing to have an observer, and at my first meeting with her was extremely welcoming and forthcoming, telling me at our first meeting about her struggle to have her children. She had had many rounds of IVF, all of which failed, but then further treatment led to the natural conception of her first child. Sam had also been conceived naturally. Louise told me that the IVF had made her extremely sick, but that she was overjoyed to be a mother. Louise described the events surrounding Sam's birth:

> The baby had been ten days overdue, as she was very keen to give birth naturally, but she never went into labour and had to have a caesarean. ... She told me a woman on her maternity ward had a very hungry baby, and her milk had been slow to come in, because she had also had a caesarean, and no one had suggested giving the baby a bottle for a few days, though he clearly needed it. She had tried to breast-feed Rebecca, but had not been able to, and so had not tried to breast-feed Sam.

Louise appears not to have considered breast-feeding Sam after the difficulty she had had feeding her older child, and here she seems to associate the caesarean with an inability to produce sufficient milk for the baby. During this first visit, Louise told me several times that she was anxious about Sam's weight. This theme would reverberate through many of my subsequent observations.

Joan Raphael-Leff (1991) describes how difficulties in conceiving can result in a mother's need to constantly monitor a pregnancy, in case a lapse of concentration could result in the baby "vanishing". Over the months I wondered whether Louise had a similar fear of Sam "vanishing", and for the first 12 months of his life, the timings and durations of all his feeds were recorded in a notebook, which was always prominent on the kitchen table. Louise always made sure I was fed, too, presenting me with a cup of tea within five minutes of my arrival and often offering me pieces of toast or cake. Selma Fraiberg has pointed out the presence of "ghosts in the nursery", "visitors from the unremembered past of the parents, the uninvited guests at the christening" (Fraiberg & Fraiberg, 1980, p. 164), and I found myself wondering if Louise's IVF babies who never were may also have played their part in her worries about Sam "disappearing".

Louise's husband worked long hours, and I admired her tenacity as she dealt with all the night feeds alone and was often very tired as a result. She employed a maternity nurse for the odd night, so she could have some unbroken sleep during Sam's early months. As is often the case with young mothers, she seemed quite isolated at times, and I found myself wondering about her mother, or whether she had friends who came and offered support. Louise's older child was nearly always at morning nursery during my observations, and although her father was a frequent visitor, a year passed before I met her mother. Louise let me know that she could sometimes experience her mother as quite intrusive, and during these times I wondered if she might lose contact with internal and external figures who could help her to mitigate her worries. It may be that this was one of the reasons she was so welcoming to me.

The early months

In my early observations, Sam appears to be a contented baby. He is often sleeping peacefully or is exploring his world happily, and Louise follows his cues. In an observation when he is 4 weeks old, Louise, is gazing at him asleep in his Moses basket and asks me if I think he has grown since my previous visit. She is concerned he is still not eating enough. She moves a muslin cloth away from his face, muttering, "Let's just make sure you can breathe." Her older child is at nursery, and when Sam stirs a few minutes later, she expresses a desire to feed him because they have time to themselves and will not be interrupted. She hesitates, looks closely at Sam, and tells me that he is not really awake, only dreaming, and leaves him to sleep on. Two minutes later Sam turns his head, stretches, and half opens his eyes.

> This time Louise went over to him and picked him up gently, placing him against her chest, with his face on her shoulder. She cuddled him and stood kissing his cheek gently, talking to him, saying, "You are such a lovely baby." She walked over to the sofa, all the while kissing him. Sam had gone back to sleep, and she commented, "Well, I suppose we can indulge this for a while, since your sister is out." Sam lay prone on her stomach with his head on her chest facing to the right, just tucked under her chin. He seemed very peaceful. Every few moments Louise turned to kiss her baby's cheek and rub his back.

Despite her concern about Sam's weight, and her desire to have the time to concentrate on feeding him without interruption, Louise, through thinking aloud—perhaps using the opportunity of having another person in the room to receive her worries—was able to give in to Sam's desire to remain blissfully asleep in his mother's arms, and to allow herself to enjoy their closeness. Sam is experiencing his mother's ability to identify with his needs and "hold" him, helping him to discover that external reality can be used for reassurance, adapting the environment to his needs (Winnicott, 1960).

At 8 weeks, Louise is trying to space out Sam's feeds, in order get him to take more milk at each feed. Sam is hungry and has been crying for a few minutes, his eyes wide and his face an angry pink.

> Louise, sounding exasperated, said "You can't be hungry. You really can't be. You only fed a second ago." She told him she was going to put him in his favourite position and walked to the other sofa under the window. She put Sam down on his back and stroked his feet, but Sam's cries intensified, his mouth widened, and tears started to form at the corners of his eyes. Louise quickly picked him up and said to him that she was going to give in and feed him—his milk was coming.

This seems to illustrate what Winnicott describes as "primary maternal preoccupation", a state of mind in which the mother is able to "drain interest from her own self on to the baby" (1960, p. 15). In Bion's (1962a) model of the container–contained relationship between mother and baby (see Appendix, "4. Containment"), Sam has been able to make his feelings clear, and Louise's maternal reverie has allowed her to process his distress and return it to him in a bearable form, a stage in Sam's development of a capacity to think.

During Sam's early months I witnessed many examples of his and Louise's mutual delight in each other. Klein points out that for the bottle-fed baby the bottle can take the place of the breast if there is a "close physical nearness to the mother and the infant is fed and handled in a loving way" (1952a, p. 99). Louise is cuddled up on the sofa feeding a 16-week-old Sam. Sam begins to frown, and Louise lifts him up, pats his back, and he burps.

> Louise sat looking at him, moving her face close to his and cooing at him. Sam gave a massive wide-mouthed smile and gently waved his arms, squawking as he did so. She tilted him towards her face and began to blow raspberries with her pursed lips. Sam smiled and squawked but every few seconds managed to purse his lips and make a weak blowing sound in imitation of her. . . . Louise stopped blowing raspberries and moved him close so she could kiss and nuzzle his neck. When she moved him back their faces remained close, and he smiled at her and cooed.

Sam and Louise's idealization of each other is clear—it is this projection of "love feelings" that Klein (1952c, p. 69) believes will allow Sam, and all babies, to internalize "the good breast", the good internal object that helps them feel all is well with the world and good inside. Meltzer (1987) has also written of the aesthetic reciprocity between mother and baby, this "love-at-first sight on the part of mother and baby" (p. 13), which is "crucial to their continued hopefulness" and the ability of the baby to tolerate the ambiguity of the maternal relationship.

Sam continued to develop well during these early months, putting on weight, although he was certainly not a greedy baby. He remained delicate in appearance—was extremely lively and curious, and rarely cried. Louise continued to express concern about Sam's lack of interest in food, but at the same time their ability to play together advanced. By 4 months it was clear that Sam was an active participant in their games. Brazelton and Cramer (1991) note how the synchrony of mother and baby can develop so that the two behave as if dancing together, each following the lead of the other. This was certainly the case with Sam and his mother.

> Sam looked up at her; she smiled, and he smiled back. She turned him round and stood him on his feet holding him up by his hands and then folded his arms down and up, stretching him out. He seemed to enjoy this and was chatting away, making little cries and squawks. When she had finished, she sat him down facing her again and leant forward and kissed him, imitating his baby

> noises. She then began to sing "Row, row, row your boat" to him, very softly, rowing him backwards and forwards as she sang. Sam looked entranced. Each time she sang about an animal noise, and made the appropriate roar or scream, his eyes and smile both grew wider, and his little body seemed to quiver.

Sam and Louise not only imitate each other but are able to anticipate each other's responses in a long sequence. Sam is learning that he has agency in eliciting responses from his mother as well as having an influence on the structure of the game, and Louise is extending his repertoire through play.

Difficult times

There were inevitably times, however, when I noticed what Stern (1977) called "missteps" in the dance. Sam was waking several times a night, and Louise was exhausted. In his 5th and 6th months, I noticed Louise worrying more about his weight. On several occasions I saw Louise attempt to coax Sam to take more of his bottle. On this occasion Sam has fed continuously for several minutes and then turns his head away from the bottle, apparently satisfied.

> Sam seemed very relaxed and floppy and was making a-a a-h sounds continuously. He put his fist in his mouth and began to suck it. Louise thought that he might want some more milk and put the bottle in his mouth. He gave two or three sucks, scratching his head with his left hand while he sucked. Louise said he did this often, and she wanted to stop him but didn't want to distract him from feeding. After a minute Sam stopped sucking and turned his head away. Louise took the bottle and sat Sam up. He gazed at me and put his fist back in his mouth. He twisted to his side and arched his back. He settled back, and Louise opened her hand in front of his face. Sam took his hand out of his mouth and held onto her hand with both of his hands. She moved her hand towards him, and she squeezed his cheeks. He smiled and continued his chatting. Louise picked up the bottle again and offered it to him, but Sam would not even have it in his mouth, immediately turning his head away.

Louise accepted Sam's refusal to have more bottle with good humour, but might Sam have been trying to find a balance between expressing his own desires and attempting to show concern for his mother as he reaches the stage of Klein's (1952c) depressive position? (see Appendix, "2. Paranoid–schizoid and depressive positions"). The infant perceives and introjects his loved object as a complete person, and a subsequent drive for reparation ensues. Sam accepts the bottle again, but in the seminar group we wondered about his head scratching. Might he be scratching his head to distract himself, or was it possibly as an expression of frustration that he must drink? Is his hand in his mouth as a way of recreating the pleasure of sucking or as a barrier to taking more milk?

As a result of his devoted early care Sam, has taken in a lot that is good, and he is a tolerant and adaptable baby, but during these few months I noticed that, at times, there were inevitable tensions and anxieties in the relationship. At the start of another observation in the same period, Louise looks strained and unwell and tells me that she is exhausted and has a cold. I notice that the feeding notebook is open on the table. Sam is delighted to see her when he wakes up from his morning nap, stretching and smiling up at her from his cot. Louise responds, cooing at him, but suddenly leans down and gets a mobile out, placing it above Sam. Sam frowns but starts to engage with it. Two minutes later Louise yanks it away, and Sam looks disconcerted.

Downstairs, Louise gets more toys out for Sam, and this pattern of interaction continues.

> First, she put a cuddly sheep on his stomach and pulled a cord so it played "Baa Baa Black Sheep". Sam seemed pleased to see this toy, giving a little shudder. As soon as the song stopped, Louise took the toy away, and started to drop a large frog with lots of coloured legs onto his stomach from a height.

Sam pulls the frog towards him and begins to suck it.

> Louise let him do this for about twenty seconds and then put him on his back and put on a dinosaur hand puppet and began to move it in front of his face. Sam put his hands on it and reached with his mouth to put one of the puppet fingers in his mouth. He sucked on it, but Louise took it away and began to tickle his tummy and his thigh with her gloved hand.

Louise continues to give and take away a succession of toys from Sam in an uncharacteristically abrupt way. He attempts to engage with all of them, either reaching for them or sucking them. He is playing with a rattle when Louise intervenes again:

> Suddenly she took the rattle from Sam, who looked startled. She pulled the baby ring towards her and put Sam in it. He immediately began to cry. She adjusted him, and he stopped crying, his eyes suddenly attracted by another of the black-and-white spotted panels. Louise then laid him back, so he couldn't see the panel, and he began to cry again. Louise picked him up and decided he must be hungry.

It seems that Sam can no longer tolerate continual disruption of his play and becomes distressed. I wondered whether Louise, feeling burdened by exhaustion and her cold, was unable to bear gaps in her interaction with him; it is almost as if he might fall through the gaps and vanish. Louise also seems less able than usual to tolerate Sam's separateness from her at this point, perhaps associating separation with loss. Louise has momentarily lost her usual very evident capacity for reverie, in Bion's (1962a) model, and is unable to allow space to play or experience frustration just now. I felt exhausted by the end of this observation: like Sam, I was unable to keep up with the changing toys and felt overwhelmed. I was also worried about Louise and wondered whether her mother or a friend could come and look after her. Louise interprets Sam's distress as hunger, perhaps unconsciously clinging to what she perceives as her main resource in her fight to ensure not only her son's survival, but his connection to her.

Sam's illness, perhaps unsurprisingly, seems to trigger similar behaviour in Louise. When Sam is 8 months old, he has a high temperature. Louise has given him medicine, but he is too unwell to play and is sitting on the sofa in his vest and nappy, watching the pictures on the television. Louise picks up a shaker and waves it in front of Sam, joking that she is getting in the way of the television.

> Sam hesitated, trying to keep his eyes on the TV, but then took the shaker and turned it round in his hand before sticking the narrow end in his mouth. His eyes went back to the TV. Louise hid a ball under one of the stacking cups on the sofa. Sam gave a big yawn. Louise called to him and took the cup away, revealing the ball. Sam glanced down. She did it again, and he gave a small smile, reached forward, picked up the green cup, put it in his mouth, and sucked it, again looking towards the TV. Louise thought maybe he should get dressed and picked him and leant him across her knee. Sam began to cry, face grimacing and arms out to his side. Sam continued to cry as Louise put on his trousers.

Sam appears to be working hard to humour Louise, who in this situation seems to find it difficult to tolerate any gap in her interaction with him, this time leaving him little space to be ill. I wondered about her persistence in dressing a sick baby when this appeared to be uncomfortable for Sam. It occurred to me again that Louise was struggling with her own feelings about Sam's illness, and she seemed to have temporarily lost any good internal figures to help her make sense of this. At times, it is clear that Louise is able to tolerate a sense of Sam as a separate individual, with his own appetite and agenda, and at other times, particularly under the extra stress of her own or Sam's illness, her anxieties come to the fore, understandably, as she perhaps becomes more worried about his survival.

The passage of time

Sam was weaned at 24 weeks, and Louise seemed to find the addition of solid food to his diet reassuring. As with the bottle, there were times in his 8th and 9th month when I thought Sam might be taking food to please his mother rather than because of his own hunger, often touching his lips with a piece of banana or a piece of cheese but then dropping it on the floor. Often Louise would then eat the food herself, as Sam looked on bemused.

Sam was allowed plenty of space to explore and develop. Louise was attentive and responsive. She talked and read to him constantly and very noticeably in their verbal interaction treated him as a person in his own right. At Christmas they gave me a small gift, and Louise told me that they had discussed it together and decided that Sam would give it to me himself. As Sam became less physically dependent on her, she seemed to find it easier to relax about his ability to survive, and was even able to acknowledge that he was thriving. Sam, it seemed, was becoming less allied with the ghosts in the nursery as he grew more robust, more corporeal. Sam coped well when Louise left the room and was able to make his interests clear during their play—he was particularly fond of balls and balloons. Louise followed his interests and encouraged him to explore and learn. Louise was proud of and reassured by his steady development and his acquisition of new skills.

At 12 months Sam began to crawl, and again this physical ability to move away from Louise seemed to help her trust in his capacity to grow and develop. She joked that she was becoming dispensable. She consulted a dietician about Sam, as if trying to gain some objectivity about his weight issue, and told me that the dietician had urged her not to worry about him—in fact at no time did Louise tell me that any health professional was concerned about Sam. In the meantime, Sam began to be more forceful about setting his own agenda.

At 13 months, Louise tries to interest Sam in his balloons:

> Sam ignored them and crawled over to a beaker of water, picked it up, had a drink, and then dropped it. Louise picked up the beaker and held it out to him. Sam batted it away quite aggressively with one hand. Louise held it towards him again and again he batted it away with some force.

Sam has enough confidence in his relationship with his mother to first ignore and then admonish her for attempting to interfere with his plans.

Sam also began to play games with Louise in which he tested boundaries. Whenever Louise told him not to put play dough or small plastic fruits in his mouth, Sam would inevitably touch them to his lips, simultaneously raising his eyebrow and a laugh from his mother. At 15 months Sam is walking and loves to kick balls round the living room. As he pursues a ball, his head comes close to the door jamb, and Louise tells him to watch his head.

> Sam stopped and turned round, looking at her. He grinned and then gently bumped his head on the jamb. He looked up at Louise and raised an eyebrow. Louise said she was telling him to be careful, and Sam gave a little smile and, once more, inclined his head and gently bumped it on the jamb. Louise laughed, told him he was cheeky, whereupon Sam walked towards her. She reached out for him and pulling him towards her, gave him a big kiss.

The teasing quality to their relationship shows the development of what Stern (1998) calls an infant's "intersubjective relatedness". Sam's sense of self is developed enough for him to recognize that his mother has a separate mind and that they can share experiences—teasing is impossible unless there is a shared apprehension of how the other will react. Louise, for her part, seems delighted by his cheekiness; she can really see that he's developing an autonomous character and identity.

By 14 months Sam was very advanced verbally, had many words, could identify the colour yellow, and loved joining in when Louise read to him. He was also able to tell Louise what food he liked, and I saw him eat a wide variety of snacks during my morning visits—some mornings it seemed as if he did nothing but eat.

When Sam was 16 months old, Louise told me:

> He didn't really have a problem with food any more; he was just Sam, a grazer who likes to have lots of small meals. He had probably always been like this, but now she recognized that this was his nature.

I was deeply moved and felt huge relief for them both.

A vaccination at 17 months seemed to trigger a return to Louise feeling that Sam's very existence was threatened, and Sam was also deeply affected when Louise went into hospital for several days and they were separated. However, by and large, Louise's delight and pride in Sam's enjoyment of life predominated, and they continued to share many special moments, appearing deeply in love with each other:

> Sam crawled out from under the table and went round to Louise and then pulled himself up on her crossed legs and climbed onto them. He leant his head right into her neck and put his little hands on her shoulders. She put her arms round him and bent her head into his neck and kissed him. They rocked backwards and forwards several times, each of their heads remaining buried in the other's neck. After a long cuddle they broke apart, and Sam turned to me and grinned. I was struck by how at one they seemed.

Conclusion

At times, during the first 18 months of his life, I wondered whether Sam's mother's worries might impinge on his emotional development. However, ultimately, I came to see that he was not a compliant baby but, rather, a child with an advanced capacity for concern (Winnicott, 1963a), a result of having a mother who was present and receptive to his efforts. Louise's own positive projective identification (Likierman, 1988) with Sam and her ability to allow him to feel enough frustration to develop a capacity to think meant that he was adaptable enough to cope with the missteps in the dance. Together, they found a way to accommodate each other. Louise was also generous to me and encouraged Sam to develop a trusting and affectionate relationship with me and with other visitors to the house.

It seems fitting to end this story with a scene that I recorded in Sam's 18th month. Sam has been playing near the stairs and is holding two small plastic balls. He gives one to Louise, and then comes towards me, with a smile, and holds up the other ball in front of my face.

> Sam then turned and walked to Louise, who gave him back the ball she was holding. Sam took both balls to the bottom of the stairs and sat down with them in his hands. He stood up and sat down again on the stair. He paused and looked ahead of him, and then glanced towards us and grinned. Louise said people still mistook him for a girl, because he had such delicate features. Sam stood up and then sat down again, still holding the little balls. After a pause, he did it again. We both laughed.

Louise accepts Sam's delicate features as part of who her child is. Sam is in close contact with his mother, and they share a mutual delight in his new skills, which he is exploring by himself. His sense of humour and playfulness entertains us both. The two balls he clutches are an indication that he is enjoying the attention of his mother and his observer, but it is perhaps most symbolic that he is clutching his mother's ball—a ball that has been offered to her as a gift and then returned to him as a gift.

Louise's receptiveness and attentiveness to Sam, together with Sam's own accommodating nature, his capacity to communicate his desires, and the reassurance afforded by the passage of time, seem to have won out over the very real and understandable worries that Louise felt about her son and his survival. Sam appears to be thriving, and it has been a privilege to watch his first months of life unfold.

Acknowledgement

We are grateful to Sam's parents for giving us permission to include Jenny Abbott's paper here.

CHAPTER THREE

An exploration of a nursery song, "The Police Dog", as a container

Tsutomu Ichige

In this essay I consider a Japanese nursery song, "The Police Dog", from a psychoanalytic point of view. This song is so well-known and popular that it is familiar to every Japanese person, as if it had existed in Japanese culture from the very beginning.

The aspect of the song that primarily interests me is something I noticed during my infant observation when the mother sang the song to her baby in response to the infant starting to cry. It seemed to me that on several occasions when the mother was tense, the song was more to calm the mother than to soothe the baby.

In this essay, it is not my aim to consider the composer or the lyricist. Instead, I focus on how this song, which has been sung throughout generations, is experienced by a mother and child, paying particular attention to what I see as its function for the mother.

First, I consider the mother's experience with regard to the lyrics. Next, I consider the musical aspects of this song and how its rhythm and cadence support the mother in her relationship with her baby. I then describe how the music can help to contain the mother–baby dyad and can help them re-establish equilibrium in their relationship when its stability has been challenged by the infant's primitive anxieties, particularly annihilation anxiety.

DOI: 10.4324/9781003564867-5

Before introducing the nursery song, I would like to present an extract from my infant observation where I became interested in the part this song played in the mother–baby interaction.

It was the eighth observation, which took place early in the new year, three weeks after the winter holidays, when the baby was 11 weeks old. At that time the baby, Amy, liked to play at kicking her mother's breast.

> While the mother was clearly in pain, she grasped one of Amy's feet in each of her hands, accepting them gently. She sang the nursery song, "The Police Dog", for Amy. The mother was more cheerful than in the last observation of the previous year; she was obviously relaxed, was enjoying communicating with her baby, and was speaking more to her. This was possibly because during the winter holidays Amy had started to smile at her mother, so she had gained greater confidence in their relationship.
>
> In the latter stages of this observation, when Amy was put down in her cot, she started to grizzle. After her mother changed her nappy, she calmed slightly, but she soon grizzled again. Her mother picked her up from the cot, then put her on the cushion on the floor and sang the song for her again. Mother's voice sounded pure, gentle, and beautiful. She said she wondered if Amy was listening to her singing, as the baby was moving her body in the rhythm of the song. She said that Amy might acquire a sense of pitch and rhythm, then she smiled at me. However, I thought that Amy still appeared anxious. She kept grizzling, turning her face to the side, bending her right arm, and bending and straightening her left arm repeatedly. Her mother continued to sing the song, although this did not soothe Amy, and she did not stop crying. Her mother tried to remember another of Amy's favourite songs, although she stopped because she supposed Amy did not know the songs she was going to sing. She said to me, "Amy might want to express something, but she cannot." She then drew Amy's attention by making a non-verbal high-pitched sound with her voice and started the kicking game by grasping both Amy's feet. "This sometimes improves Amy's mood, but not every time", the mother said. Amy was lying on her back on the cushion, gazing at me. She smiled just for a moment, but immediately her facial expression returned to being tense. Amy's mother held her up very naturally and swayed her body rhythmically while holding Amy in her arms. Once her mother realized that Amy had calmed down, she put her in the cot again.

When the mother first sang "The Police Dog" in this observation and while she played the kicking game with Amy, accepting Amy's aggression playfully and appearing to deal with her own pain and unconscious aggression, it seemed to me that she was able to feel confident as a mother.

When Amy started to grizzle, her mother sang the song again. I think that in this tense situation she might have been attempting to recover the previous good relationship with her baby, without being aware of that. Although the tense atmosphere gradually increased, she continued singing. When she tried to remember another song but could not recall one, it seemed to me that what she was truly looking for was a common language and memories of her good relationship with Amy.

After mother sang the song, she was able to express her feeling that she could not give her baby what she really wanted; she stopped singing and instead, she attuned with Amy by making more primitive sounds and created a rhythm with the kicking game. It might be, in other words, that she changed the song into a more primitive form for Amy. Through such interaction she might have been unconsciously attempting to accept not only the baby's distress, but also her own. Then she was able to hold Amy, and the baby could calm down.

In this context, I thought the nursery song played a role for the mother in soothing her and helping her to recover from a period of tension in the relationship between her and her baby.

Introduction to the song, "The Police Dog".

Poor little kitty cat has lost her way
Where is her house and where will she stay?
If you ask her address she cannot reply
If you ask her name little kitty starts to cry
Meow meow meow meow
Meow meow meow meow
Just ask her name and kitty starts to cry.

The police dog is deep in trouble now
All he could answer was
Bow wow wow wow
Bow wow wow wow.

Poor little kitty cat has lost her way
Where is her house and where will she stay?
If you ask the crow he won't know what to say
If you ask the sparrow she'll just fly away
Meow meow meow meow
Meow meow meow meow
Just ask her name and kitty starts to cry.

The police dog is deep in trouble now
All he could answer was
Bow wow wow wow
Bow wow wow wow.[1]

This song, with music by Megumi Oonaka and lyrics by Yoshimi Sato, was published in 1960. The main protagonist in the lyric is the police dog, who finds that even though he attempts to ask the little kitty about her identity, she can only cry. This leaves the police dog in a quandary, and this interaction between them is amusing and heart-warming. It makes me feel as if I hear the dog really saying, "It is me who wants to cry." The police dog who should not cry finally starts to sob, "Bow wow", and I find this really honest and human. In the relationship between the dog, cat, crow, and sparrow, we see that language cannot facilitate their communication. This song seems expressive of the situation where the animals are trying to understand each other but can't—they are upset, they want to help, but they have totally different tongues.

The element of a lost child in the song and in the mother–baby relationship

I am interested in what I see as a parallel between the relational dynamics portrayed in the song and dynamics within the mother–infant relationship; in the following sections I explore various aspects of the inter-psychic and intra-psychic processes suggested.

This interaction between the police dog and the little kitty seems to replicate the situation where a mother picks up a baby's distress when the baby starts to cry and then attempts to understand the baby's pain by asking, "Are you hungry, does your nappy need changing, or are you sleepy?"

The theme of this song is "lost child", and I think the primary "lost child" can be found within the mother–baby interaction. In the paper "The Infant's Response to Entrapment between Contradictory Messages in Face-To-Face Interaction" (Edward, 1978), the still-face experiment, a situation is described where the mother does not respond to her baby in her usual animated way but, instead, just presents the baby with a lifeless, completely still expression. It has been observed that a 2-month-old infant will attempt to gain her mother's attention in several ways, until the infant exhibits hopelessness and just resorts to crying. In the still-face situation the baby loses the mother through the disappearance of her lively facial expression and her sudden withdrawal of any ordinary interaction. This means that the baby loses the mother's smile, gaze, and warmth in reality, and also the ideal mother figure in fantasy. The baby then feels alone. Therefore, the baby has to look for both the internal and external mother, a situation described above as the primary "lost child". Winnicott (1967, p. 112) states that, in the mother's face, "what the baby sees is himself or herself", and he suggests that the mother's mirror-role leads the baby to find himself or herself and to exist. We could think of a lost child, not as losing its way physically, as the kitty does in the song, but, rather, as experiencing the absence of the internal and external mother—an experience that will be accompanied by a feeling in the child of losing him or herself.

Bion (1962b) explained that if an infant's capacity to tolerate frustration is inadequate, the infant cannot perceive "no-breast" and "instead there takes place a hypertrophic development of the apparatus of projective identification . . . all thoughts are treated as if they were indistinguishable from bad internal objects" (p. 112). The police dog is constantly asking the little kitty about her identity, but she can only cry. It seems that she is absolutely overwhelmed by frustration and distress and is unable to know who she is. The kitty is now in a regressed state: this situation of being "a lost child" thus evokes annihilation anxiety in her rather than separation anxiety. It can be said that her very existence is exposed to a crisis.

The crisis of the mother's existence

As I am particularly interested in exploring the mother's experience, I would like to pose the question of whether the mother might suffer a crisis of existence, just like the little kitty. Since the police dog starts to cry because he could not manage the distressing situation, we might infer that the kitty evacuates her annihilation anxiety into him through projective identification (Klein, 1946). Projective identification (see Appendix, "3. Projective identification") is an unconscious phantasy in which aspects of the self or of an internal object are split off and attributed to an external object (Spillius, Milton, Garvey, Couve, & Steiner, 2011b). Bion extends the application of this concept to interpersonal communication within the early mother–baby relationship, where the infant communicates his distress nonverbally through evoking a similar state of mind in the mother. The fear evacuated from the infant is *actually* experienced by the mother through projective identification, so, as Bion (1967b, pp. 114–115) described, "If the infant feels it is dying, it can arouse fears that is it is dying in the mother."

Linking the police dog and the kitty's interaction to a mother–baby relationship, I think it could be said that the mother has also become a lost child through experiencing the fear evacuated by the baby. It is interesting in this context that mother does not feature in this song—in other words, the mother herself might also be looking for a mother figure.

When intense raw emotion is projected into the mother by the baby, she can temporarily lose her sense of her identity. This challenge to her sense of herself comes on top of her still recent experience of becoming a mother, which is, in itself, an unstable situation that forces her to reconstruct her identity and will undoubtedly still be in the background. In the case of a mother with a high tolerance of frustration, while she can tolerate a crisis of losing her identity, she also has to look for several aspects of herself: her previous self as an individual, herself as a mother, and a good internal maternal object that helps to calm her down. In this case, it could be said that the internal good object means internalized "alpha-function" (Bion, 1962b).

Mother's internal dynamics

As well as understanding the parallel between the relationship of the police dog and the little kitty and a mother and baby—both inter-psychic relationships—I believe it might also be possible to make sense of it in relation to a mother's internal dynamics—the intra-psychic relationship. The internal state of tension created in the mother as a result of the infant's evacuation of distress into her could be regarded as a chaotic state between the parts of herself represented by the police dog, the superego, and the part represented by the little kitty, the id. Freud's view (1923b) was that the superego is formed through the "identification with parents". Therefore, this state might be described as the coexistence of the internalized parental aspect and the infantile part of herself. The reason I am avoiding the word "conflict" is that it does not convey the chaos of this internal state. The mother, who does not appear in this song, might herself experience difficulties in dealing with this situation and in finding the ego that is to organize the internal chaotic state.

Having considered unconscious processes during a period of emotional turbulence in the mother–baby relationship, the following sections examine in detail how effective music can be in soothing both mothers and babies and the role it can have in facilitating the restoration of a harmonious mother–infant relationship. I go on to consider what it might be about the content and structure of the police-dog song that can help mother and baby restore a harmonious relationship after a period of intense and destabilizing anxiety.

The place of music in repairing relationships

According to Graham Music (2017), singing improves an infant's mood, sleep, eating, and learning and is central to how infant emotional life is regulated. Shenfield and colleagues showed that maternal singing modulates 6-month old infants' arousal by lowering the cortisol level in their brains (Shenfield, Trehub, & Nakata, 2003) and was later found to be more effective than maternal speech at inducing recovery from distress in 10-month-old infants (Trehub, Ghazban, & Corbeil, 2015).

Before infants develop language, musicality is essential in communicating with them and attracting their interest. Infant-directed speech (IDS) is common in nearly all cultures and is characterized by the use of a higher pitch, longer hyperarticulated vowels, shorter pauses, and more repetitions than in usual speech (Music, 2017). Infants show an interest in the rhythm, prosody, and tempo of speech long before they understand the meaning of words (Malloch & Trevarthen, 2009).

From a psychoanalytic point of view, Winnicott viewed musical notes as transitional phenomena (Winnicott, 1953). In the mother–baby relationship, when the baby starts to cry and the relationship changes from being a previously undifferentiated/closely identified state to the baby and the mother facing sudden separation, they can become a "lost child" and a "lost mother". Thus, the mother might sometimes use music as a transitional phenomenon to alleviate the pain caused by separation and to help her to accept it. This might be based on the mother's experience of using music to soothe herself or perhaps her experience of having found her own mother's song soothing early in her life. Indeed, more primitively, it could represent babbling when she was an infant or the intra-corporeal beat during the embryonic period. In addition to learning from the experience of singing being passed down from mother to child, this soothing function would also be inherited and passed down through the generations.

The focus of my argument here is the annihilation anxiety that the mother and baby experience on a level deeper than separation anxiety. When the mother has taken in her baby's annihilation anxiety, is emotionally destabilized and is losing her integration, to what extent might music soothe her and help her to recover, and what impact might this have on the mother–infant relationship? In my view there are two general qualities present in such a situation, which I go on to consider.

The first quality is consistency. Music is a conglomeration of sounds, tones, and pitches. One note cannot be deemed music, as music must be composed with a certain rhythm, and it has an order and a structure. As people experience music, they could well have the experience of synchronizing their own internal physical and emotional rhythm naturally with the tempo and beat of the music they are listening to. Therefore, in the situation where the mother or the baby is fragmenting as a result of unbearable distress—that is, playing chaotic music in the relationship—I suggest that this type of actual music might help both mother and baby reconstruct and recover their own individual states of integration and therefore their capacity to re-establish a harmonious relationship. Within their relationship, the bond is held by a certain reciprocal rhythm, and this underpins their connection. Following a period of disturbance in the relationship, music might help them become more in tune with each other again on a nonverbal level, the level of connection that is fundamental in the mother–infant relationship.

The second quality is discharge, which I see as related to the action of singing and which therefore benefits the mother. In order for the mother to contain and digest the frustration and destructiveness projected into her by the baby, I see it as necessary for her to discharge or sublimate her own aggression. In the situation I describe, speaking and singing might be an effective way to deal with the aggression. Thus I believe that music can contribute to the recovery of the relationship through the consistency of its rhythm and the opportunity it gives the mother to manage her aggression through discharge.

The nature and function of repetition

Repetition, which seems to be of a specific type in the police dog song (Mine Kitamura), is a basic characteristic of nursery rhymes and is something that helps children understand and memorize them easily. In addition, it has been pointed out that it can be effective in improving memory function (Blum, 2013).

The police dog song contains layered repetition: it is useful to hear or read the original words:

Maigo no maigo no koneko-chan
Anata no ouchi ha doko desuka
Ouchi wo kite mo wakaranai
Namae wo kite mo wakaranai
Nyan Nyan Nya Nyan
Nyan Nyan Nya Nyan
Naite bakari iru koneko-chan

Inu no omawari-san Komatte shimatte
Wan wan wa wan
Wan wan wa wan

Maigo no maigo no koneko-chan
Konoko no ouchi ha doko desuka
Karasu ni kite mo wakaranai
Suzume ni kite mo wakaranai
Nyan Nyan Nya Nyan
Nyan Nyan Nya Nyan
Naite bakari iru koneko-chan

Inu no omawari-san Komatte shimatte
Wan wan wa wan
Wan wan wa wan

The song starts with repetition of the first words, "*Maigo no Maigo no*"; line 3 (beginning *Ouchi wo . . .*) is echoed by line 4 (*Namae wo . . .*) and this is followed by the cry of the kitty and the dog. The words of the second verse are an almost exact repetition of the first verse—only 9 of the 120 letters are different. As is typical of many nursery rhymes, the song is made up of a straightforward pattern of short, regular phrases, and there is frequent repetition of the simple four-quaver rhythm throughout.

With its repetition of the first word, the simple phrase structure, and the chorus, there are several similarities to the song "Twinkle Twinkle Little Star", a very well-known song that has traditionally been sung by mothers across cultures to soothe their babies.

Twinkle, twinkle, little star
How I wonder what you are
Up above the world so high
Like a diamond in the sky
Twinkle, twinkle little star
How I wonder what you are.

When the blazing sun is gone
When he nothing shines upon
Then you show your little light
Twinkle, twinkle, all the night
Twinkle, twinkle, little star
How I wonder what you are.

Repetition has various qualities, and I believe it can also have a range of effects on mental states, some of which I explore briefly below.

Repetition is predictable; its predictability can lead to a sense of security, and since it does not require complex psychological work, it can induce a relaxed state. This can be very useful for certain populations, such as people on the Autistic spectrum, as they commonly like to use repetition to find a sense of security in a world they can experience as excessively unpredictable. It is easy to recognize and imitate a repetitive pattern, and because it is easy to take in, the repetition can be effective in shifting attention away from distress. Moreover, the use of onomatopoeia in the Police Dog song makes the sound visual, so both the ears and internal eye are busy, thus adding an inherent element of distraction.

In addition, repetition produces a rhythm, and I believe that if a comfortable rhythm is connected to a comfortable memory, a similar rhythm will evoke comfort. It might replicate the mother's bodily rhythm during the intrauterine period, or it might evoke for the baby the experience of having been rocked in his mother's arms or in a cradle.

I think there is also a way in which repetition can create a space to ponder. When the mother is singing a repetitive melody, the repetition could lead to the suspension of the sense of things moving forward in the ordinary way, thus opening up a space to ponder—for something to be considered or reflected on. I believe that, through that process, the repetition can help the mother digest her intolerable emotion. It gives pause for reverie (Bion, 1962a) and thought.

A final and important feature of repetition is that it involves an ending that precedes the beginning of a new measured unit; there is a point at which one rhythm comes to an end and the same rhythm starts anew, and this can be seen to represent the cycle of death and rebirth. This might be experienced unconsciously, as an indicator that massive unbearable destructiveness is not endless, but finite. Furthermore, the experience that a certain rhythm still exists, even when the subject's emotion has changed dramatically, is related to object constancy. This might contribute to the capacity to tolerate distress, and even if the subject loses touch with her good objects, the continuing rhythm might help her to recover a more integrated state of mind, or at least a good part of the self.

The significance of sufficient regression in a mother role

Finally, we arrive at the chorus section, which seems the most characteristic in this song. Although the chorus is the most joyful section for both children and adults—particularly, perhaps, for adults—it could be said that it facilitates regression. This might not only be because this section is made up of the animals' calls, but it also consists of the vowel sounds "a" and "w", and the consonant "n", all of which are close to the infant's linguistic competence. Thus this part of the song could become the release point for the mother and the baby.

A mother will frequently sing or speak to her baby using similar language to her infant's voice. While singing the song, she both maintains her maternal function but also regresses emotionally to an extent, and in this way the song helps the mother tune in to both her own infantile self and the baby in her arms. Therefore, it could be said that the ability to regress to some extent is a necessary capacity for a container.

Should a container be in a major or minor key?

Although the theme of this song is "lost child", it is composed in a major key, which would traditionally give expression to an optimistic or happy theme. It may be a challenge for a singer to attempt to keep the balance between the sad content and the optimistic major key, which is perhaps similar to the mother keeping and holding pain in her mind while, at the same time, not being overwhelmed by a painful experience.

To empathize fully with the infant, it is vital to understand the infant's experience through being open to his distress, communicated through projective identification. However, if only offering empathy, the container could just stay in sympathetic vibration with the infant's painful emotion, leading not only to the container being emotionally overwhelmed, but also reinforcing the infant's pain. The process of psychological digestion is also an essential aspect of the containing function.

In general, a sad song is sung in a minor key; but this is not a straightforward correlation, and there are also songs such as this one or parts of songs, exploring painful experiences, that are written in a major key. If this major key evokes only good feelings where pain is denied (a manic defence), singing the song could work as a temporary measure, but not as a container that could facilitate growth. In my opinion, this is an important point and is linked with whether or not the mother is able to digest the frustration evacuated from the baby and act as a container for the baby's distress.

On listening to this song, unlike some songs in a minor key, I do not hear anyone who feels deeply sad. Instead, I imagine that the mother figure who can tolerate the difficult situation and can bear the strong feelings is there, somewhere in the background. She is supportive and watching over the kitty and the police dog, smiling slightly. That is the object and support that the mother herself needs if she becomes a "lost mother" in the emotional turbulence, and also the alpha function and healthy part of the mother's self.

Thinking of a song as functioning as a container, there are many complexities in whether it is preferable for it to be in a major or minor key, one of these being that unless a piece or song is very short, it is likely to include passages in both major and minor keys. There is no single prescription, even for a very short song—this might vary depending on the relationship portrayed, the degree of pain being expressed, and the quality of containment needed. If the person who needs to be contained is more immature or vulnerable, we could say that the container is be required to promote his or her own resilience and positive emotion within the relationship. Following this argument, as this song is a nursery rhyme and explores the young child's strongest fear of being separated from the parent and getting lost, I think it makes sense here that the major key is used, promoting the sense of a resilient container.

Conclusion

In this chapter a nursery song, "The Police Dog", is explored from the viewpoint of a mother–baby relationship, highlighting the mother's experience.

When the baby is exposed to intense frustration or distress, the mother can experience fragmentation as a result of the baby's projective identification, and she might also become a "lost mother". If she can discover an internalized mother as alpha function in her internal world and organize herself, she can recover and in so doing recover her capacity to contain her baby.

For the mother singing the song, the chaotic state that she is experiencing with her baby is reflected back to her through the song, and she can re-introject it in a simpler and more playful form, as a container–contained experience. This may help the mother to regain her capacity to think about the baby and thus restore equilibrium in the relationship.

The musical aspects of this song, with its lynchpins of rhythm, consistency, and repetition, help the mother reintegrate several aspects of herself. The song can hold and bond mother and baby—even a fragmenting mother–baby dyad. The processes described can contribute to the mother recovering her maternal function and repairing the relationship with her baby that had fractured momentarily.

Note

1 https://www.youtube.com/watch?v=OzD59YsLqXA)

CHAPTER FOUR

"Mother-less": A psychoanalytic observation of an installation by Cathy Wilkes

Deirdre Ingham

I first came to experience the work of Cathy Wilkes in 2013, at the 55th Venice Biennale, where her installation, *Untitled (Possil, at last) (2013)*, was exhibited. I was drawn to it without knowledge of Wilkes or her work, but nonetheless it spoke to me and pulled me into its psyche. Such was the emotional and psychological quality of this work that I continued to observe it from within, long after I had separated from its physical presence.

In this chapter I attempt to communicate what I experienced and continued to experience through my personal relationship with Wilkes' work, and in doing so aligning it to the psychoanalytic practice of infant observation and psychoanalytic ideas that strive to understand another's experience. It is therefore not an analysis of the artist but, rather, a reflection upon what her work communicated to me. It is a conversation between the work and what is referred to in psychoanalysis as my "inner world" (see Appendix, "1. The inner world and the good object"). Of course, there may be some overlap between the unconscious of the artist and the unconscious of the observer,[1] but unlike Freud (1914b), who approached Michelangelo's *Moses* as a psychobiography of the artist, this chapter is more concerned with the experience of engaging with art. For this reason it is also necessary to give some thought to the psychoanalytic observational approach that has imbued the observer's experience.

DOI: 10.4324/9781003564867-6

The art of observation

The way in which I related to Wilkes' work was very much informed by my experience of psychoanalytic infant observation[2] as originally taught by the Tavistock Training and described in Chapter 1. In the 1950s the child analyst Esther Bick developed the role of infant observation as a method for training child psychotherapists. It now forms a central part of many psychoanalytic trainings, with its tenets serving to inform practice. Outside the sphere of psychotherapy, its application is also widely recognized and can include, but is not limited to, a psychoanalytic understanding of art, literature, music, theatre, politics, and society.

At times misconstrued as being solely a task in learning about child development, its wider concern pertains to the world of relationships, inner and outer. The observer learns to observe, not just what is in front of them, but equally what is evoked inside them by what they see. In other words, the observer also learns to observe themselves. Michael Rustin (1989) emphasizes the need for the observer to be able to take in what is in front of them when he says, "The observer has to be a receptive register of emotions in others and herself" (p. 66), and, in line with this paper, so does the observer of art. Such observation of the internal and the external gives rise to meaning making and an endeavour to understand the other.

According to Winnicott (1963b), artists are people driven by the tension between "the urgent need to communicate and the still more urgent need not to be found" (p. 186). It seems to me that one can extend and map this idea also on to the experience of the observer of art. What we see in a work of art may be a discovery of something hidden within ourselves, which can, in turn, be given expression in the observer's response. In the practice of psychoanalytic infant observation, following the hour-long observation, the observer must write a detailed account of what they have seen and what they have felt. The observer creates a written piece that is their interpretation of the scene played out before them. It is akin to the artist's drawing of a life model—or, indeed, to the writing of this chapter.

Psychoanalytic infant observation requires a stillness in the observer that allows for the mother–infant relationship to emerge in front of them. At times the whole scene is taken in, and at other times small fragments, gestures, and words might capture the observer's attention. The observer may become interested in how the infant feeds; how the mother lays the infant down; how the eyes can follow; or how the infant's milk drips from the corner of her mouth after time at the breast. The observer's emotional lens allows for an apprehending of the whole, as well as of particular details that capture her curiosity. This; too; echoes how the observer engages with the art object.

While the observation of art and its relationship with psychoanalytic infant observation is embedded in this chapter, it is also worth acknowledging the process of making art as having a corresponding observational property. The artist, whether drawing from life or assembling objects, as with Cathy Wilkes, is engaged in the observing of life outside herself and from within herself. There is dialogue with what she sees and what she feels, culminating in the art object. Of course, this is a somewhat reductive description of an otherwise intense and complex process, but it highlights the function of close observation as having a resonance in art making, art observing, and the practice of psychoanalysis.

The artist's voice

Originating from Northern Ireland, Wilkes moved to Glasgow to study Fine Art, and, after qualifying, has continued to live and work there.

In a video produced by The Tate, Wilkes speaks about her work, illustrating her contemplations on the inner and outer realities she ascribes to objects (The Tate, 2008). Much of what she describes in her relationship with the world of people, objects, and experiences parallels the language of psychoanalysis—for example, she speaks about internal and external objects: inner worlds, shadows, and the psychoanalyst's attempt to understand another's experience. Thoughts of her inner world, her memories and realities, create a sense that Wilkes is intuitively working across the conscious and the unconscious realms, as in the psychoanalytic experience. However, in her reflections upon her work she makes reference to the direct influence of a more philosophical perspective, through the work of Friedrich Nietzsche. Pondering the objects she uses, she probes their relationships, both internal and external, to herself and others.

These contemplations are continued in her personal notes, shared by the artist with the author of this chapter. Wilkes ruminates upon the story of the infant Moses—or, more specifically, the moment when Moses' mother Jochabed lets go of the infant Moses in his basket. The quality of the ruminations below resembles that of the free association of thoughts and feelings revealed on the psychoanalytic couch.

> Even during the most intimate experiences when I have extended beyond myself, far out of my limits, my body and mind; the births of my children, the deaths of my parents, separation has remained unbridgeable. There's no expectation that an audience will participate. And no need for someone to fully understand. At the same time,

> through contemplation and communion, all objects can become transcendental. I fixate on the sensation and vision of Jochabed's fingers, and the bulrush basket which has her baby inside. Her fingers rest on the basket, and then she withdraws them. According to her conscience. I won't leave this sensation alone and I keep going over it, repeating the picture in my mind, pushing forwards with my fingers into nothingness. The suffering of Jochabed, and the ebb of the water. Minds make everything continuous and whole. As much as I fixate relentlessly—and that may be about object relations—I also conceive of wholeness which makes everything present in the same thought.
> [Personal communication to Kate Robertson, 2023]

In comparing her work to the image of an infant, born from inside her, and then the painful task of separation, Wilkes vividly brings to life the intimacy of her creative process. At the very moment of separation Wilkes seems to be reflecting upon whether the infant was let go of, or whether he was taken from the hands of the mother through the ebb of the water. Such ruminations on these uncertainties and separations appear embedded in much of her work. Are they narratives of the external world, or are they expression of her internal world? Are they the world of the living or the dead? The observer is never quite sure, but one could imagine that the resulting impact might also lie in the internal world of the observer.

What is particularly striking about Wilkes' metaphor of Moses is that in the original story Moses' mother released Moses to the river as his life was in danger. Such was her fear about Moses' safety, she was prepared to let him go without knowing how, or if, he would be found. The moment when her fingers are "withdrawn" appears to encapsulate something for Wilkes that is essential in her communication. Perhaps the parallel here is when her work moves into other spaces and is received by the world. The conflicting ideas of whether her "art infant" is taken or whether it was let go of is evident. The association that is conjured in my mind is that of the young women in mother-and-baby homes who lost their infants under the notion that they would be safer with another mother. These infants were both given up and stolen, as was Moses basket both let go of and taken by the water. For Wilkes' art infant, once this separation has occurred, it is then met by the mind of the observer—or, using the Moses story, the arms of an-other mother, the observer.

The phrase "separation has remained unbridgeable" perhaps emphasizes the sense of unrecoverable loss that permeates Wilkes' installation and, as referred to by her, is likely to be part of the process of the making of her art. Through this unbridgeable and unbearable separation comes a repetitive working through in her mind—an attempt, as Wilkes says, to bring the experience into a whole existence in her mind.

Untitled (Possil, at last)

Following on from the Venice Biennale, further versions of this installation have been exhibited in Glasgow, Liverpool, and Europe. While all versions have the same title and are assembled with broadly the same objects, there are also some subtle differences that are brought about through the relationship with the space and the relationship to other works placed in proximity. At Tate Liverpool it was less easy to identify the boundaries between the installation and her other pieces of work in the exhibition. The installation seemed to either have expanded to take on new dimensions, or have merged with earlier pieces with similar qualities. The merging resulted in a seeping and leaking effect. Such merging evoked uncertainty regarding where *Untitled (Possil, at last) (2013)* ends or begins, or what belongs inside or outside, as was also evident in the original installation exhibited at the Venice Biennale.

This fluidity presents the observer with a sense of precariousness and elusiveness, like that of memories that alter depending on the context in which they are remembered. Despite this, Wilkes' work continues to hold on to a powerful sense of loss, mourning, and deep despair. The seeping between images and memories did not seem to change the meaning or the impact but felt more like a searching, or a further attempt to join up and make sense of experiences. A search to communicate and find a mind to be homed in—a mind to hold it and a mind in which to be remembered and understood.

While the observer's personal response to the installation was formulated prior to the writing of this chapter it is interesting to note the points where it touches the artist's own voice. In the earlier quote by Wilkes she states, "There's no expectation that an audience will participate. And no need for someone to fully understand." Later, she adds, "I also conceive of wholeness which makes everything present in the same thought." Through these words she seems to allude to the audience's/observer's mind as a further attempt to hold and attempt to make sense of the separation.

Maternal loss

Wilkes' installation (Figure 4.1) consists of five figures—four children and one male figure (Figure 4.2), who is slumped near an empty brown bottle. The figures are unformed, rudimentary, and offer only the suggestion of a person. Genders are not absolutely clear, nor are their relationships. One can easily infer a family unit, but, as with much of Wilkes' work, there lies

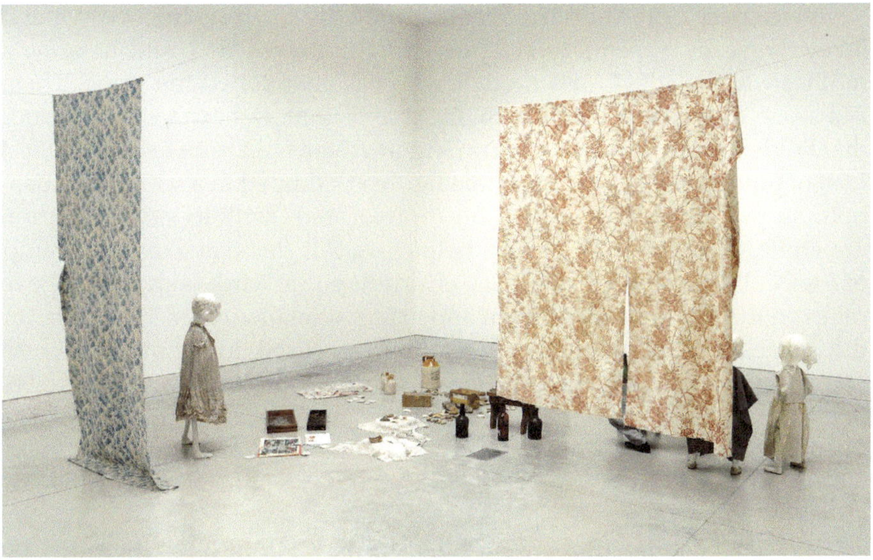

Figure 4.1

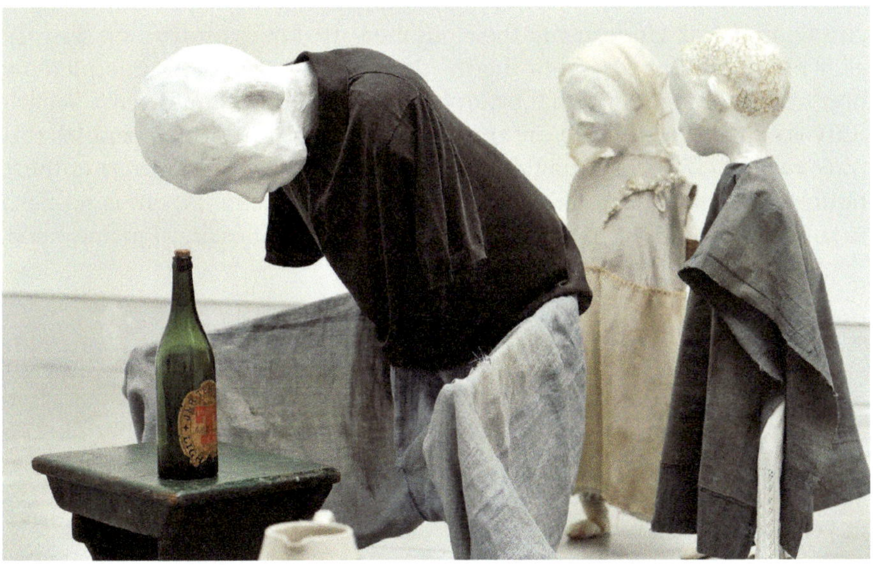

Figure 4.2

uncertainty. Objects appear scattered across the space: a brown bottle, a milking stool, faded textiles, and broken pieces of earthenware, all objects possessing an historic quality, as if speaking of the deep past.

While the figures and objects appear striking, the sense of what is not present seems to hold equal significance in this piece. It is at times the negative space or the absence that captured my interest. On a very literal level, the scene appears to lack an actual mother. One could imagine a mother who has died, or a mother who has abandoned the scene. There is a sense of this loss being permanent and final, rather than an absence that holds the potential for a return. Again, there is an echo here of Wilkes' idea of unbridgeable loss. The male figure is slumped in a seemingly alcoholic stupor at the loss, or possibly "intoxicated" with loss. The children are alone, bleak, and observing helplessly. All this climaxes in feelings of loss, collapse, and emptiness. Considering this work with a literal eye relies on the world of attachment and external relationships. However, for the purposes of this analysis my reading is focused on the installation as primarily an expression of the internal world of object relations. This does not negate a more narrative reading, as both may operate simultaneously. Therefore, on a less figurative level and perhaps more interestingly, I also look at the maternal loss as it is echoed in the symbolic use of the materials and the more abstract aspects of the piece.

The lack of a maternal presence makes itself felt through the structure of the figures. Seemingly constructed from papier mâché or felt, the man and the children are draped in faded antique cloth that appears to be like curtain material. Underneath the cloth there are knees protruding sharply, as if piercing the body from the inside (Figure 2). Something is piercing him from within, an internal trauma desperate to reveal its secret. A curiosity is evoked, and the observer wonders what else is hidden beneath this pink curtain skin. One imagines no flesh or muscle on the bones of these figures. They seem starved and bereft of any protection; there is no flesh to softly wrap and cushion their structure. Their bodies are skin and bone.

Breast-less

According to Donald Winnicott, an infant manages separation from the mother through adopting a transitional object, which holds qualities that are akin to the mother/breast. One such physical quality is that of softness, and often a soft toy or blanket may become the comforting object in the mother's absence (Winnicott, 1971b). Such a soft quality is not evident in Wilkes' piece. The work feels devoid of any such softness or comfort, and there appears no attempt to recreate a symbolic sense of the comfort of the maternal through any of the material objects present in this installation. I found myself wondering if perhaps this is not necessarily symbolic of a lost maternal object that was known but, rather, a mourning of something that was never fully experienced or known and subsequently not concretely remembered.

This experience is suggestive of Bollas' idea of the "unthought known" (1987, p. 34), whereby an archaic experience of maternal handling and care is remembered inside us, but not as a concrete memory—rather, on a sensorial level. The mother, through the process of her bodily and psychic care, transforms the infant's experience and in doing so becomes a "transformational object" (p. 14) to the infant. According to Bollas, "If he is distressed, the resolution of discomfort is achieved by the apparitional-like presence of the mother. The pain of hunger, a moment of emptiness, is transformed by mother's milk into an experience of full-ness" (p. 33). This transformation of feeling, through the milk and the handling of the mother, is what Bollas describes as the earliest human aesthetic (p. 32). Bollas stresses that this is less about the mother as a person and more related to the infant's repetitive experience of her, and this experience remains inside us throughout our lives—known, but not thought. The adult later searches unconsciously for a familiar transformational object through relationships as well as through aesthetic experiences such as art. In these moments the observer of art enters into an "an intense affective experience" that has its origins in the early transformational object (p. 17). Wilkes' installation, through its presence and absence, held me as described by Bollas.

In a later version exhibited by Tate Liverpool, the installation includes child figures lying on the floor of the gallery. Their heads are in contact with the cold, hard concrete floor. There is no pillow/breast, and the image feels stark and painful—so much so, that one wonders whether the children are, in fact, dead, or deadened, in order to manage this pain. An even more powerful response is the imagining of what is not there—the pillow—and the desire it evokes in the mind of the observer—a wish to summon it physically and to place it under the head of the child lying on the concrete floor. Melanie Klein states that softer, more comforting objects represent the comfort of the mother or the breast: "We find that things to sit and lie upon, as well as beds, occur regularly in children's analyses as symbols for the protecting and loving mother" (Klein, 1929, pp. 213–214). There is no object to sit on other than a small milking stool, and this is utilized by the adult figure. There are no beds, no cushions, pillows, nor blankets. There is only the silent timbre of the absence of softness, love and maternal qualities.

Arm-less

After a slow advent in the mind of the observer, Wilkes' installation reveals what feels like a secret. The figures are arm-less, unarmed, and lacking protection. As in the entirety of this installation, this facet is steeped in ambiguity. We know neither if arms were had and lost, or if they were never formed. The limbs that allow one to hold another, or to hold oneself together, are absent. In turn, there are neither hands to hold, nor to be held. There is no reaching for another, only space between, each figure appearing in their own desperate isolation.

Winnicott's idea of holding refers not only to the physical holding of the mother's arms, but also to the emotional and psychic experience of the environment. It is both a concrete description and a metaphorical one. Not only do the arms hold, but so do the voice, the face, and the eyes. The armless children in Wilkes' work create an emotional sensation in the observer to hold them, as they have never been held.

In totality, the work conveys a lack of holding in the absence of arms, the lack of softness and sense of collapse in the male figure. What is curious, however, is that I felt that the piece had enormous capacity to "hold" me as the observer. I mused upon these armless figures and endeavoured to peer into the gaps in the cloth where arms should be, in an attempt to find a trace, a stump of an arm, or to find evidence that they had been absorbed into the torso in order to hold oneself from inside. Perhaps I was drawn in, hoping to discover the potential for holding and something that could be developed, as its absence was unbearable. This was particularly the case in relation to the children, whose desperation begged the observer's arm-like mind to hold them, as if held in arms. They needed to be held in mind.

Face-less

The children in Wilkes' work have faces that feel unformed, almost foetus-like (Figure 4.3). It is as if emotional development has been arrested, that the gaze while at the breast has never taken place, having not been held by maternal eyes. Alternatively, and in the spirit of this work's ambiguity, one could observe this as an expression of regression in the face of desperate loss. Either reading presents the viewer with faceless figures that have only black dots for eyes, no orifice for a mouth, and no nostrils to breathe. It is as if every possible bodily aperture between inside and outside is sealed. Nothing can be introjected, nor projected, thus leaving the figures locked inside themselves. This ultimately gives the work a sense of an unawareness of the observer's presence: its gaze is not returned, nor are we breathing the same air. The observer is glimpsing some ancient history, a step back in time.

Through his work with adults, Winnicott (1967) developed a theory that considered the mother's face as being an emotional mirror for the

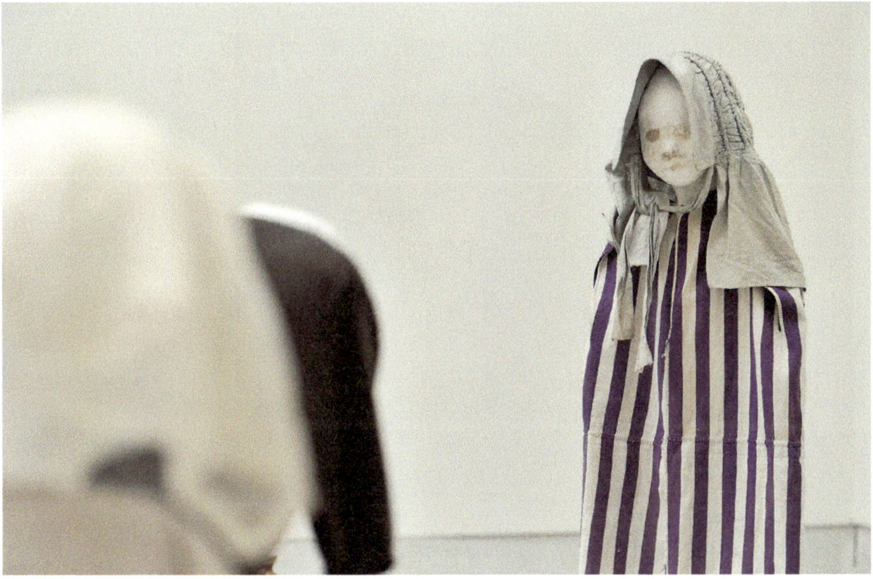

Figure 4.3

infant. He wondered what the baby sees when looking into the mothers face) and suggests that the baby sees him/herself. This process of reflection is essential in the emotional development of the infant but can at times be disrupted. When the mother reflects her own defences or her own mood, the infant's "own creative capacity begins to atrophy" (p. 112). A lively and loving maternal face lends itself to a more affective understanding of the infant's emotional state. Alternatively, the flat and inanimate facial expression will also be taken as the infant's own. Within Winnicott's writing there is an acknowledgement that this experience has to be repeated over a significant period of time for it to be taken on by the infant: the mother's face is not taken in by the infant through a one-off event.

If one imagines the maternal experience of Wilkes' children, it would be that of a depressed and withdrawn mother. Their faces reflect a blank, lost, distant feeling lacking the internalization of the mother's face. Perhaps if there ever was a mother, she would have been absent even in her presence.

Skin-less

Evocations of skin permeate the piece in the form of cloth and papier mâché, with faded textiles covering and draping the figures. Large sheets of domestic material loosely divide and cut up the space (Figure 4.4).

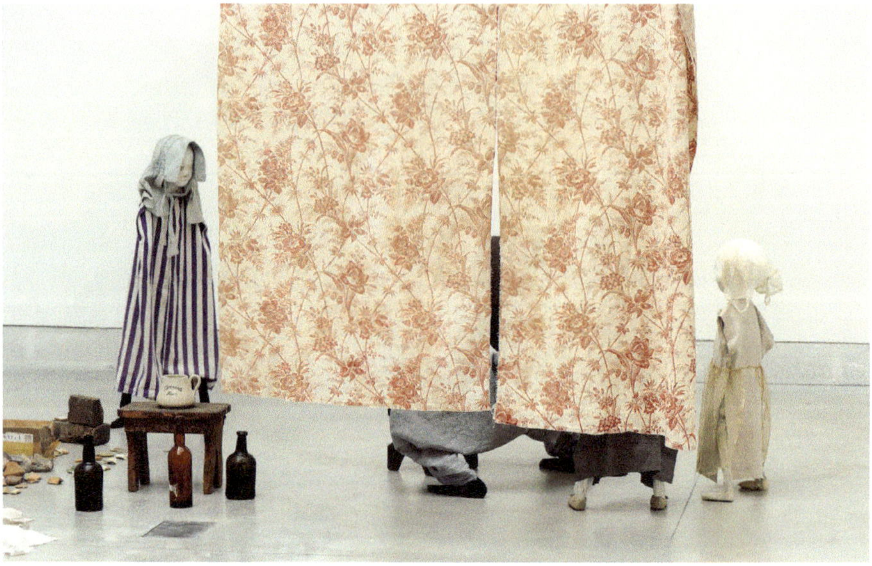

Figure 4.4

Little direct representation of skin can be seen as the material covers most of the body. The material itself appears to represent a skin that offers a vague and loose delineation between the outside, inside, and underneath. The skin's ordinarily protective quality is not evident in this covering. Its looseness gives way to gaps and spaces, drafts and the cold.

A closer observation of the cloth reveals its warp and weft, the rhythmic coming together of these threads forming the holding and protective function of clothing. At times the warp and weft are so tightly together that there is no discernible difference between them; at other times they appear so loose that there is the potential for seepage or a rift. Like the coupling of the parental couple, in its perfect resonance, it comes together to form what is needed for the child. However, in *Untitled (Possil, at last) (2013)*, it seems to provide little protection, containment, or holding. The material seems to have found a second-hand function, having been discarded from its original domestic function, perhaps of a curtain. The cloth does not originate there but has, rather, been bequeathed, like a maternal ghost, providing an inadequate replacement for the skin formed through a relationship with the maternal mind.

In her 1968 paper, "The Experience of the Skin in Early Object Relations", Esther Bick explores the skin's integral contribution to the early emotional development of the infant. For Bick, the infant is thought to possess a bundle of bodily sensations, with no sense of inside and outside.

The skin operates as a container that provides the infant with an experience of being physically, and therefore psychically, held together. The skin's containing function comes into being with the attention of the mother, which, if dysfunctional, could create what she calls a second-skin defence in the infant. One such example of this is the child who adopts a more muscular containment in form of her strength.

We could think of Wilkes' cloth as a form of second skin that is, in itself, an extremely inadequate attempt at holding the self together. It is loose and lacks the firmness of holding; it is compensatory to the protective skin, which would have grown with the help of the maternal mind. Such a sad and desperate attempt at being held emphasizes once again the despairing and desolate theme underlying this installation.

Place-less

Wilkes' chosen title for the piece reflects the familiar feeling of uncertainty—*Untitled (Possil, at last)*. We are unsure whether it is named, unnamed, or perhaps there is something that just can't quite be named in this piece. "Possil" perhaps refers to the Possil Pottery of Glasgow, which initially created stoneware and later stoneware beer bottles. Here the piece is given a more social dimension and evokes echoes of the loss of the pottery in 1942. The pottery employed, as did most potteries at the time, many women and possibly even children. It's loss is likely to have had a huge impact on the livelihoods of the women and their families working in them. Therefore, the name of "Possil" used in the title could bring in yet another sense of loss, poverty, and deprivation, albeit on a societal level, but equally resonant of the personal loss for the families.

The material of pottery and clay also hold archaeological significance in relation to women. According to Neumann (1963), pottery and the clay from which it is made has deeply feminine (and therefore maternal) associations. The pottery in this installation is broken, shattered, and strewn across the space, with seemingly no hope for repair. The name of "Possil" has echoes and reverberations across time and space. It has a relationship with the work of women, the body of women, and the loss of place that functioned as a provider in Glasgow. In this aspect of the installation Wilkes seems to be drawing from the context within which she works. But this place no longer exists, it has gone. Even the potential imagining of the containing walls or pots are in pieces on the ground. The work, not having the frame of a painting or the plinth of a sculpture, finds its place within the looser frame of the structure of the gallery and, as previously discussed, through the mind of the observer.

The materials of the maternal

The materials an artist uses and how they are used holds a fascination for me, whether the artist is a child in my role as an art or child psychotherapist, or a formal artist. The relationship with the materials allows for the materialization of something new. In Wilkes' piece I moved my observational position, so that I could both take in the whole piece and zoom in to the detail and the materials from which the piece has been made. Such zooming in allows for a more abstract and sensorial response to the minutia of the work. As an observer of Wilkes' work, the materials that particularly resonated were the use of cloth, the broken clay, and what seemed to be papier mâché and felt used for the heads of the figures, all of which created an urge in me to engage physically through touch—something forbidden and impossible in the gallery space, as well as psychically. This inability to touch created a distance, as if witnessing a ghost-like memory.

For Bollas (1992), evocative objects embodied what he calls a "sensational print" and are recognized in a "sensational knowing" (pp. 34–35) by the other or, in this case, by the artist or observer of art. We are drawn to them as they resonate with our inner states, they speak to us as they hold the sense of our early experience with the transformational object. Following this line of thought, the artist chooses materials according to her inner world, as these objects and materials speak to her of something familiar. The observer of art is, in turn, equally drawn to the materials in images as they, too, resonate with her own inner state, perhaps for reasons different from those of the artist.

The "sensational" qualities inherent in these materials are held together by the sense of something archaic, distant, and partially remembered. The observer could, through her mind and body, imagine the roughness of the cloth, the sharpness of the broken pots, the coldness of the floor. The heads of the children beckoned a wish to be stroked and smelled, like one would smell the head of a new-born infant. Those qualities invited the observer into a maternal interaction.

Conclusion: time-less

Throughout this chapter I have referred to an overarching atmosphere of something deeply ancient and archaic contained within this installation. It is difficult to place it within a particular time, but its haunting quality reverberates of the old. However, for me as the observer, I can equally feel a sense of the present—or, more specifically, the past in the present. In this way the piece is timeless and summons the notion of loss that continues to breathe within its aesthetic. I am reminded of the seminal and often quoted paper by Fraiberg, Adelson, and Shapiro (1975), "Ghosts in the Nursery: A Psychoanalytic Approach to the Problems of Impaired Infant–Mother Relationships". The paper begins with an almost poetic account of the intergenerational transmission of trauma: "In every nursery there are ghosts. They are the visitors of the unremembered past of the parents, the uninvited guests at the christening" (p. 387). The use of the description "unremembered" seems to me at the core of my aesthetic response to this installation and swaddles all the aspects of maternal loss described above. The maternal loss may, of course, not be an actual loss but, rather, a loss or an absence of a quality of feeling and experiencing.

My intent here has not been to interpret, nor to psychoanalyse, the artist but, rather, to describe my aesthetic response to the work she created. Much like the artist and her materials, this chapter has become the embodiment of my aesthetic relationship with *Untitled (Possil, at last) (2013)*.

Image credits

Cathy Wilkes, *Untitled (Possil, at last) (2013)*; Mixed media; Dimensions variable. Installation view "The Encyclopedic Palace", Venice Biennale, Venice, 2013. Courtesy of The Artist and The Modern Institute/Toby Webster Ltd, Glasgow. Photo Cristiano Corte https://www.themoderninstitute.com/artists/cathy-wilkes/exhibitions/the-encyclopedic-palace-venice-biennale-venice-2013-06-01/4653/

Notes

1 The observer's response may also echo the response that other observers of the art may experience.
2 It is important to differentiate psychoanalytic infant observation from other forms of infant observation used by other professionals interested solely in the physical development of the infant.

CHAPTER FIVE

The is-ness of things: reflections on observation used in contexts where words are hard to find

Olivia Sagan

Although it feels fresh, like yesterday, it was almost twenty years ago that I undertook the Psychoanalytic Studies course at the Tavistock, an integral part of which is an infant observation. Learning to observe without notes, assumptions, intervention, or plan was a challenge, but it opened up a vista for me of both the possibilities and the demands of free-floating attention (Bion, 1970a) and negative capability (Keats, quoted in Bion, 1970a, p. 125). Later, I found that the Buddhist concept of Sartori, or Zen Kensho, with its evenness of passivity, insight, and receptivity, added further dimensions to these concepts—as well as further challenges. It is not within the bounds of this chapter to go into these concepts in detail, but I do give a vignette of how powerful they have been in enabling me to observe observation—and be human first and foremost in my critical and analytic work as a teacher, counsellor, psychologist, and researcher. My observational experience nearly two decades ago laid a touchstone for me to return time and again to the words of the late great psychotherapist and Buddhist, Nina Coltart. She insisted that "Bare attention has a sort of purity about it. It's not a cluttered concept" even when, or especially when, conditions are far from conducive to the paying of attention (Coltart, 1998, p. 176).

The observations I undertook of Kazim, a refugee child (Sagan, 2003), in a North London nursery taught me first-hand two important things: First, the infinite layers of being, cognition, emotion, and activity involved

DOI: 10.4324/9781003564867-7

in observing an action and *refraining* from interpreting it, let alone judging it, allowing its witnessing to "wash over" you until something of its essence has settled and resonated. While Kazim went about his aggressive "trashing" of a domestic play scene in which two other children were happily engrossed, for example, what I felt once I allowed the frustration and my impulse to "do" *subside*, as I watched his apparently senseless and macho intervening on another's child's delicate and homely play—was sheer pain: something of loss, of envy, too, and yearning. These messy and unwelcome feelings were core to understanding Kazim a little, and a key to his experience as a refugee child coming from a war-torn part of the world in which he had witnessed horrific scenes of violence and senseless destruction that could not possibly begin to be processed by so young a child.

Second, emerging very quickly in my observations as Kazim struggled with language, both with his native tongue and with English, was the power, fickleness, and inadequacy of words—yet their potency, too, and their power as currency. Brought sharply to my attention, too, was how poor we are at "listening to silences, the omissions, the stutters and the slips" (Sagan, 2003, p. 14). As I observed Kazim's struggles and his rejections of language, conversation and listening, and how, like the old pop song I used at the time suggests, "you say it best when you say nothing at all . . .", I knew that much more than spoken language was being contested by this small boy. The arena of Kazim's silences, blurtings, misappropriations (the nursery teacher would often insist he say "soweee" when it was clear he was uncertain about the offence or, indeed, not sowee at all) was busy, tense, and fraught. In Adam Phillips' words (1999, p. 46), I was, indeed, wondering "what speaking and listening are like for the child (being penetrated, being soothed, being taken in, spoiling and so on)."

Yet I also learned that psychoanalytic theory was rich with attending to precisely these powerful speech and silence moments. The work of Winnicott, Klein, Bettelheim were starting points, as was the classic Freudian *Fort-Da* analysis. Later, I encountered the Lacanian story of the triad of loss, anxiety, and desire. Feminist scholars such as bel hooks, Deborah Britzman, and Lyn Stanley brought into sharp relief the power struggles fought in the bloodied language arena, and the debris left there as voices of oppressor and oppressed battled, with only one of the two being heard time and again. This journey took me, later still, to phenomenology, the insight of Ricoeurian rescripting; the power of "story not yet told", offering the possibility of producing a better story, "more bearable and more intelligible" (Ricoeur, quoted in Wood, 1992, p. 30). The journey took me, too, to Hannah Arendt's poignant, heartfelt words on wordlessness and isolation. Like Bion, and like Klein, for whom thinking was a hard-earned prize, its seeds nurtured through a successful containing experience in infanthood, Arendt observed how an inability to *think* lay at the root of, in Arendt's argument, the banality of evil (Arendt, 1994).

Each theory and each theorist has delved deeply into enduring political and moral questions of who comes to voice and who comes to be heard, and through which words—crafted, fashioned, and honed, by whom. As we grapple with a new era of fake news, mis- and dis-information, thinned out, misappropriated language, and the relentless proliferation of verbiage on an unimaginable scale, an era in which the ability to think without resorting to groupthink has taken on a whole new edge, these questions remain alive and with a new urgency. In the sections that follow I come back to these enduring lessons of observation and language, and I say more about how they evolved in my work.

Research: the journey begins

Author and anthropologist Zora Neale Hurston pithily described research as "formalized curiosity", adding that "It is poking and prying with a purpose" (Hurston, 1942, p. 91). The infant observation experience on the Psychoanalytic Studies course was hugely influential in formalizing my curiosity and gifting me the rich, reflective, attentive space I needed to gradually appreciate that my natural instinct to poke and pry could serve a purpose. It became plain to me that research was nothing if not observation.

On the course, the two, observation and research, worked in tandem. The skills of observation and application of theory and, crucially, that of free-floating attention in which assumptions and categorization are held in abeyance as much as is humanly possible were becoming interwoven strands in my developing stance and identity as a researcher. The central quest for both observation and research came to be to observe while refraining from making judgements or drawing on assumptions—a quest I later found central to the phenomenologist method, developed by Husserl (1973), of epoché or "bracketing". In this method, I (the thinking person) disengages from belief or disbelief by holding off on assertions or questions about the existence of things that extend beyond their appearance as observed. While I came to question the possibility of epoché in the research process, I value it as an aspiration, but I seek rather, to achieve "phenomenological sensibility" (Finlay, 2014). This sensibility enables me to "be responsive to the phenomenon" and able to capture "something of its 'is-ness'" (Finlay, 2014, p. 121) in what the philosopher Komesaroff (1995) would call a microethical moment. This "is-ness of things" requires observation, first and foremost.

I was teaching in a psychiatric institution (Sagan, 2002), offering study skills in specific subjects, usually one to one, to residents who ranged from those being housed in a rehab block with some community access to those housed 24/7 in the high-security ward. Their crimes varied in severity. For the most part, the residents were under the age of 35, poorly educated, with a high proportion being men identifying as African Caribbean, who came from socioeconomically deprived backgrounds. Many had multiple diagnoses and addictions, along with complicated patchwork histories of abuse, trauma, criminal activity, and/or self-harm. Many were withdrawn, some uncommunicative, almost all low in verbal fluency. I found this a troubling but fertile ground for observation, not least of the sometimes "bizarre dynamic between psychiatric patient and teacher" (Sagan, 2000, p. 137), in which the ebb and flow of projective identification sometimes left me feeling wasted, unheard, impotent—providing a highway, perhaps, into the experience states of so many in the institution. It often, too, fascinatingly, left me speechless, lost for words, confused. Here's an entry from my research at the time (Sagan, 2000), after a particularly difficult session with a black female resident.

> She initially responds well to the incorporation of more literature by black women writers, but this is soon trashed, both verbally and by her indifference to tasks and discussion. She often says she does not understand the words, the meanings, the metaphors. We are about to reach a peak in her attacks on the sessions; [uncanny occurrences take place]. Locked doors fail to open as I fumble with keys, pens run out of ink, I bring the wrong books to the sessions, I cannot think straight.

Experiences such as this enabled me to reach a deeper understanding of Bion's (1959) conceptualization of the no-thought experience and how certain virulent projections actually constituted an attack on thinking. This was important in giving me a better understanding of what was happening in the here and now, in some challenging and tense situations—in this case, for Petra my student, for me, and to acknowledge the "thing" sitting heavily between us in our sessions. This "thing" was a Gordian knot of projection, speechlessness, defensiveness, fear, envy, and threat of collapse—all further shot through with the problematics of a white professional working with a black resident and the weight of the freight that that, in itself, carried.

Through the observation and my early research based within the white walls of the psychiatric institution with its perpetual rank background smell of urine and sweat, I learned about Bion's theory of containment, which plays such a role in understanding infant needs and the role of the caregiver, and which was seminal in my working towards a better understanding of Kazim in the observation work on the course. This was also to become crucial in my understanding of the learning and teaching dynamic, as both my research and, later, my counselling practice progressed—both focused on the individual from backgrounds that were severely, multiply, complexly deprived. Teaching psychiatric patients, I observed and sensed how a container can be offered by the session itself, "as if the teaching setting mirrors the analytic setting in the requirements for regularity and consistency in order to provide a sense of containment where learning can take place" (Thompson, 2001, p. 31).

Also brought to my attention was how learners could find containment in the material, space, and paraphernalia of the sessions, as well as in the words, in the sentences, the clumsy but quiet fine motor skills of learning to write, the colour and stretch of maps in geography, the cadence of a new language, the symbolic patterns in mathematics, the softness and give of fabrics, the reliable repetition of computer blips and dings. The learning, like the teaching, was so much more than "a class"—rather, a deep exploration into what "the student is trying to get right" (Gardner, 1994, p. 118). And there were a lot of wrongs to get right, it seemed. Personal unconscious battles and lessons remembered, repeated, perhaps being worked through (Freud, 1914g). As Pitt and Britzman reminded me, "Learning is uncannily organized by repetitions of past investments and conflicts—or, in short, new editions of old conflicts" (2003, p. 761). This repeating and revisiting often took form in ways that were neither easy nor pleasant. At times they provoked outbursts, withdrawal, and fear when, far from feeling contained, these spaces, objects, words, and textures formed "bizarre objects" (Bion, 1957, p. 39) by which "the patient feels himself [*sic*] to be surrounded". The spaceships, aliens, and gaping black holes of one of my student's avid but troubled SciFi readings and comics were often right there in the room with us, or so it seemed.

Time and again my quiet, unassuming training in observational skills brought me back to the here and now and to a steadfastness, perhaps, rather than a calm, in which I learned to "park" me, not outside, not divorced from the here and now, but parked as an intrinsic albeit non-active, but participant part of "it". And *that* me could think, could hold eye contact, could breathe, and could be—be there for whatever drama was ensuing. And in this quiet, steady, yet sometimes very difficult experience of observing and being I saw, time and time again, a struggle for words: the myriad ways in which Kazim's trashing of a play scene was enacted, when thought was impeded and when words, even if they were to be had, were inadequate approximations at best or slippery misrepresentations, and how people found their way and ways around this gulf, with greater or lesser success. The trouble with words, as Dennis Potter observed, is that you never know whose mouths they've been in. So, words were often abandoned, given up on, never to be trusted or employed. In the busyness of everyday life, who has the time, after all, or the willingness or patience to sit with the mumbles and the stutters, the monosyllabic delivery, the impeded phonemes and malapropisms, the rude, the rough, the guttural, the spat out? The unspoken easily, quickly, conveniently, becomes the unheard.

Counselling: a close observing of unfolding and refolding narrative

After I left the Psychoanalytic Studies course and began my training as a counsellor, my work in community settings expanded. I worked exclusively in areas of high deprivation, and my caseload was soon to include individuals (mainly women) from what was then termed BAME (Black and Minority Ethnic) backgrounds, with a large number of refugees, asylum seekers, and people to whom the powerful and polysemous adjective of "displaced" was attached. Each came, superficially, to talk about their problems, with some rudimentary belief or hope that doing so would help with distress, with anxiety, with fear, with trauma, with paralysis. But again I observed how words sketched a story, at best, unable to fill in the textured, nuanced areas in which the crux of the narrative and its resolution or rescripting lay. Armed with all the skills of a newly qualified counsellor, the tools of her trade and the trappings of empathic listening, mirroring, rephrasing, reframing, and gentle Socratic questioning, it was the single skill of *being* that allowed me to be human.

Sitting with one client, Loren, I observed her folding and flattening her tear-drenched tissue, getting the corners just so, the creases pressed by her fingertips into invisible lines, the folds as crisp as folds in a wet piece of cheek-mopped paper could allow for, and wondered what she was so desperately trying to tidy away, to fold into a neat compression, to clear and to soothe, and how hard it was for her to find the words to say it. I became acutely aware of the power both of words and of silence (Sagan, 2024) and how some people "grow up with life-denying meanings and are hostage to toxic stories that adversely define and constrain their identity and self image" (Roberts, 2000, p. 435).

I listened carefully as Océanne—who, I knew from her notes, had been brutally and repeatedly raped in her loved but lost Democratic Republic of Congo homeland—spoke for weeks, sweating and breathing heavily, about the theft of her battered second-hand car, rather than about anything else. I grasped something of her pain at its loss: the breaking into its prized (by her) interior, the taking of it, the absence, now, of being able to drive, independently and safely, to work and back, knowing the proxy value of this story, and how, in time, if I heard the story often enough, attended to its detail carefully enough, listened closely enough to Océanne's repeated torment of losing her car, then her story would move in time to another chapter. And it did. And when we got there, there were few words through which to tell of its horror, but we were both better prepared. In time we were able to explore, too, how her story and its insufficient words had become stuck in Océanne's chest, lodged hard as a knot in her thorax, cicatrized in her throat, and had played a role in, or even caused, her audible respiratory difficulties, which I could hear, as a constant reminder of what I still could not. Medical sociologist Arthur Frank pointed out (2004, p. 19) that there are occasions "when we must respond to another person, and the nature of that response declares our moral self" and in hearing stories heaved up from the depths of a person's pain, the response of close, quiet observation and the suspension of clamouring for meaning is the only moral response.

Over time, then, my observing developed further sharpnesses: my listening between the lines, making fewer assumptions, fewer rushes to complete, to categorize, to narrate, developed, too, more competence in *negative capability*. And what emerged time and again was that although we are, to quote the philosopher Yuval Harari (2015), a narrative species, *verbal* telling is often the hardest thing we humans can do. When our articulation is low, our vocabulary limited, our thought impeded, our trauma strangling, or our trust in the listener eroded as a result of layer upon layer of testimonial injustice (Fricker, 2007), then that already hard act of telling is a daunting and unnerving task. And it is lonely. This last point was a further enduring lesson rooted in my psychoanalytic observation studies: for, as I watched Kazim and tried to make sense of his senseless attacks, I was struck by the loneliness of trauma, experienced alone: one is subsequently alone to process it and to find words in which to think it, let alone speak it.

Frank (2004, p. 9) remarked that "The resonance of stories is what they give beyond what they ostensibly tell." The stories I was told, those I heard or helped co-construct in portacabins, draughty breezeblock community annexes, church halls, and borrowed offices stayed with me, made me wonder, ask, pursue. What was it about our telling, moving voicelessness to voice, silence to words, that was so powerful? I wanted to observe the very process by which people came to words, and wanted to watch them, as they acquired some.

Later research

An application I made to the Local Authority for some additional funding to run an evaluation of local opportunities for adults with mental health difficulties to learn how to improve their below L2 literacy skills was declined. But an off-the-cuff remark that it "read more like a PhD" sowed a seed: I would do the PhD, then. As a single parent with three-part time jobs, undertaking a PhD was clearly not the best of ideas. Yet, fuelled by the auto/biography (Stanley, 1992) of the question and by the injustices I perceived to be rife for this group of people, I started one, and within a year had a cohort of people I was to observe and interview, and, indeed, come to know, for the following four years (Sagan, 2008a). One of them was Marge, who was baffled that I could be interested in her, exclaiming gruffly, "Dunno what you want to know about me for . . .". Here's a vignette from one of our interviews:

> 65 years old, painfully riddled with arthritis and with a history of mental illness stretching "prob'ly as far back as I remember, lass", Marge is late for our session, and for a variety of reasons, I am irritated. I had cycled here in the rain, having hastily dropped my daughter off at school; my journey had been fractious, battling along grimy streets alongside impatient and insular drivers. I was cold, depleted, restless, and now my interviewee was late. Then I heard her shuffling her way along the corridor.
>
> Marge pushes the door open with her bulk, her stick and her bags and makes fleeting eye contact with me, a strained, apologetic look on her harassed face. She shuffles stiffly towards the table, grunting a little and struggling with her stick, the task of moving, and her bags. Time slows down. Once seated, she carefully places her carrier bags around her, each in some deliberate spot. I hear her wheezing and offer her a cup of tea as she wheezes, "no, you're awright, lass . . ." and places her stick to rest against the grubby Formica table. She looks at me, and simultaneously her stick, ill-held by the table, begins to slide to the floor. She bends her painful bulk and retrieves it, replacing it in exactly the same spot. She heaves her chest, her face reddening with the effort of it all. I thank her for coming, but before I get to the end of the sentence, her stick slides away again and clatters once more to the floor. Marge

> looks at me, unsmiling, embarrassed, perhaps, and perplexed but, most of all, tired. She bends again, struggling, and retrieves the stick. She replaces it in exactly the same spot. I lean instinctively towards her, the stick, and towards saying something—but I am stopped, suddenly, mid-movement and mid-utterance. And *there* it is. A moment of suspension between the inevitability of doing and the necessity of being. I sit back and watch the stick fall a full three more times, before Marge looks at me, questioningly, and I, unspeaking, make an open-handed, soft gesture of offer, to which she nods. I take the stick and lie it on the floor, from which position it has nowhere to go. Our interview then progresses, with Marge shooting the stick regular side glances.
>
> It was only later that the penny dropped: that in enquiring about Marge through an interview in which I urged her to tell me about her life (Sagan, 2008a) she had, in fact, not told me but shown me. In a rare encounter in which I had observed and stayed with rather than intervened, she had told eloquently of the discomfort, the loneliness, the relentlessness, breathlessness, and chore of a 65-year-old's battle with arthritis, mental illness, and compulsive obsessive behaviour.

The longitudinal study of my PhD with a small group of adults with enduring mental health difficulties showed me how little the "talking cure" paradigm and its corollaries, be it autobiographic writing, oral history, or counselling, featured in the lives of my participants. Despite the power of autobiography and agency over self-narrative being repeatedly highlighted as key for mental health recovery (for a recent systematic review of this claim see Llewellyn-Beardsley et al., 2019) these people, with their backgrounds of poverty, hard graft, abuse, alcoholism, physical illness, and disability, were not practised in any form of talking about themselves. Yet they were expert at marginalizing themselves with the same swiftness as they were marginalized by others. This absence of narrator/listener threw into stark relief some of the loneliness of a life lived not expecting to be heard, or found interesting or valid.

I grew fascinated by how learning to write basic autobiographic pieces in simple vocabulary, stunted grammar, and erroneous punctuation might be a step towards a narrative self and an imagined listener (reader). My quest became one of "compassionate inquiry" (Britzman, 2003, p. 149) into "questions of loneliness in learning, the loneliness of learning and the learning of loneliness" (Sagan, 2008b, p. 44).

I wondered if loneliness, as Fromm Reichmann (1959, p. 10) suggested, was "such a painful, frightening experience that people will do practically everything to avoid it", rendering loneliness all the more poignant for being unsaid and unthought of in the solitary confinement of our hyper-social times. Loneliness, in these sharing, shared days of networks, social media, blogs, vlogs, and online, exposed lives, and the ubiquitous culture of autobiography, oral history, and genealogical excavations into who we are to whom, has become the ultimate taboo (Sagan & Miller, 2018). Within this milieu, the language of alone ness was collapsing loneliness, isolation, and solitude, and popular discourse was busy hollowing out all three, leaving us lost for ways in which to think about being alone as anything other than terrifying—the "naked horror" of Binswanger (1958). Drawing on the powerful work of Melanie Klein as she struggled with her own loneliness, and whose final words before her death were written on this loneliest of subjects (Klein, 1963), Deborah Britzman (2003, p. 149) reminds us that loneliness is also "a fragile bridge necessary for thinking to cross from the emptiness of loss and anxiety to the poignant work of mourning and reparation."

This questioning, about the imbrication of loneliness, mental ill health, and the voicelessness that often follows on the heels of not being heard, was to continue to the present day (Sagan, 2020, 2022) and were recurring strands in the tapestry of narratives shared with me by a group of long-term mentally ill visual artists, who were part of a later project, which was to further make use of observational abilities.

Art, imagery, and film-making

Throughout my teaching, counselling, and research I was struck by both the generosity of people in sharing their stories and the messiness and pain they often encountered in doing this in words. I observed people struggling in myriad ways to tell their story: from Kazim trashing the playhouse home he never had, to a psychiatric resident deeply intent on simple sums, his adding trying to bring something apart together, to a client able to repeatedly describe her brother's suicide in minute detail but unable to speak about any of the overwhelming emotions she herself felt about his death, or a middle-aged couple with learning difficulties and mental illness joyfully discovering "ways to say I love you" (Sagan, 2011b). Kleinman observed the toxic stagnancy that "arises in part by telling dead or static stories, situating the individual in a wasteland" (Kleinman,1988, p. 438), trapping you in a version of a story that hounds and depletes you (Sagan, 2011a). And if the story didn't entail loneliness, then the frustration of not telling it or of not having it heard, ever, certainly did. Yet, as I first glimpsed on the Psychoanalytic Studies course through observation, people *would* tell their story and the frustration, fear, and relentlessness of it, all the time. For this is what we, the narrative species, do, finding a way, despite all odds sometimes, like the Victorian-era seamstress Agnes Richter, who painstakingly stitched her autobiography into every inch of the jacket she fashioned from her Heidelberg psychiatric hospital uniform (Hornstein, 2012). There is a long tradition of people finding the words, somehow, with which to tell their story, stretching back at least to Greek mythology. In one such example, Philomena, having been raped by Tereus, then defiantly threatens to tell the world. When Tereus' response is to cut out her tongue and imprison her, Philomena, traumatized and alone, weaves a tapestry—one that would tell her story.

One of the ways in which we tell our story, remember it, explore it, and even display and shout it has, since time immemorial, been through the making of art, to which I turn now.

In 2009 an Arts Council grant enabled me to work with a group of mental health patients who were involved in a hospital arts project. What began as a small undertaking grew rapidly into a multimedia participatory arts project, with a large group of service users being peer-trained to film, edit, interview, transcribe, photograph, and/or critique their/our work. The final film was, and is still, shown around the country, in mental health groups, colleges, and arts events, including a sold-out viewing at the Tate Modern. A book collected the interviews, observations, and images (Sagan, 2014) and explored the reparation and connection sought, yearned for—and sometimes won through art-making.

I interviewed, spoke, engaged, joked, cried with, and observed tens of adults with enduring mental health difficulties, all of whom passionately felt that making visual art helped them in a number of ways. I looked at their work as they spoke about it, I observed them make it, trash it, or love it. Some spoke at length, many times, and sent me email updates and further reflections, keeping in contact long after the initial project had ended, some to this day. Most, though, spoke haltingly and sometimes reluctantly. What I heard was that their artwork told the stories they couldn't and had not been able to, through therapy, hospitalization, rehabilitation. There were stories they couldn't remember (but which were brought back through the making), stories they couldn't articulate (but were given form through the images), stories they wanted to leave behind (and could move on from once given form), stories they wanted to share with others (perpetrators, loved ones, faceless institutions, unknown strangers who faced similar traumas), and, memorably, critical difficulties in interaction and trust, which were slowly, painstakingly confronted through being, for example, the film-maker, protected by the lens, connecting at a distance felt to be safe (Sagan & Sochos, 2015). Some art products were harrowing;

some were given a funny spin; some, deeply ugly and dark, were woven into sunlit vistas, grainy atmospheric photographs, stitched patterns, and bizarre sculptures. Each told something that words could not, to viewers who could now see something, at least, of what they had not been able to hear.

This project, which I was trusted to be part of and which was difficult on personal, political, and ethical levels (Sagan, 2011c), taught me further lessons in observing: lessons of observing the telling, the making, the recollecting, and the chosen ways of displaying—with the art object as an intersubjective third (Froggett, 2008). Much of what I observed and heard resonated with the psychoanalytic theory of the Psychoanalytic Studies course, now embedded in my thinking: theories of play, of making and unmaking, of our reaching out "towards an object, with perhaps the expectation of a response; a medium that allows itself to be transformed; and a 'finding' or creating within that medium of significant forms that reveal the subject to himself" (Wright, 2009, p. 144), theories, too, of deep woundedness through "deficiencies of response" (p. 49) of the early environment, and the epistemic injustices of repeatedly being "unseen".

This long, at times unwieldy project taught me, too, further lessons in me observing me observing: observing my own drive to repair and to connect and to make sense of a story at times senseless. For, as I learned on the course, observing others is nothing if not a prolonged observation of the observer. The gazer becomes the gazed at. And what I saw was often troubling, messy, and painful—but, in the same way as my artist participants had found, from that trouble and mess and pain some semblance of order, connection, voice, beauty, and calm could, even if only temporarily, be reached.

Slippery tales

Kazim taught me to watch. Probably an inveterate observer anyway, growing up as I did, minutely watching the shifts in atmosphere, temperature, pressure, and storms of my father's climate, always ready to run for cover, looking on, observing, watching was what I have always done. And I do still, watching these words form on the page, knowing their truth or fiction to be relative, their meaning open to multiple penetration, interpretation, or indifference, their import temporary, their presence fickle. What's important is to have the language, the words, and speech to play with, and to have, at least sometimes, someone to listen with an open-hearted generosity (Frank, 2004). And we don't all have these: questions of privilege and safety arose as I watched Kazim, questions too of entitlement and lack; the early woundedness of storytellers (Frank, 1995), and the strategies they thereafter develop through which to show and tell.

As I write, loneliness is considered an epidemic (Holt-Lunstad, 2017), one further ignited, it would seem, by the sudden onset isolation of the COVID-19 pandemic and its enforced limits on our lives and social spheres. And part of my understanding now of the lonelinesses described to me in my research implies the absence, early on, then repeatedly, of a listener. Despite, or perhaps as a result of the global worry about loneliness, our narrative species has perhaps never been more vocal. On a dizzying array of platforms and multimedia, forms of self-disclosure, first-person testimony, and the lived experience are legion, now common by-phrases for people talking about their lives. The value of such stories is now embedded into practice documents, while policy has been reconfigured to specify the value of the voices and lived experiences of service users and patients. We are all busy listening. Through the stories, particularly of the ill and the recovering, we are told new stories and new versions of old ones, and these form counternarratives that offer diverse representations of survival that reclaim the ground from the clinical language that has for too long colonized experiences of distress. Yet there is a dark side to this use of voice and of stories (Pascal & Sagan, 2018), as words, and the narrative and discourse in which we frame and re-imagine ourselves, are tightly welded to power and its asymmetries.

We are also in an era of fake news, misinformation, and post-truth, where fact-checking has become an industry, though not one we necessarily trust. This post-truth world has emerged, it is argued (Lewandowsky, Ecker, & Cook, 2017) as a result of societal shifts, such as the decline in social capital, growing economic inequality, increased polarization, a disbelief or scepticism about science, and an increasingly fragmented media landscape. It is also perhaps an inevitable part of the evolution of post-modernism, which, as David Bell states:

> dispenses with any conception of truth, claiming that no distinction can be drawn between what is claimed as truth and preference or fashion. Where there is no conception of truth, its various counterparts, namely deceptions, lies, and misrepresentations also lose their foothold.
>
> [Bell, 2009, p. 90]

And this leaves us with an even greater need, perhaps, of negative capability, as the uncertain or untrue ground shifts beneath our feet—or does it—perpetually. But before we rush forward into a moral panic regarding these headlines, Harari (2018) reminds us that fake news is not new. In his book, *21 Lessons for the 21st Century*, he reminds us that "When a thousand people believe some made-up story for one month, that's fake news. When a billion people believe it for a thousand years, that's a religion, . . ." (p. 234). Ah, words and their power. So we are not only a narrative species, but a post-truth species, whose very potency depends, according to Harari, on creating and believing fictions. All the more reason to pay quiet attention, to observe and to listen between the lines at what is being said, what is not being said, and what is always only an approximation of the unsayable.

There is a famous video of two teams playing basketball that is used as an awareness test. The viewer is asked to count how many passes the team in white makes. Whether you get the answer right or wrong is immaterial: you will most likely have missed the moon-walking bear who blithely walks across the court. I show my students this video as a starter point for a discussion on observation in research: how much we miss when we are busy looking for something else. How much we don't hear, too, in people's stories, as we race to complete, confirm, dispute, or corroborate the narrative. So it is only when we are able to listen between the lines, to hear between the pauses and to allow the simple is-ness of things to unfold, that we begin to hear the story that Kazim was busy telling anyone who would listen.

PART II

POETRY

One of the themes that infuses the thinking on the Psychoanalytic Studies course, and the work included in this book, is the relationship between psychoanalysis and the artefact or art form being explored from a psychoanalytic perspective. As described in the Introduction, the way this relationship has been understood has developed over time and continues to evolve both within the course and in psychoanalysis more widely.

In Chapter 6 Judith Edwards, who led the seminars on poetry and psychoanalysis for many years, addresses the relationship between the two disciplines: a dynamic relationship vividly captured in the chapter's title, "This Is Not for Tears: Thinking"—Poetry and Psychoanalysis in Orbit". Edwards draws attention to how early analysts tended to treat a poem like a clinical session, analysing the poem's maker. She considers that to be a mistaken approach and explains how we are now much more concerned with the artefact created, which is a thing in itself, "has a life of its own", and can illuminate states of mind for the reader. As addressed in the Introduction, the process of uncovering and exploring states of mind suggested by, or expressed within, an artwork is inherent in the approach taken in the Applications strand of the course.

Drawing on the work of Ogden and others, Edwards highlights the links between psychoanalysis and poetry but also their distinctiveness, aiming to draw on each to illuminate the other, while wishing, as she says,

DOI: 10.4324/9781003564867-8

neither to blur their distinctiveness nor over-simplify their similarity. As in the varying distances between a pair of celestial bodies in orbit, there are points of greater closeness and greater distance between the two disciplines, and throughout the chapter Edwards elegantly draws out the nuances and subtleties of this complex relationship.

Edwards emphasizes that for genuine learning to take place, what she calls "direct confrontation" with the works is needed, so in these seminars the focus is on the text of the poem and the experience of listening to it being read aloud. "Direct confrontation" is a striking phrase, perhaps suggesting considerable challenge in the live encounter. As for the observer in an infant observation or the analyst in a psychoanalytic session, the aim is for the listener to set aside theoretical preconceptions and be open and receptive to the live emotional experience conveyed through the poem. This receptivity inevitably involves exposure to the most difficult, distressing, and disturbing feelings as well as what might be more easily metabolized, and in this way the encounter is inevitably a challenging confrontation that can stir and disturb.

In the seminars, Edwards encourages "a form of listening that responds to sounds and multilayered meanings", a quality of listening that surely mirrors that of the analyst who, following Bion's exhortation, puts aside memory and desire (Bion, 1967a), thus allowing evenly suspended attention to his patient's material. In this way, in both settings, space is created in which meaning can emerge. A further parallel is suggested in the evocative quote Edwards includes by the film-maker Robert Bresson, who advised, "Don't run after poetry: it penetrates unaided through the cracks." We might wonder whether this could be paraphrased for the aspiring psychoanalyst as, "don't run after the unconscious: it permeates unaided through the cracks", as unconscious material will come to the fore in the clinical setting, regardless of conscious intent, through non-verbal communication or the process of free association, to be received and worked on by the analyst's mind. Again, this highlights how these non-clinical students are nonetheless learning something of the psychoanalytic approach through being encouraged into a particular quality of listening and becoming increasingly aware of and alert to their emotional experience.

As in the other art forms or artefacts explored in this book, Edwards suggests that poetry can illuminate states of mind, but, perhaps because it expresses those states of minds in words, it also has the particular capacity to make thoughts coherent or thinkable. She suggests that "the two phenomena of poetry and psychoanalysis may be mutually illuminating, in terms of states of mind in us all".

Another theme highlighted in the chapter is that of "the space in-between". Here, Edwards explains that psychoanalysis and poetry are both concerned with inner and outer experience and the area of meeting between the two, the space that Winnicott formulated as "the transitional space—the location of cultural experience" (Winnicott 1971a, p. 95). Again, this brings to the fore a thread that runs through many of the activities described in this book: infant observation takes place within the observational space, the physical and mental space created between the observer and the observed infant, mother–infant dyad, or family; experiencing an art installation takes place in the geographical and imaginative space between the observer and the work; a play or an opera unfolds in the space created between the performers on the stage and the audience; a novel comes to life in the space between author, text, and reader. In different ways, these are all spaces where the live emotional and cultural experience unfolds and meaning can be perceived.

Edwards notes that both psychoanalysis and poetry are concerned with two overarching areas: registering and containing powerful feelings, and the negotiation and management of loss. Both these areas are central in the two subsequent chapters, which form the remainder of Part II. The pain of loss and the process of mourning (see Appendix, "8. Mourning") are at the heart of chapters 7, " 'Of Mutability', Mourning, and Containment" by Anne Kane, and 8, "Resistance through Mourning: A Poem by Mahmoud Darwish, 'In Her Absence I Created Her Image' " by Elina Matter. Both authors were, at different times, students in Judith Edwards' seminars.

During a period of huge impending personal loss, Kane found that Jo Shapcott's series of poems "Of Mutability" provided containment and a framework within which feelings and experiences that were almost unbearable could be borne and worked through. In Chapter 7, she explores the title poem of the set, drawing on Klein's work on mourning and the importance for emotional growth of working through loss and mourning. Bion's ideas about containment and thinking also underpin her argument. Kane examines in detail the shifting states of mind suggested in the poem, but she also notes that there will be a range of different views about a particular poem or group of poems. Each individual will respond to them differently, and the poems will mean something different to each person who encounters them. What we offer here and in the other chapters is one psychoanalytically informed perspective: that alternative readings and meanings are always possible.

Elina Matter's Chapter 8 sets a detailed analysis of the Palestinian poet Mahmoud Darwish's poem, "In Her Absence I Created Her Image", in its historical context and within the field of "poetry of resistance". This widens the exploration of loss and mourning into the political realm of exile from the homeland, but, as Matter emphasizes, the poet captures an experience of exile that is also beyond the political realm—the experience of inner exile from the self and a deep longing for a home within the self that is perhaps familiar to us all. As in the previous chapter, Matter makes use of Klein's ideas about mourning and draws further on Segal's development of those ideas in her work on the creative process and aesthetics. The author highlights the internal creative process whereby Darwish's poetry can be understood as being inextricably linked with his process of mourning and emerging from his need to repair his internal world. Through his own experience, he and the other resistance poets create a space in which readers can experience their own anxieties and experiences of terrible loss in more bearable form.

The link Matter makes between the Palestinian strategy of resistance "Sumud", meaning steadfastness, and the importance both symbolically and concretely of the mother in the Palestinian struggle, is compelling and leads to further exploration in relation to Bion's concept of containment.

Edwards wonders whether the two disciplines of poetry and psychoanalysis can come into fruitful dialogue, asking whether we could think of poetry as "some sort of hotline to the unconscious". In their explorations of poetry within the clinical setting and outside, these three authors amply demonstrate not only a fruitful dialogue, but one that enriches both disciplines and illuminates deeper meaning without the need, as Bresson might say, to "run after" it or to pin it down to one interpretation.

CHAPTER SIX

"This is not for tears: thinking"—poetry and psychoanalysis in orbit

Judith Edwards

This writing has been five years in the making, since I have been running a series of seminars about poetry and psychoanalysis at the Tavistock Clinic for non-clinical students. The title comes from a poem by John Berryman, "Dream Song 29", and it sums up how, in this seminar, we have tried both to feel what we feel in an authentic way when reading a poem, and think about the links it may have with the central core of the students' study, which is psychoanalysis. Are the two disciplines in any way complementary? Can unconscious phantasy be tapped into via the medium of poetry? In this chapter I hope to show that while there are profound differences between poetry and psychoanalysis, there are also similarities, as the work with students has highlighted. I also include three brief clinical vignettes.

***

John Berryman [1914–1972] was a key figure in what was subsequently called "the Confessional School" of poetry. The title of this chapter comes from his "Dream Song 29" (1964, p. 77), which, while having been open to many interpretations, the poet himself considered to be "up to the listener . . . funny or frightening or both" (quoted in Linebarger, 1974, p. 124). So the aim of the seminar series has been to look at poetry through a psychoanalytic lens, thinking about both current poetry as well as poems from various previous writers who have left us a body of work to consider, linking this with clinical material where appropriate. This is indeed about

DOI: 10.4324/9781003564867-9

"thinking" as well as "feeling", as Henry says in "Dream Song 29". The two disciplines are in orbit in the way they can be seen to circle around one another, each informing the other in a way that can provide further illumination to both, orbiting around the central body of the human psyche. We thought in these seminars about manifest content and possible latent content, but without making explicit one-to-one correspondences and without attempting to analyse a poem, a poet, or the students in the seminar.

Following an introductory session, each subsequent week, in the company of an additional visiting lecturer (including practising poets), we found ways of considering poems and psychoanalytic texts, looking at possible means of exploring the territory between them. We considered the role of rhythm, meter, language, and voice as they combine to illuminate states of mind. Apart from a short list of background reading, no texts (except the poems) were sent out to accompany each seminar. True learning takes place through direct confrontation with the works, not by seeing them through the lens of any particular theorist. This is the way learning has taken place in these seminars—a kind of playing with the ideas that may (or may not) connect the two disciplines, of poetry and psychoanalysis. Students over the years have found this both refreshing and liberating. The learning has continued after the seminars had ended, as students have told me or the course staff have subsequently stated. They have come onto the course from a variety of professions: some are practising clinicians, or psychologists and psychiatrists, and some specialize in art forms such as photography or painting.

Student reactions: these themes are universal

Many students have come to the seminars in a doubtful state of mind. As one overseas student said, "I'd better tell you right now, I've always hated poetry"; and she ended up saying something more nuanced: "Well, now I'll give it a go, at least." Many reactions tended to be more positive: students liked sharing poems they themselves had written (which was one suggestion I had made) and meeting those who actually practised the craft of poetry. As another overseas student suggested, it was important to tolerate not understanding everything and waiting until meaning emerged. There was a general consensus that there could, indeed, be a potential space opening up between the two disciplines, where new thinking could take place. One student said that while she had previously had "a contempt" for poetry (linked up with Marianne Moore's cry "I, too, dislike it"; 1935, p. 131), it had now become "a secret pleasure". Another student had "put up with" her mother reading poetry to the children—"When Daddy Fell into the Pond" (Noyes, 1952) was one she remembered—but now she felt grateful and would do the same for her own children. "This seminar far exceeded my expectations", she said. Some students had bought volumes of poetry for the first time (Heaney and Larkin being favourites). One middle-aged student had read no poetry since school and was struck by my thought offered to the group that it's interesting to think how a poem reads you rather than vice versa, as this can change over time. As another said, it is important to allow the links to be "slippery" rather than make one-to-one correspondences.

But the poet Philip Larkin had a different view, and one student said he very much liked that contrary opinions about poems and poets could be expressed over the weeks of our meetings. "Poetry is like everything else", Larkin said in one of his letters (1992, p. 39); "If you're not 2/3 of the way there already, you'd better not start." This forthright view also chimed with another student, who said that up until then she had considered poetry "pretentious", but she was opening a door to new understandings now.

In the last seminar of the 2016 sequence, a Chinese student offered us a poem from his own culture, by a woman poet writing in the eleventh century, and read it out loud in Chinese. It was a moving experience for us all, hearing these strange-sounding syllables, which were nevertheless full of meaning, and he then let us know what it meant in English. He told us she was considered the greatest female poet in Chinese history (the poem is quoted at the end of this chapter). This was, indeed, our last seminar and seemed to sum up how universal these themes are over time—as the student himself said, written by someone many centuries ago who had lost hope and seemed lost in an endless process of mourning, perhaps melancholia, in a world where all helpful objects had died, externally and perhaps internally too. Here we could see, in this poet's words, the themes of leaving, silence, loss, and non-existence being played out in a few short lines. The span of the seminars had enabled us to consider poems written in different states of mind, from joy to despair, and poems to be read by us all in different states, too, with different reactions. It has been a true "playing with ideas", as Winnicott recommended (1971b, pp. 63–64).

What is poetry?

The poet and rapper Kate Tempest,[1] who won the 2013 Ted Hughes Award, said:

> a poem is a half-finished thing until it's heard . . . it's physical and belongs in the body as much as in the mind . . . it doesn't have to be read in a big, theatrical fashion, it can be very quietly whispered to yourself, just to get the sense of the sound, the shape . . .
>
> [Tempest, 2016]

With the advent of the internet and screens in seminar rooms, during the seminars we have been able to listen to such poets as the aforementioned John Berryman and Sylvia Plath read their own poems, as well as reading them ourselves in the group. And since Bob Dylan won the Nobel Prize for Literature (in 2016), we listened to his song, "Forever Young", thinking about both the manifest and latent content there for us all to mull over, linking this with acceptance or denial of our mortality. There has also been an emphasis on considering poems from different cultures around the world—and the students themselves have come from as far away as Chile, Uruguay, and Hong Kong, as well as Europe, bringing poems in various languages, including Chinese, for us to think about.

In a sense poetry sits halfway between prose and music, and, as the poet Ted Hughes said, "we can all do this. We are all story tellers and all poets, it is a question of keeping your eyes and ears open, and your heart too. And listening to the music of the words we use" (1967, p. 10). Linguists and neurologists have suggested that poetry speaks to a primitive part of the brain, in the right hemisphere (Zeman, Milton, Smith, & Rylance, 2013). Rhythm and rhyme helped oral bards remember verses before the invention of writing. When we respond to poetry, we engage a part of our being that is more primitive and in some way "purer" than the more intellectual left hemisphere. We are in one sense getting to the latent content beneath the manifest, in both disciplines.

The congruences between poetry and psychoanalysis have long been recognized. There are many affinities between the poetic process and the psychoanalytic process. We explore a number of these affinities during these meetings; for example, at their best, each has the capacity to find symbolic form for as yet un-apprehended emotions or psychic states. Each is concerned with how powerful feelings can be registered and contained; how loss can be negotiated and managed. Each is about the value of engaging with inner and outer experience and the meeting ground between the two, in the space that Winnicott (1971a, p. 95) called "the location of cultural experience", and finding some way of communicating such experience is the matter of both inner and outer. Can the embodiment of paradoxical truths be expressed in language that moves and breathes? Poetry writes itself into the self and may differ in each re-reading—rather like a psychoanalytic engagement between two people becomes part of the self, so that over time the transference can be modified. In these seminars, I aim constantly to draw on one to illuminate the other, while not wishing to blur the distinctiveness between them, nor to oversimplify their similarity. Both analysts and poets live in a world of symbolism, imagery, and heightened language, shifting fluidly between conscious and unconscious processes, exploring conflict and conflictual states in the perennial search for meaning.

"I, too, dislike it [poetry]: there are things that are important beyond all this fiddle", said the poet Marianne Moore (1935, p. 131). But, she went on, if you read it with a "perfect contempt" for it, you can find something genuine. So her contempt was not for poetry in general, and she herself, of course, was a poet. She mistrusted "the poetic" and demanded poetry in "all its rawness". Then she says, if you demand this, too, you are interested in poetry.

Links between the two?

Tom Stoppard's definition of poetry as "the simultaneous compression of language and expansion of meaning" (quoted in Ogden, 2001, p. 206) is a good way to start thinking about the links between poetry and psychoanalysis; in other words, a lot is packed into as few words as possible in poetry. It's also important to bear in mind that texts are in a sense living things, whose meanings shift from one reader to the next, and between reader and text. As put so succinctly by another Nobel-prize-winning poet, Cseslaw Milosz, the purpose of poetry is to remind us how many "others" we have inside our "selves": "For our house is open, there are no keys in the doors, and invisible guests come in and out at will" (Milosz, 1968, p. 240).

How is a poem written? Some poets need to "drive to the interior", as the US poet Elizabeth Bishop once said (somewhat like free association in analysis, which then, in time, reveals what is "underneath") (Bishop, 1952). Others do not set the scene but plunge right in, wresting meaning from circumstances, forcing a pattern on the chaos of lived life.

Seamus Heaney said in a BBC Radio 4 *Desert Island Discs* programme in1989 that poetry was the way small children managed their fears even if they're only "menaces in the imagination . . . solitude and fear of the world, that's where the poetical being resides". He said you needed to write and read poetry too, to develop "the inward touch"; and he maintained that "all life of poetry is the life of fear". He admired robust poetry but also wished for "almost unwritten poems like haikus of sweetness and delicacy". And it was Robert Bresson, the film-maker, who made images speak so potently, who said "don't run after poetry: it penetrates unaided through the cracks" (quoted in Quandt, 2012, p. 35). So if we are reaching for what Marianne Moore called "the genuine and the raw", can we make links with the discipline of psychoanalysis and its search for meaning? Potentially, literature and psychoanalysis have been linked from the beginning. Freud read widely, wrote excellently himself (e.g. his work on Leonardo da Vinci, 1910c), and was interested in all forms of the writing arts: "what he [the artist] aims at is to awaken in us . . . the same mental constellation as that which in him produced the impetus to create" (Freud, 1914b, p. 212). Poets and philosophers discovered the unconscious, and Freud insisted that what he discovered was the scientific method by which the unconscious could be studied (Trilling, 1951)—rather like the way that Columbus could not be said to have "discovered" America, but he mapped it, which had not been done before.

Early analysts may sometimes have made what we might see now as the mistake of treating a poem like a clinical session and analysing the poem's maker: they were more interested at that time in being archaeologists of the past and reconstructing from the fragments they unearthed. It is true, of course, that the poem and its creator cannot be fully separated, but also that a poet and her/his craftsmanship produce this third thing: a work of art that has a life of its own, which, at its best, can provide illumination for the reader.

Later evolution in the art and science of psychoanalysis drew practitioners to think about the transference and countertransference (see Appendix, "7. Transference and countertransference"): what is happening in the to and fro, and the here and now of a session, where *how* a particular narrative is told is the key element to be attended to. So now we can perhaps think about poetry as illuminating states of mind, hidden aspects of the personality, making thoughts coherent, or thinkable, as Bion says (1962a, p. 83). Freud's "evenly suspended attention" comes into play when the craft of the poem is so assured that it becomes a background object, and the poem becomes, as it were, a thing in itself. As Thomas Ogden suggests:

> we are known as we had not known ourselves, because up to that point we had not been ourselves as fully as we are becoming in experiencing the poem, and as the poem experiences us.
>
> [Ogden, 2001, p. 177]

As he also says:

> the experience of writing is the place where a writer is most alive, it is the place where he lives . . . it is up to the reader to listen for and do what he or she will between the resonances: between the life of the writer and the life of the writing . . . in this way, we as readers are not only eavesdroppers on but also participants in the "conversation" between the life and the work.
>
> [p. 119]

A good poem, then, makes one feel alive and invigorated, and what my hope has been in these seminars is to follow the path where the two phenomena of poetry and psychoanalysis may be mutually illuminating, in terms of states of mind in us all. As the poet Robert Frost said, "a poem would be no good that hadn't doors". This was a phrase that resonated with many of the students in the group and is indeed memorable in terms of something new that may happen when we let a poem read us (quoted in Ogden, 2001, p. 53).

However, to quote Ogden further: "a critical divide separates the two activities; psychoanalysis is a therapeutic activity while reading and writing poetry are aesthetic activities" (p. 104)—do we agree with his rather radical separation here? He goes on: "an attempt to draw one-to-one correspondences between the two represents, I believe, a form of reductionism that obscures and distorts the essence of these two quite different human events". That, at least, seems clear. Analysts are, as he says, trying to communicate with the patient in a way that will hopefully produce emotional growth: "the poet on the other hand is answerable only to the art that he (or she!) is attempting to create. His/her failures are lines that lack vitality and imagination and are devoid of feeling" (p. 104).

But what we have been thinking about in the student group is something that may indeed be common to both and lie at their hearts: a form of listening that responds to sounds and multilayered meanings, so that we may meet parts of ourselves in new ways.

In Maria Rhode's Sixth Annual Meltzer Lecture (Rhode, 2013) she quotes the poet A. E. Housman, who had a simple test for whether a poem was the real thing: if he recited it to himself, did it make his beard bristle when he shaved? We can all perhaps resonate with this experience of involuntary shivers down the spine when something "hits us where we live". She also acknowledges her debt to a recent paper by Andrew Briggs for a related quotation from Robert Frost. Frost said that "his poems always started as a lump in the throat that searched for an idea, which then demanded the search for adequate words to describe the feeling" (Frost, 2013). He was also "interested in the use of words as spoken in the mouth to convey meaning" and wanted his poems to be read aloud, so that they could be "felt as shapes in one's mouth and sensations in one's body" (p. 87). All the factors mentioned by these poets—the importance of rhythm, of shapes in the mouth and of involuntary bodily responses—link with the aspects of language that Donald Meltzer explored, as well as with converging findings from child development.

Imagination and states of mind

A perennial question is: how do we value the products of our imagination? Genesis says that God caused a flood to wipe out what he saw in man: "every imagination of the thoughts of his heart was only evil continuously" (Chapter 7, verse 5). Plato (380 BC) would have banned certain poets from his ideal state, because they called into imaginative being emotions, opinions, and situations of which he disapproved. He thought imagination was subversive, dangerous to the status quo. Yet he maintained a strange ambivalence to it: "Poetry is nearer to vital truth than history", he said, showing an attraction as well as a resistance to poetry, as witness the story in *The Republic* of a beautiful woman who is rejected, and yet he (in the person of Socrates) also wants her back (p. 15).

In contrast, English nineteenth-century Romantic poets such as Samuel Taylor Coleridge and William Blake have seen in human imagination the highest good—even a divine manifestation of our being. Does imagination in poetry have a truth-telling function, either daily truths or eternal truths? Or is it merely a kind of lie or evasion of the truth? Or does it depend on the writer's state of mind? This idea lay behind the speaking title of Britton's chapter, "Milton's Destructive Narcissist or Blake's True Self" (Britton, 1998b, p. 166).

That is one dimension, but a second and more profound level (and often the two are linked) involves the nature of the reports that imagination/poetry gives us on *internal reality*; news from the internal world, or at least new thoughts about it. Distinguishing between the inner and outer worlds is only the beginning. There is, then, the more difficult task of evaluating its quality, its meaning, and its degree of emotional integrity. The poet's task consists of engaging with experience, suffering it, and producing something from this engagement that offers a "something" to the reader, too, which enables the growth of the mind. Private experience can then become universal.

Can there be a link with the task of psychoanalysis here? Can we discern the appearance of psychoanalysis' major conceptual ideas in poetry—splitting, projective identification, denial and resistance, introjection, idealization, denigration? In a book making links between psychoanalysis and poetry, I chose three Yeats poems that seemed to me to represent something about the differing states of mind we are all prey to as we struggle with the human task of going-on-being (Edwards, 2003).

David Tuckett, then editor of the *International Journal of Psychoanalysis*, in writing about "clinical facts" in 1994, talked about how it sometimes seems impossible to put adequately into words the combination of thoughts, feelings, and events that lead to one particular train of thought (he is, of course, talking about a clinical session, but I think it is also helpful in terms of what one tries to puzzle out about poetry too):

> A great deal more takes place in a session than we can deduce from a verbal transcript alone—even if the session were tape recorded and fully annotated to take account of gesture, tone of voice and so on. The words used by the participants and how they said them is central to a degree, but the essence of the situation is that the immediacy of the meaning of what is said is subjective, and also the unconscious meaning is to be inferred according to highly subjective principles in which the apprehension and comprehension of affects play a leading part.
> [Tuckett, 1994, p. 866]

In other words, taking this into account, you might also say that there's a huge amount going on when each of us reads a poem, and as a result it reads us in a particular way, and was written, too, in a particular way, which also involved both conscious and unconscious factors in the writer's mind.

This is a huge subject, of course, and there is an enormous amount that is beyond my remit here—for instance, the relationship between poetry and political climate where, in the most repressive regimes, poets find they have to struggle to convey truths in ways that will not result in persecution but nevertheless articulate those truths. Here we have Plato's idea of imagination as subversive writ large. This, of course, could also be linked up with Klein and the development of symbolic thoughts (Klein, 1930); repression of thoughts then goes on to appear elsewhere as symbols. Perhaps this necessarily rather brief discussion will be continued elsewhere, either by me or by someone else taking this subject forward.

In such circumstances, where persecution becomes the spur to finding a code that readers will understand but that will not break the censorship constraint, simplicity becomes the goal, the "rawness" that Marianne Moore was speaking about, or "to speak in plain words" as Melanie Klein also put it when describing her work with children—what Freud before her had termed "calling a spade a spade" (Kahr, 2017, p. 84). Zbigniew Herbert, the Polish poet, wrote about this too in his poem, "A Knocker". He talks ironically about those poets who can grow "gardens in their heads" when writing poetry. He describes conversely his own imagination as "a wooden board", which he strikes, and "it answers yes–yes, no–no" (Herbert, 1985, p. 42).

I think this would have passed Marianne Moore's test of being genuine and raw. The question for the poet here is what he has inside, beneath what she called "all this fiddle". The Scottish poet Iain Crichton-Smith lived on the island of Lewis in the north of Scotland, where, as he says, "they have not time for the fine graces/of poetry, unless it freely grows/ in deep compulsion" (2011, p. 22). As Alvarez (2003, p. xiv) says, "in order to find out what is going on in a work of art, the critic must let go of his own sensibility and immerse himself in that of the artist, without theories and without preconceptions". Bion (1962a, p. 91) was, of course, making the same point.

Poetry and observation

It has taken more than 200 years for science to catch up with the eighteenth-century English poet William Wordsworth, who saw the development of imagination as a product of the nurturing, loving relationship between mother and child. It is now well known that the human brain more than doubles in size and complexity during the first year of life, and that right-brain development is experience-dependent (Schore, 2001). Wordsworth (1799) was mapping this very development:

> . . . the babe who sleeps
> Upon his Mother's breast, who, when his soul . . .
> Claims manifest kindred with an earthly soul,
> Doth *gather passion* from his mother's eye.
> Such feelings pass into his torpid life
> Like an awakening breeze, and hence his mind,
> Even in the first trial of its powers,
> Is prompt and watchful, eager to combine
> In one appearance all the elements
> And parts of the same object, else detached
> And loath to coalesce.

. . . anticipating Melanie Klein's 1946 formulations about part-objects, splitting and eventual integration by more than 100 years.

> Thus day by day
> Subject to the disciplines of love
> His organs and recipient faculties
> Are quickened, are more vigorous; his mind spreads . . .

. . . what a wonderful phrase; and a process observers of very young infants see developing in their observations.

> Emphatically such a being lives,
> An inmate of this active universe . . .
> Such, verily, is the first
> Poetic spirit of our human life.

And then, as Allan Schore, the neuroscientist, said: "the early social environment, mediated by the primary caregiver, directly influences the final wiring of the circuits in the brain that are responsible for the future socio-emotional development of the individual" (1994, p. 30).

John Stuart Mill, the philosopher and social reformer [1806–1873], found Wordsworth's poems a huge help when he went through a mental crisis: "they expressed not mere outward beauty", he said, "but states of feeling, and of thought coloured by feeling—they seemed to be the very culture of the feelings which I was in quest of" (1865, p. 19). In the early twentieth century, W. B. Yeats wrote: "We make out of the quarrel with others, rhetoric, but of the quarrel with ourselves, poetry" (1924, p. 492). He talked of "the ordinary man" being "a bundle of accident and incoherence" but the same ordinary man/woman, when he struggles to render the incoherent more tolerable and accessible, emerges with a poem as a poet, and the finished work he sees as "something intended, complete" (Yeats, 1994, p. 228; quoted in Edwards, 2003)—at least for that moment, at that time—and this may then find an interface with the internal worlds of others and speak to them too. This is where Winnicott located what he called the aforementioned area of cultural experience: the space between people, what he called "the transitional space", which first develops as the infant starts to experience and manage the separation from mother. Experience, in all its multifarious forms, both agonizing or uncomfortable as well as happy and sometimes beatific, becomes contained in works of art such as poetry and, hopefully, transformed, much as Bion said: a mother contains and transforms the terrors and fears of her baby, by receiving them, thinking about them, and returning them in a more manageable way. Poetry survives an individual's death, said W. H. Auden (1949, p. 27) in his poem, "To the Memory of W. B. Yeats", and is modified "in the guts of the living": a digestive and assimilative process that, one hopes, produces growth. Auden also wrote in memory of Sigmund Freud and the psychoanalytic method, and his words indicate something of the same process of re-membering (Auden, 1966, pp. 168–169).

In *The Use of Poetry and the Use of Criticism*, T. S. Eliot says:

> It is reasonable, I feel, to be on guard against views which claim too much for poetry. Poetry may make us from time to time a little more aware of the deeper, unnamed feelings which form the substratum of our being, to which we rarely penetrate; for our lives are almost constantly evasions of ourselves.
>
> [Eliot, 1933, p. 15]

We can link this with Freud's assertion that we are emphatically not "masters in our own house"—that our conscious mind is just the tip of the iceberg. And since we do not fully "own" ourselves, we can reflect on signs that may mean more than they immediately tell—that is, on our own symbolic products as well as the products of those who came before us, which set up reverberations inside the individual mind. As Harold Bloom (2000, p. 32) said, "poetry is the crown of imaginative literature, in my judgement, because it is a prophetic mode". He says that an important way to really experience poetry is by memorizing poems: "Once a staple of good teaching, memorization was abused into repeating by rote, and so was abandoned, wrongly." He suggests that if you memorize a poem, it becomes somehow part of you—almost as if it expresses a part of you that is universal.

Hearing poetry read aloud is a pleasure and a huge treat. Again, it sets up, as it were, a dialogue between one's own internal voices (and I do not mean madness here) through its rhythms and cadences in a very powerful way. It feels, as John Stuart Mill suggested, "overheard" rather than simply heard; words that "set the darkness echoing", to quote Seamus Heaney—a way of strengthening the self through identification, and recognition, in that "transitional space", which is, as Winnicott suggested, "the location of cultural experience" (1971a, p. 95).

So, we can wonder about a poet's own path to writing poetry, how each one may think about the nature of their poems, what supports as well as interferes internally—the "internal saboteurs"—during the process of writing, and the place of unconscious or non-conscious elements in the process. Questions still arise: Are poems written with a real or imagined audience in mind? What do they contain, for the writer and for the reader? Can the two disciplines of poetry and psychoanalysis come into fruitful dialogue, given that both start with words and with a shared interest in language, both internal and external, silence and its relationship to words, and the ambiguity of mental states? Do both disciplines encourage us to be better listeners, both to ourselves and others? Does "the music of what happens" (Ogden, 2001) occur in the silences between words, a truth that inhabits the spaces in-between, what Bion called "alpha-function" and then the mystery of "O"? (Bion, 1970a, p. 26). Can we live with some degree of mystery and the tolerance of "not knowing" rather than rushing to premature conclusions? Could we think of poetry as some sort of hotline to the unconscious?

Poetry and clinical work

Over the past years, several clinicians within the student group have talked about their patients' poems as well as their own. I do not talk about these in this chapter because of confidentiality. Here I include three vignettes from other sources. These are necessarily quite brief because of space considerations, but each is referenced further for the interested reader. My own only example over many years of clinical work occurred with my first intensive patient, a young adolescent called "Joe", who was emerging from an autistic state:[2]

> In one session he talked about Dad keeping him in order, reminding him of things, "That's what dads do, isn't it?" I linked it with our work and with me as a sort of monitor of his states, and he said, "Yes", lapsed into silence for some time, took off his watch, tapped it and shook it. I said he was trying to find out things about me and how I worked. There was a lot more silence, and I found my thoughts wandering. I said how hard it was for him today to keep his thoughts in the room. Later he started to make a timetable of sessions, saying, "It's funny, I can do this really well here, but not at school, where there's a lot of noise". He talked of the "peace and quiet", looked at his work, and said, "It's a map—no, in fact it's a contents page. I'll make a book, is that OK?"

It seemed as if the ideas of mapping his states of mind in the therapy had given him an internal space in which to start "the book", a narrative that had begun in a formless and terrifying void, but which could now move forward, although painfully and slowly, out of the abyss. As he announced to me rather grandly, "I don't have keys any more, I have thought."

In the next session he told me about a poem he'd written about space, then could not remember it, and now felt hopeless. We stayed with this feeling, and I suggested that sometimes it was hard for him to have the idea that he *could* recover from feeling low and scared. In the session following his memory lapse, however, he stood in the middle of our room and shyly declaimed his poem, about a silver surfer in space. I saluted his creativity and his memory, as well as the idea that he had things inside him; he was not alone. I did not write the poem down, but he had remembered it by heart, and indeed it was a moment filled with new hope. It described the surfer, adrift without a breathing line in space. And suddenly, the spaceman remembered he was connected to the line, and he could return to his ship. Slowly, a new narrative was forming for Joe, and this small poem seemed to sum up his feeling that he was no longer "adrift without a spacesuit", as Bick so memorably described the newborn baby, but someone who had agency, and was connected by links to "the mother ship", where there was also a Dad to help him remember things. In a sense I had become in his mind a combined object, which then vivified and helped him retrieve his thinking, much as in the way in the first year of life we now know that an infant's brain grows new neural networks, and brain size increases by 100%, needing the offices of good caretakers.

Bianca Lechevalier-Haim's patient "Julia" wrote the following poem when she was 14 years old, and again emerging from an autistic state:

> I will be responsible
> for watching over the snow dogs
> I will follow my footsteps
> And listen to the howling in the evening
> And if I get lost in the night
> The wolves will help me if I call on them softly
> And the wolves will once again become my good friends.

Julia, two years earlier, had seen herself only in "a looking glass" in "Las Vegas", as though her psychotherapy were a card game in which she was to have all the aces. As Lechevalier-Haim notes:

> on the one hand the analyst has to avoid being plunged into despair: on the other, to acknowledge that levels of development exist, and to have due regard for defensive organisations in the service of life, while also not following a wish to ignore the adolescent's destructiveness.
> [Lechevalier-Haim, 2001, p. 91]

Lechevalier-Haim talks of her "true amazement" at the growing evidence of Julia's increased capacities for thinking and for loving, and the development of a more benevolent superego (as with Joe above). Julia's poem appeared towards the end of their time together. Our work as analysts and psychotherapists has been greatly enhanced by bridges that have been built between the findings of child developmentalists and psychoanalytic workers, and also the work of poets, as suggested here. These may help us unpack complex situations and enable a moving on in our patients.

My third brief example comes from Thomas Ogden's (1999) paper, where he presents a close reading of a Robert Frost poem and a detailed discussion of an analytic session, side by side. Using examples from both, he then thinks about the relationship between the way he listens to the language of Frost's poem, "I Have Been One Acquainted with the Night", and the way in which he and his patient listen to one another. He tries to listen to the sound and feeling of "what's going on" in both the poem and the session, without trying to dig down into the poem or "beneath" the patient's reporting of a dream. He suggests that if the analyst attends to his own experience of reverie and "what's going on" for him, correspondences will emerge:

> it seems to me important that we develop a capacity to use language that does justice not only to the task of understanding and interpreting conscious and unconscious meanings . . . our language must be equal to the task of capturing and conveying in words a sense of "what's going on here" in the intrapsychic and intersubjective life of the analysis. [Ogden, 1999, p. 980]

Thus our own reverie experiences can point the way towards new understandings, of poetry, patients, and ourselves.

The Chinese poem

聲聲慢

尋尋覓覓, 冷冷清清, 淒淒慘慘戚戚。
乍暖還寒時候, 最難將息。
三杯兩盞淡酒, 怎敵他, 晚來風急?
雁過也, 正傷心, 卻是舊時相識。

滿地黃花堆積。
憔悴損, 如今有誰堪摘?
守著窗兒, 獨自怎生得黑?
梧桐更兼細雨, 到黃昏, 點點滴滴。
這次第, 怎一個, 愁字了得!

Longing, longing, missing, missing;
Lone, lone, bleak, bleak;
Sad, sad; sorrowful, sorrowful; forlorn, forlorn.
At this season, now warm now cold,
It is most difficult to keep well.
How could a remnant of soft wine, two or three cups
Withstand the wind that comes rushing up at dusk?
The wild geese have passed over,
While I feel heartbroken, and only to know
There are my old friends of the past!

Yellow flowers are piled all over the ground.
Withered as they are,
Who cares to pick them?
I am staying alone by the casement,
How terribly dark!
Tick-tack, tick-tack,

The rain drips onto the phoenix tree in the gloaming.
Such a scene is
Too much for the single word "Sorrow".
[Li Qingzhao (Chinese: 李清照, 1084–1155]

Conclusion

What I have explored here is ways in which unconscious phantasy can be tapped into when one reads a poem as well as when one writes one, even if these phantasies are not explicit in poem, poet, or reader. As one student in the seminars observed, she had learned that one had to wait until meanings emerged, rather than force them upon oneself or upon a poem. How very similar to the analytic process. Analysts and therapists who read and listen to poetry being read are training themselves to resonate with dreams, with free association, and the primary process that reveals conflicting states involved with wishes and desires. I would like to end by quoting from Ogden's (2006) paper "On Teaching Psychoanalysis". He is, of course, talking of analysts in training, but I think one can extrapolate from what he suggests in order to reflect on how to introduce and amplify psychoanalytic concepts to students over a wide range of fields, including that of poetry, in a dynamic way. He talks about reading poetry as "a form of ear-training": words create experiences to be lived by the reader. To paraphrase Ogden, this is "a form of emotion-training" in how to think about painful emotional states. "In sum, teaching psychoanalysis is a paradoxical affair; someone who is supposed to know teaching someone who wants to know what it means not to know" (p. 1083).

In these seminars we have engaged in a "form of emotion-training", which has given us all new insights and differing points of view.

Acknowledgement

Unpublished poems by Bianca Lechevalier-Haim's patient "Julia" and "The Chinese Poem" are published with kind permission of the author and translator.

Notes

First published in 2018 in *British Journal of Psychotherapy, 34,* 2 (2018) 270–284 and is reproduced by kind permission of John Wiley & Sons Ltd.

1 Kate Tempest came out as non-binary in 2020 and is now known as Kae Tempest.
2 For a fuller account of this treatment, see Edwards, 1994, 2016.

CHAPTER SEVEN

"Of Mutability", mourning, and containment

Anne Kane

This chapter is based on an essay written several years earlier, while I was a student on the Tavistock Psychoanalytic Studies course. That essay, about work by the poet Jo Shapcott, was written at a time of considerable personal uncertainty, as my partner had just received a diagnosis of metastatic breast cancer—a primary cancer had returned and spread. The "return" was particularly traumatic, manifesting through a sudden and acutely painful spinal fracture. The metastatic cancer could not be "cured". In interviews, Shapcott questioned the notion of "cure", and this is echoed in her work; it was just one of the ways in which I found these poems to be a place of understanding at a time of crisis. It seemed to represent a form of truth-talking—grappling with profound change or loss—which rendered her poetry moving and powerful. Instead of cure, the many unknowns of my partner's metastatic diagnosis had to be lived with and the likelihood of a reduced life span tolerated, if a thinking life, for the remainder of what time was left was to be possible. It did turn out to be possible, for both of us, I believe: full of moments of terror and sadness, but also of aliveness, work, pleasure. Another poet, Audre Lorde, touches on this difficult and particular point in life in her beautiful poem, "Today Is Not the Day" (1997). Written as Lorde neared her death, from a breast cancer that had metastasized, the poem speaks to living with acute uncertainty, unflinching, knowing, and yet being able to live in the day that is not yet "the" day.

DOI: 10.4324/9781003564867-10

Shapcott's collection of poems was part of realizing the possibility of coping with the uncertainty of that time. The collection came to me as a gift from my partner around the time of the cancer's return. My memory is imprecise, blurred by anxiety: was it before or after the diagnosis? They were part of living in the shadow of an aggressive cancer and amidst the aches and pains that finally were diagnosed as its metastases. What I remember is the important communication that the gift meant to me. These poems—of incomprehension, fear, aloneness, relief, joy, beauty, uncertainty, mortality—facilitated, and came to symbolize, a process of containment of my anxieties. At least, that's how I think of it now. Reading them, emotionally absorbing them—in different ways at different times—discussing them, writing about them, and drawing on them since supported an apparatus for thinking (the most dread-ful) thoughts and experiences, and hence to more or less bear them. Lorde—in words that uncannily mirror Bion's on the development of thinking—says: "Poetry is the way we help give name to the nameless so it can be thought" (2017, pp. 2–3). As a reader, Shapcott's poem(s) was/were a container capable of rendering fear more thinkable and bearable at varying moments: though emotionally thinking, or naming, fear (of dying), "nameless dread" (Bion, 1962b, p. 116), in these moments, was not the outcome.

"A poem . . . may alter its meaning as it moves from one place or time to another", says the literary theorist Terry Eagleton (2013, p. 117). In this way the meaning of "Of Mutability" changed for me over the years. In the depths of grief, these poems became a sort of bad object. The idea that they had once represented, of going on amidst uncertainty, rang hollow: instead of solace, they offered accusation and mockery. As my own "jagged", "raw" cells (in Shapcott's language) eased and the inner good object recovered, somewhat, over time, and I could better bear the loss, I could encounter these poems with less foreboding. While they were never the same again, identified as they are with fundamental loss and its concomitant anxieties, they became more whole objects, a mixed bag—a source of pleasure, but always run through with a sense of pain.

One stepping stone in this process was the experience of returning later to discuss some of the poems in *Of Mutability* with a new group of students on the Psychoanalytic Studies course (and similarly later, in the discussions around this book). In the discussion there were, of course, a range of different views. Hearing these, thinking and discussing together, helped these poems become something else for me. This mutability is, Eagleton suggests, part of the essence of a poem. Another compatible, way of thinking about it is that there was sufficient capacity for reverie in the group to receive my painful feelings about the poems, for these to be understood, digested, communicated by and in the group, and reabsorbed by me, changed. As these feelings and history were not explicitly discussed, this was an unconscious process. Such a seminar group is not a therapeutic group as such, but the experience was such in part: in this sense, it was a containing space, one that allowed emotional experiences to be part of thinking.

Again, as Eagleton suggests, the nature of poetry—its rhythms, symbols, condensed and multilayered meanings—facilitates this kind of communication. Different meanings may arise, jostle, synthesize or not, representing alternative possibilities. The poet Kate [now Kae] Tempest spoke to this labile character:

> the beauty of a poem is that it has a life beyond the sum of its words. So reading about one moment in my life can become about a moment in yours, or a moment that hasn't happened yet, or a moment you have forgotten about.
>
> [Tempest, 2014]

Moments (these poems and thoughts about them) communicated between us, consciously but especially unconsciously, could become, could come to mean, something else, shedding emotional light on their past meaning or allowing for different emotional futures: for moments that haven't happened yet, in an ongoing reparative process.

Of Mutability

In her paper, "Mourning and Its Relation to Manic-Depressive States", Melanie Klein addresses the emotional growth that can result from working through painful situations in life. Mourning is not only, for her, about bereavement but stands for the kind of "mental work" that may be involved in encountering "painful experiences of all kinds". Such pain has "something in common with mourning. It reactivates the infantile depressive position; the encountering and overcoming of adversity of any kind entails mental work similar to mourning" (Klein, 1940, p. 360) (see Appendix, "2. Paranoid–schizoid and depressive positions"; "8. Mourning").

With this in mind, this chapter considers a work of poetry—"Of Mutability", by Jo Shapcott—which was written following the poet's experience of potentially life-threatening illness. The illness—the cancer that was or is inside the body of the subject, is implicit but is never named as such in the work—presents losses, ones the poet alludes to and some the reader may read into the text. That is to say, loss relating to illness or impairment can be complex. It may include the sense of loss of a previously assumed certainty of good health and expectation of a certain lifespan, and the sense of identity, or self, bound up with these. Or illness that leads to discrimination may result in the loss of employment and the injury to one's identity and financial security that this may mean. It may involve the loss of friends struggling with their own anxiety in response to illness or impairment (Watermeyer, 2013). As Shapcott's work illustrates, such "pain" or "adversity" offers itself up to consideration by Klein's insights on mourning.

Bion's ideas on containment and thinking (1962a, 1967b) provide another angle on the work. Shapcott explained that the experience brought about a "changed sensibility" and required her to "carry out 'reconstruction'" of her brain (Crown, 2010). Referring to Virginia Woolf's essay "On Being Ill" (2009)—which, in its meditation on the solitary and existential force of illness, Shapcott's poem seems to speak to and draw upon—Shapcott said that the "horizontal" perspective enforced by lying in bed ill allowed her to "see life anew". She said "I've had to remake myself as a poet". With such ideas in mind, I believe the work illustrates the psychological, as well as artistic, value of being able to tolerate uncertainty: to tolerate the uncertainty represented by serious illness, the frustration of the absence of the certainties one could previously more easily presume, the dread of the unknown and of not knowing. Put in Bion's language, such toleration can produce thoughts and, in turn, thinking, rather than damaging pathological reactions (Bion, 1967b). One's ability to tolerate such frustration depends on having built up an inner mechanism through an early container–contained communication or relationship. We can see this mechanism at work in the poem.

These ideas about loss, mourning, the experience of feelings of dread and their working through help to reveal latent meanings of the poem, "Of Mutability", and of the collection of which it is part. They can deepen our understanding of why it is emotionally satisfying to the reader. The work can be seen as moving through the kind of "reality-testing" Freud (1917e [1915], p. 244) described as taking place in mourning, to where, in Klein's framework, the person feels their "inner world" (1940, p. 353) threatened, along with the external object loss, to the acceptance of loss and a slow and uncertain consolidation and enrichment of the mourner's inner world.

Context

"Of Mutability" was published in 2010. Jo Shapcott was diagnosed with breast cancer in 2003 and went through the grinding process of surgery, chemotherapy, and radiotherapy that can take around a year. This was her first major work for ten years and won considerable recognition. Reviews referred to Shapcott's "recovery" from cancer or even that she was "thankfully, fully recovered" (Anderson, 2011). Shapcott took a different view, saying,

> The distinctive thing about breast cancer is that you're not cured, you're only ever in remission. You become aware that the body is going in one direction: towards disintegration. That's true for all of us, of course—but now it's at the front of my mind, and that means living with a changed sensibility.
>
> [Crown, 2010]

One can infer that while some reviewers took refuge in denial of loss, Shapcott did not feel the need—rather, she was able to tolerate and contain the anxiety of her cancer diagnosis and allow and recognize a "changed sensibility".

Shapcott's awareness is consistent with the facts. Breast cancer is the most common cancer in the UK, with a one-in-seven lifetime risk that a woman will be diagnosed with it. Although improved treatment means that nearly eight in ten women now survive more than ten years (Cancer Research UK, 2024) the variability of the disease, the limits of medical knowledge, and unevenness of access to timely and adequate health services make for varying outcomes. Many find it hard to stop worrying about recurrence, and some respond by "plunging into life" or making sure they do things that "may not have materialized if it were not for the fact that I was diagnosed with cancer" (Healthtalk.org, 2012).

Shapcott rejected suggestions that "Of Mutability" is an autobiographical account of her cancer experience, but she says it is "emotionally autobiographical" and concerned with the "boundaries between the body and the world" (Crown, 2010). The early death of Shapcott's parents arose in interviews: when she was 18, her mother had died of cancer, and her father of a heart attack one month later. She says it was from the time of these losses that her "interest in the body, its edges, its weaknesses" emerged. One is drawn to Klein's point that, as distinct from the infant who "loses" the "good" object even while—in ideal circumstances that are not be realized for many children—the carer is there, later grief of the grown-up is of "the actual loss of an actual person". They may be helped in the face of this loss by having established a "good" object (or a core sense of oneself we might say) inside—objects to which Shapcott perhaps turned her "interest", with curiosity, creatively, and, it is suggested, with concern (Klein, 1940, p. 361).

Applications to the poem

"Of Mutability" is the title work of a collection of 45 poems that spans an arc of mourning and would be interesting to consider psychoanalytically as a whole. "Era", the second poem in the collection, is about denial amidst the shock of diagnosis. "Procedure", at the other end, speaks of reparation and life going on. What follows is an in-depth analysis of the title poem, which I consider a sort of microcosm of the whole. It is the voice of someone looking back, from, as it were, the—for that moment—achieved depressive position and able to communicate meaning she has drawn from emotionally thinking about her pain. The dates in the title poem and "Era", respectively, suggest the vantage point of the former as the first major annual check-up after treatment has finished, which would mark a significant moment of uncertainty.

> Of Mutability
>
> Too many of the best cells in my body
> are itching, feeling jagged, turning raw
> in this spring chill. It's two thousand and four
> and I don't know a soul who doesn't feel small
> among the numbers. Razor small.
> Look down these days to see your feet
> mistrust the pavement and your blood tests
> turn the doctor's expression grave.
>
> Look up to catch eclipses, gold leaf, comets,
> angels, chandeliers, out of the corner of your eye,
> join them if you like, learn astrophysics, or
> learn folksong, human sacrifice, mortality,
> flying, fishing, sex without touching much.
> Don't trouble, though, to head anywhere but the sky.

Structurally this is a sonnet. The rigid and brief form encases tones that shift dramatically, particularly between the first and second stanzas. The voice changes abruptly from the distanced "Of" in the title, to the first person of the first stanza—where the text implies diagnosis and isolation—to the direct address to, and inclusion of, the reader (and the inner object) in the second stanza. Whereas the first stanza (of the persecuted ego voice) forms a slow, pounding (heart-)beat rhythm, which brings attention to the inside and medicalized nature of the body being discussed, the second stanza (addressing, and defending, the object) moves in a more rapid, excited—or manic—rhythm. This stanza seems to direct the gaze outwards, but to a complex cacophony of images that contain multiple meanings.

This tone ends with a depressive, or realistic, bump in the last line, which nevertheless suggests hope has won ("sky"). These features suggest an attempt to control frightening, unpredictable unknowns. On the one hand, we could conclude the struggle lost, because the poem evokes uncertainty. But the vitality of the outer world is identified with as the poem develops, and this life-force seems drawn inwards, with the last line prioritizing the living of life *amidst* uncertainty. One could say that the structure of the poem utilizes, but ultimately rejects, rigid (manic defensive) control and is, instead, able to tolerate and look at the pain of loss and accept that good and bad can co-exist.

To consider the text in detail.

> Too many of the best cells in my body
> are itching, feeling jagged, turning raw
> in this spring chill.

Klein explains how in mourning early psychotic anxieties are revived (Klein, 1940). This regression means that the person feels that their inner good objects are lost and "bad" objects predominate. These first three lines of the poem express this dynamic. Dramatic opposites are presented, suggestive of a persecutory state of mind, with splitting of objects into good and bad. The negative "too many" is set against the positive "best cells"—the feeling is one of encroachment. These "cells"—the building blocks of the body—could be taken to represent both the external loss imposed by illness and the unconsciously feared lost inner objects, such as described by Klein when she says that a child, having incorporated his parents, "feels them to be lived people inside his body in the concrete way in which deep unconscious phantasies are experienced—they are, in his mind, 'internal' or 'inner' objects" (Klein, 1940, p. 345).

Here, Shapcott describes cells (objects) that are being horribly affected and "turning raw". The ego's attempt to protect them through idealization—they are the "best" cells—is unsuccessful. The emphasis also remains on the persecuted ego: the main voice emphasized is "my body"; the "cells", a word that also suggests imprisonment, are the ego's. The ego is being punished. As a whole, the lines bring to mind the (often objected to) warlike metaphors commonly used when speaking of cancer (Judd, 1995; Sontag, 1990) and the ways these may reflect an unconscious sense of attack and battle.

Then there is a "spring chill"—a phrase that again speaks to paranoid–schizoid processes of splitting by juxtaposing life-giving "spring" to deathly "chill". From a literary point of view, Empson (1977) described such use of opposites as illustrating a fundamental division in the author's mind. In making "spring" and "chill" adjacent, good and bad are also brought closer together than in the first line of the poem, suggesting that the power, or need, to split and keep apart good and bad is waning slightly.

> It's two thousand and four
> and I don't know a soul who doesn't feel small
> among the numbers. Razor small.

The attempt to bring good and bad closer together appears to have been premature, as these lines continue to show persecutory fear: time is passing (a reminder perhaps of the finite nature of life and the writer's sense of this reality) and the ego and all the person's inner objects feel "small", on the verge of being overwhelmed by the "numbers", the persecutors. "Numbers" could also be understood as a reference to a cancer patient's test results, one year after diagnosis and treatment onset. With "Razor small" (given stress by the upper-case R) the threat is big, acute (threateningly sharp) and close to the object. The allusion to treatment (cutting, and also removal) is reinforced.

> Look down these days to see your feet
> mistrust the pavement and your blood tests
> turn the doctor's expression grave.

This section sees a shift, with manic defences strengthening and battling with recognition of the fear of loss as the depressive position gets nearer, suggested by the change of voice from "I" to "your". This shifts the emphasis from the ego to an ego-and-object relationship. The change in subject to "your" both addresses the internal objects in these lines: "feet" and "blood tests" and addresses the reader, drawing us in. We could say that through projective identification the writer (or ego) of the poem communicates the intolerable feelings to her objects.

Reinforcing the interpretation that the pain of loss is getting more conscious, and manic defences are being mobilized, is the phrase, "look down". This has a hint of "look away": denying the fear just felt. The feet (standing for the object dialogued with) cannot trust—cannot be safe in—the outside world. Is fear denied and reality turned away from? Klein says "without partial and temporary denial of psychic reality the ego cannot bear the disaster by which it feels itself threatened when the depressive position is at its height" (Klein, 1940, p. 349). Or, as Eliot expressed it, "human kind / Cannot bear very much reality" (1983, p. 14).

We can see that danger remains near—the "grave" of the doctor's expression echoing death and burial. However, concern is increasingly clearly for the object—"*your* blood tests"—not the ego alone. There are two further meanings that add to this and also indicate a process of containment to mitigate this anxiety. First, the phrase, "Look down these days" has a reflective sense to it and can be interpreted as the ego trying to test reality. Second, it is in the imperative form, indicating communication, which is both internal (steadying the inner objects) and external (to us, the readers). The ego is trying to tolerate the anxiety from this danger, communicate it, and allow it to be thought about.

> Look up to catch eclipses, gold leaf, comets,
> angels, chandeliers, out of the corner of your eye,
> join them if you like, learn astrophysics,

The second stanza opens with a complete change of tone. Using Bion's concept of containment, we could say that now we see that intolerable fears have become modified by their communication to and "sojourn in": the inner and external objects in the previous lines. The object that is reintrojected "has become tolerable" (Bion, 1962a). We (the inner objects being recreated and the reader) are told to "look up". This can be taken as a positive injunction: to be hopeful. But the images suggest something more complex as well. The object is told that it can have just a glimpse of hope: "catch . . . out of the corner of your eye". The images to be caught—eclipses, gold leaf, comets, angels, chandeliers—are beautiful, sparkling, stellar ones. They suggest wonder at nature and the cosmos. But again, there is also a suggestion of difficult thoughts of one's finite time and place in nature: the other-worldliness of "comets" and mention of "angels" can be read as suggestions of death. One could interpret that the communication established has modified the raw fear expressed in the first stanza and produced thought and the beginning of thinking. The thought may be that this terrible thing can, in fact, be borne, and look, there are all these wonderful things to be seen and be part of.

Yet fear remains, and bearing this in mind, these lines could simultaneously be interpreted as slightly euphoric. This brings to mind Klein's view of elation in the context of normal mourning as a "passing state" between sorrow and distress, which "are manic in character and are due to the feeling of possessing the perfect loved object (idealized) inside" (1940, p. 355). Klein says that such idealization is disturbed by hatred, and this helps us to understand the line: "join them if you like, learn astrophysics". Again, this suggests two meanings: first, an injunction to embrace life; alternatively, as a sort of omnipotent, almost angry, phantasy, suggesting, perhaps, that if only something very difficult can be learned, the badness and threat will be controlled, and the good object will be safe.

Woolf's essay "On Being Ill" offers another juxtaposition. In words that Shapcott echoes, she writes that the necessity to stop, to draw in, required by illness offers the opportunity to "perhaps for the first time for years, to look round, to look up—to look, for example, at the sky". Yet the wonder of nature is followed by an awareness of one's irrelevance to that natural world: "Divinely beautiful is also divinely heartless" (Woolf, 2009, p. 105). Or:

> learn folksong, human sacrifice, mortality,
> flying, fishing, sex without touching much.

These lines evoke sadness, as if the pain of the situation, the loss, can now be acknowledged. The images are mystifying, but this feels appropriate—as if, through projective identification, the reader is being informed about the frustration of the unknowable and of things not being as expected. Can the reader receive this communication and tolerate these perhaps frustratingly complex images?

They are ambiguous images. There is so much in the world, on the one hand. Yet we are told to learn things that, as they all can't literally be learned, particularly "mortality", have, in this context, a connotation of "learn to accept". Placing "mortality" between "human sacrifice" and "flying" could be thought of as suggesting that if only an offering of someone *else's* life could be given, one's own could be salvaged: one could "fly" or thrive.

Segal (1952) argued that the realization and sublimation of the depressive position in art requires an acknowledgement of the death instinct, "both in its aggressive and destructive aspects", and that the "reality of death for the object and the self" must be accepted. Applying this here, we could interpret the acceptance of death of the object through "human sacrifice": the external loss, excised through surgery, and the re-lived death of the inner objects, one's earlier self. We can interpret "mortality" as the acceptance of the potential future death that this experience has put on the cards, or as Shapcott put it, the acceptance that: "the body is going in one direction: towards disintegration" (Crown, 2010).

In Bion's model, this acceptance of the reality of death, or loss, is possible as a result of tolerating frustration. This allows thinking. It shows dominance of the reality principle is present (Bion, 1967b).

Then "fishing" suggests multiple interpretations in this context: something realistic after the illusion of "flying"; rummaging around for a solution; but also, the sadness of killing something to eat (take inside), which can, however, bring nourishment and life: feeding and rebuilding one's inner world.

"Sex without touching much" is suggestive of a sad and not very intimate encounter, as if one may be leaving soon and wishes to avoid becoming too close. Following the twists and turns of the preceding images, this one suggests a closure of these lines by acceptance of loss and of letting the sadness in, and into the most intimate of moments.

> Don't trouble, though, to head anywhere but the sky.

The last line again looks upward, hopefully. Having acknowledged the loss, borne the frustration, been able to emotionally think about it, and been able to start to nourish and rebuild the inner world, life can move forward, looking to the sky. The opening "don't trouble though" here emotionally balances the "closing sky". It also balances the rhyme with "eye" four lines above and echoes the references there to other-worldly elements. Allusions that were previously, in part, connected with denial are now "contained" by "don't trouble" and the acknowledgement of loss and death in the previous lines and transformed into something hopeful but realistic.

Conclusion

A psychoanalytic reading can show how this poem succeeds in giving meaning to fearful bodily and emotional experiences. Unbearable sensations, which we may think of as Bion's beta elements, become thinkable, or alpha elements, and this alpha function (Bion, 1962a) is imparted to the reader. An example of this was, for me, provided by a young woman I heard speak about the meaning of this poem to her. She came across the collection just after learning of her father's cancer diagnosis: "it was a moment of recognition". Yet it took her about a month to realize the issue of cancer ran through the whole book: "though I felt it before that" (The Poetry Exchange, 2019). The emotional sense of the poem was taken in (felt), contained, and, over time, understood more consciously. The cycle of mourning traced in the text of the title poem is explored more extensively across the collection as a whole. Psychoanalytically, the beauty of the poem could be said to be its bringing together of something ugly or painful, expressing the death instinct, in a form with rhythm and unity, expressing the life instinct (Segal, 1952). For the reader, the poem helps us to contain our own difficult feelings about illness and mortality. We understand that it is possible to enjoy life amidst its mutability. Indeed, that mutability, with its unknowability, is the inescapable essence of living.

CHAPTER EIGHT

Resistance through mourning: a poem by Mahmoud Darwish, "In Her Absence I Created Her Image"

Elina Matter

Mahmoud Darwish [1941–2008] was a renowned Palestinian poet. Considered one of the first poets of resistance, a Palestinian literary movement that emerged in the 1960s, his poetry has given voice to the voiceless. Darwish's poetic mastery lies in the conveyance not only of a Palestinian experience of exile, but also an experience of exile beyond the political realm. As a third-generation Palestinian, I have connected most to his rendition of the universal experience of loss and exile. This is partly due to my own experiences of being far removed from the concreteness of the conflict and, instead, experiencing it intergenerationally through my father. Also, the poem I have chosen to discuss, "In Her Absence I Created Her Image" (Darwish, 2005), belongs to a collection of poems that Darwish wrote after 1997, a time during which he adamantly did not want to be read solely through a political lens. Admittedly, it is impossible to completely divorce Darwish's poetry from the political, also apparent through the rich symbolism used that connects him to Palestine. However, it is possible to denote how his expression of exile goes beyond the concrete, touching upon an inner exile from the self and a deep longing for a home within the self: "As much as he is the voice of the Palestinian diaspora, he is the voice of the fragmented soul" (Jounah, 2013, p. 172).

"In Her Absence I Created Her Image" presents this longing for a home, one that can be understood symbolically as well as literally. It reflects the painful process of mourning and what I see as Darwish's

DOI: 10.4324/9781003564867-11

attempt at rebuilding his inner world, as is discussed through Klein's concept of mourning. I have also found that through this poem Darwish reveals his creative process—in particular, the containing function of his poetry, which facilitates his ability to mourn. This is further elucidated through Bion's model of the container–contained, which highlights the sustaining function of the "poetry of resistance".

I wrote this chapter in 2020, before the horrors that began on the 7th of October 2023. Four years later, I find it impossible to feel far removed from the concreteness of the conflict. I re-read this chapter at a time when Palestinians are experiencing the most catastrophic destruction of their home, identity, and world, and I question how much more can one continue to resist. However, this chapter also reminds me how Palestinians have continued to survive in the face of adversity, as demonstrated through Palestinian resistance poetry, for 76 years. I hope this chapter provides light on Palestinian culture and history, and my take on how they have and will continue to resist through mourning.

Poetry of resistance

The significance of Palestinian resistance literature can only be understood by acknowledging the historical conditions out of which it was born—specifically, the Nakba of 1948, and the aftermath of the 1967 Six-Day-War. While the year 1948 is celebrated by Israelis as the year Israel became an independent state, Palestinians mourn it as the year of "Al-Nakba": the catastrophe. Triggered by Britain's decision to end its mandate in Palestine, the war of 1947–48 led to the systematic dispossession of Palestinians as more than 700,000 were expelled from their land and traces of Palestinian culture and identity began to be erased. This was particularly apparent in the way Palestinians were treated following the 1967 Six-Day War,[1] in which Israel gained control of Gaza and the West Bank. Palestinian life under Israeli authority was greatly oppressed, and any forms of Palestinian expression, including art and literature, was prohibited. Political activity was made illegal, and education was suppressed, with few allowed to attend high school and enter university. In response, Palestinians began asserting their identity through the development of "resistance literature". This literary category is one that is driven by liberation struggles and oppression and has emerged in various resistance movements in the Middle East, Africa, and Latin America. Barbara Harlow explores the underpinnings of this literature in her book, *Resistance Literature,* describing how "the resistance writer, like the guerrilla of the armed liberation struggle, is actively engaged in an urgent historical confrontation" (Harlow, 1987, p. 100). Harlow also credits Ghassan Kanafani, a prominent Palestinian author and political activist, for coining the term "resistance literature".

Kanafani divided Palestinian literature into two recognized branches: literature written by Palestinians living in Israel: "resistance literature", and literature written by Palestinians outside Israel: "exile literature". He was the first to bring attention to the resistance poets in a published anthology of their poems in 1966, describing the literature of resistance as "courageous, full of vitality and optimism and highly charged with the spirit of defiance" (Kanafani, 1968, p. 4). Poetry, the most popular literary form in Palestinian culture, underwent major changes during the 1960s, as it became known as the "poetry of resistance". Some discernible features of the "poetry of resistance" include the poets' use of folklore and colloquial language, breaking away from the classical Arabic tradition, as a way of relating to the humble background from which Palestinians came. Themes of exile, identity, racism, and colonialism are often explored, thus expressing the experience of a dispossessed population. Moreover, resistance poets are distinguished by the symbols used to represent Palestine. For example, elements of Palestinian nature, such as olive trees and palm trees, are often used to symbolize their organic connection with their land. Another notable symbol is that of the "mother" as a representation of Palestine; this is further explored below.

One of the most respected and admired poets of resistance, Mahmoud Darwish, experienced the Nakba of 1948 at the age of 6, during which he witnessed the complete destruction of his village, al-Birwa. This experience is one that has shaped his poetry. As he described in 1996:

> In 1948, when this great rupture of ours took place, I jumped from the bed of childhood onto the path of exile. I was six. My entire world turned upside down and childhood froze in place, it didn't go with me . . . finding the child Mahmoud Darwish who once was is possible only in the poem. Not in life.
>
> [in Yeshurun, 2012, p. 48]

Darwish and his family found refuge in Lebanon for a year, before returning to Israel illegally in 1949; they settled in Deir-el-Assad, a village adjacent to al-Birwa. They were not eligible to apply for citizenship and thus were declared present–absent aliens. Darwish began writing at the age of 17, and soon his poetry became a means by which he could convey his experience of exile. His questioning of identity is often met with in his poems, with one of his most well-known poems, "Identity Card" (Darwish, 1964), becoming a protest song, for which he was placed under house arrest. After being denied entry to higher education, Darwish decided to leave Israel for Moscow, to study political economy. After a year, he left for Cairo, where he worked as a journalist before joining the Palestinian Liberation Organization (PLO) in Beirut. This led to him being banned from entering Israel for 26 years, during which he alternated between several countries, including Paris, Beirut, Tunisia, and Jordan. In the 1990s, Darwish quit the PLO, as he was opposed to the Oslo Accords[2]; he believed the terms of the agreement were too vague and unequal and would eventually lead to an escalation of the conflict. Having quit the PLO, he was allowed to reside in Ramallah, where he lived for the remainder of his life under Israeli occupation. Darwish died in 2008 in Texas, following complications from heart surgery. Three days of national mourning were declared by President Mahmoud Abbas.

Mahmoud Darwish wrote more than 30 books of poetry, which have been translated into 20 languages. While he was known as a Palestinian national poet, he struggled with being labelled as such. He maintained that his poetry emanated from his personal experiences, and he never intended for his work to be used politically. He was first and foremost a humanitarian, who advocated equal treatment for both Palestinians and Israelis. He sought to show the humanitarian meaning of the Palestinian cause to the world and express the spirit of the people:

> Because in the end we are all exiles. The occupier and myself—both of us suffer from exile. He is an exile in me and I am the victim of his exile. All of us on this beautiful planet Earth, we are all neighbours, we are all exiles, we are all walking in the same human fate, and what unites us is the need to tell the story of this exile.
>
> [in Yeshurun, 2012, p. 50]

Resistance through mourning

From these historical conditions, the resistance poets created a space where the experience of loss could be endured. This is further explored by considering the poets' creative process, as well as the recurring symbol of the "mother" in resistance poetry.

The creative process

In Kleinian theory, creativity is inextricably linked with the working through of the depressive position. The depressive position involves the realization that the "bad" persecuting object towards which sadistic attacks were directed is also the "good" ideal object. A new set of anxieties arises: the fear of losing and damaging the good internal object due to destructive impulses. And so emerges the unconscious impulse to repair the object felt to be damaged, in order to "save the loved object, to repair and restore it" (Klein, 1935, p. 270). Anxiety and guilt are then lessened through restorative phantasies and actions, as the "child tries to recreate the other it has destroyed, first by phantasies of omnipotent reparation, later by affectionate and healing gestures towards real others, constituting the drive towards creative effort" (Glover, 2009, p. 54). The depressive and paranoid–schizoid positions being perceived as modes of mental functioning and not just as developmental stages, Klein posited that whenever a loss is experienced, the depressive position is reactivated, undermining "the feeling of secure possession of the loved internal objects, for it revives the early anxieties about injured and destroyed objects—about a shattered world" (Klein, 1952c, p. 77).

Segal furthered developed the link between creativity and the depressive position through a theoretical articulation of Kleinian aesthetics. Building on Klein's understanding, Segal explicitly reiterated that what is present in the unconscious of all artists is a destroyed world: "all creation is really a re-creation of a once loved and once whole, but now lost and ruined object, a ruined internal world and self" (Segal, 1990, p. 190). She posited that artistic activity derives from the artist's awareness of the state of his inner world, through which he expresses his anxieties and "does work similar to the work of mourning in that he internally re-creates a harmonious world which is projected into his work of art" (p. 199). Thus, Darwish's poetry can be understood as emerging from his need to repair his inner world. Mourning fuels his poetry, and, as he repeatedly rebuilds his inner world, an effort that requires the ability to tolerate the intolerable, he resists in the face of devastation. According to Darwish, "Poetry cannot conceal the truth within me. Poetry is the scandalous revelation of my secret" (in Yeshurun, 2012, p. 54). Indeed, it is because of his authentic conveyance of his depressive anxieties, his destroyed world and the gradual rebuilding of that world, that his poetry has sustained so many Palestinians. Through his poetry, readers re-experience their own anxieties in a more bearable form, and just as Darwish is able to resist, they, too, resist. Segal argues that the experience of aesthetic pleasure is derived from

> an identification of ourselves with the work of art as a whole and with the whole internal world of the artist as represented by his work. In my view all aesthetic pleasure includes an unconscious reliving of the artist's experience of creation.
>
> [Segal, 1990, p. 203]

The mother symbol and container/contained

In the 1970s, the symbol of the mother became the representation of a new strategy of Palestinian resistance against the occupation: *Sumud* [steadfastness]. This strategy commanded Palestinians to resist by remaining rooted in their land. Carol Bardenstein traces the development of the mother as a symbol for Palestine in "Raped Brides and Steadfast Mothers: Appropriations of Palestinian Motherhood" (Bardenstein, 1997). She shows how Palestinian resistance literature became inundated with female imagery that symbolized the *Sumud* strategy: "in the face of adversity, the ability to withstand, to hold out against, to outlive or survive even the most difficult circumstances and experiences" (p. 179). From a historical point of view, this symbolization was a representation of woman's role in the Palestinian struggle. Mothers fulfilled an important task in nurturing the fighters during the resistance and were commended for their ability to withstand the loss of their children:

> Mothers are seen as remaining steadfast in the traditional roles of providing, nurturing, and protecting, even when circumstances require that they substantially adapt these roles, and expand the scope of the 'family' considered the rightful recipient of their 'mothering' energies. [Bardenstein, 1997, p. 179]

Undeniably, the symbol of the mother and its link to the *Sumud* strategy is striking due to its connotation of the mother–infant relationship and can be further explored through Bion's container–contained model.

Bion postulated that when the infant projects intolerable emotions (beta-elements) into the mother, the mother acts as a container by receiving these emotions. Through her reverie, the mother receives and transforms these feelings into a tolerable form (alpha-elements), and thus the infant re-introjects the modified and contained feeling. Eventually, the infant also "introjects the containing/alpha-function itself and thus has the beginning of a means within his own mind of tolerating frustration and for thinking" (Spillius, Milton, Garvey, Couve, Steiner, 2011a, p. 510). For Bion, creative activity is based on how meaning is created out of intolerable emotions, which become contained within the creation. Interestingly, the resistance poets often present the return to the homeland as the idealized union between child and mother. Through this symbolization, their experience of loss and exile is compared to that of a child losing their mother, denoting the collapse of their inner world, as well as the loss of the containing mother. The idealized union conveys their attempt at re-finding the internal mother who symbolizes the ability to withstand the intolerable. Thus, they create meaning out of their emotional experience, much like the mother's reverie creates meaning out of her infant's emotions, and this drives their resistance.

Moreover, Bion highlighted that psychic development depends on the to-and-fro movement between the paranoid–schizoid (disintegration) and depressive (integration) positions. In Bion's words:

> Learning depends on the capacity for [the growing container] to remain integrated yet lose rigidity. This is the foundation of the state of mind of the individual who can retain his knowledge and experience yet be prepared to reconstrue past experiences in a manner that enables him to be receptive of a new idea.
>
> [Bion, 1962a, p. 93]

It necessitates the ability to withstand the dismantling of the container—a move into disintegration—before the container can be re-established. Darwish's acute description of his creative process echoes this oscillation between disintegration and integration: "our whole life is an alternation between life and death. Every time you die in a poem, you are born anew" (in Yeshurun, 2012, p. 58). Darwish articulates the role of disintegration through the experience of "dying" in the poem a destructive force. It may be interpreted as indicative of a dismantling of the container, and a necessary move from integration to disintegration. He is "born anew" as the painful experience of disintegration is contained and expressed through the creation of his poem.

Hence, resistance poetry is driven by mourning, as the poets attempt to rebuild their home internally and thus withstand its loss in the external world. Their ability to mourn is also dependent on their capacity to tolerate unmanageable emotions, which, through the medium of their poems, become contained and are given meaning. The sustaining function of resistance poetry thus lies in the poets' ability to represent previously unsymbolized emotional experience, "digested facts", which "helps the non-artist to digest" (Bion, 1990, p. 143). Darwish articulates this process in "In Her Absence I Created Her Image". The poem presents the painful work of mourning, while enabling him to mourn as he enters a dream-like state.

Mourning in "In Her Absence I Created Her Image"

> In her absence I created her image: out of the earthly
> The hidden heavenly commence. I am here weighing
> the expanse with the Jahili odes . . . and absence

is the guide, it is the guide. For each rhyme a tent
is pitched. And for each thing blowing in the wind
a rhyme. Absence teaches me its lesson: "If it weren't
for the mirage you wouldn't have been steadfast. . . ."
And in the emptiness, I disassembled a letter from one
Of the ancient alphabets and I leaned on absence. So who am I
After the visitation? A bird, or a passerby amidst the symbols
And the memory vendors? As if I were an antique piece,
As if were a ghost sneaking in from Yabous, telling myself:
Let's go to the seven hills. Then I placed
My mask on a stone, and walked as the sleepless
Walk, led by my dream. And from one moon
To another I leapt. There is enough of unconsciousness
To liberate things from their history. And there
is enough of history to liberate unconsciousness
from its ascension. "Take me to our early
years", my first girlfriend says. "Leave
the windows open for the house sparrow to enter
your dream", I say . . . then I awaken, and no city is in
the city. No "here" except "there." And no there
but here. If it weren't for the mirage
I wouldn't have walked to the seven hills . . .
If it weren't for the mirage!

Darwish begins the poem by inviting the reader into his inner world; his use of the colon right after stating that he's creating the image of his absent home can be said to represent the entry into his world. As he creates his loved home out of the earth, the only unchanged feature of Palestine, he describes it as "heavenly", which evokes a feeling of unparalleled bliss. From a psychoanalytic perspective, the image Darwish is creating could be interpreted as that of an ideal loved object. The state of his inner world is then described as he references the "Jahili odes" which relate to a form of pre-Islamic poetry that is distinguished by its nostalgic mood. The pre-Islamic poets used to begin their poems by claiming that they were "standing by the ruins" of their beloved, emphasizing the feeling of longing and despair (Seigneurie, 2011). An image is then created for the reader that mirrors that of the poet's inner world: Darwish, in the ruins, attempting to re-build his ideal home. As each rhyme pitches a tent, Darwish reinforces that it is through the medium of his poem that he will re-build his inner world.

In lines 6 to 11, Darwish presents the painful experience of absence as he is faced with the ruins of his inner world. For Darwish, the ability to withstand this state, "steadfastness", is dependent on a "mirage", a dream like state that disappears just as quickly as it appears:

> . . . Absence teaches me its lesson: "if it weren't
> For the mirage you wouldn't have been steadfast. . . ."
> And in the emptiness, I disassembled a letter from one
> Of the ancient alphabets and I leaned on absence. So, who am I
> After the visitation? A bird, or a passerby amidst the symbols
> And the memory vendors? As if I were an antique piece. . . .
>
> [Lines 6–11]

As Darwish is faced with the ruins of his inner world, he is plunged into an empty world, thus insinuating the deterioration and collapse of "his internalized good objects who became part of his inner world from the earlier stages of his development . . . are too felt to have gone under, to be destroyed" (Klein, 1940, p. 353). Darwish elicits a sense of non-being, a state in which all that was once known is now no longer known, which is further echoed by his disassembling of a letter, the mode through which he expresses his thoughts. As he questions who he is, he depicts to the reader his loss of identity and his inability to relate to himself in the present. The referral to the "memory vendors" can be interpreted as the conflict between Israel and Palestine, as Darwish analyses "the meaning of a home . . . as a struggle between two memories" (Parmenter, 2004, p. 97). It further echoes his disoriented state of mind, which reflects the Palestinians' reality. This state also brings to mind Bion's non-pathological aspect of the paranoid–schizoid position, in which the ability to experience this chaotic and unknown state—to disintegrate—is an integral capacity that then leads to a state of integration—perhaps it even presents an experience of Bion's elusive "O", which he saw as the essential basis of creative work. It is

> the ultimate reality . . . it can "become", but it cannot be "known". It is darkness and formlessness but it enters the [knowledge] domain when it has evolved to a point where it can be known, through knowledge gained by experience.
>
> [Bion, 1970b, p. 26]

It is an experience of emptiness because it necessitates a relinquishing of the known self, an entry into the unknown and the uncertain. It is through the function of this dreamlike state, the "mirage", that Darwish is able to withstand this state and remain "steadfast":

> As if I were a ghost sneaking in from Yabous, telling myself:
> let's go to the seven hills. Then I placed
> my mask on a stone, and walked as the sleepless
> walk, led by my dream. And from one moon
> to another I leapt. There is enough of unconsciousness

> to liberate things from their history. And there
> Is enough of history to liberate unconsciousness
> from its ascension. "Take me to our early
> years." My first girlfriend says. . . .
>
> [Lines 12–20]

The mirage begins as Darwish refers to himself as a "ghost" coming in from Yabous. Yabous, which refers to Jebus, is what is known today as Jerusalem in Israel. According to the Hebrew Bible, it was inhabited by a Canaanite tribe before its conquest by King David in 1003BCE. Darwish often refers to the Canaanite tribe, as it is seen as the origin of Palestinians:

> he recognized himself as the inheritor of the various civilizations that have passed through his land and extends his roots further back in time to the Arab Peninsula, to the Canaanites . . . thus boosting and enriching his Palestinian heritage.
>
> [Yousef, 2011, p. 679]

The process by which he is able to create meaning out of his emotional experience, thus beginning to rebuild his world, is marked by the removal of his "mask". In Bion's words, he relinquishes his "saturated" self with expectations, memories, and desires in order to experience the emotional self. As he drifts into a dreamlike state and walks as the "sleepless walk", he transforms the emotional experience into processed thoughts, and "access to O depends upon this dream-like state of mind, which presents one's raw primitive experiences to be transformed into thought" (Reiner, 2012, p. 2). A sense of hope is elicited, and the confusion of the previous lines begin dissipating as he begins rebuilding his inner world by providing himself with stable roots to his identity and thus regains "trust in external objects and values of various kinds", which "[strengthens] his confidence in the lost loved person" (Klein, 1940, p. 355).

The "mirage" thus represents the containing function, much like the mother's reverie. It is through this dream-like state that his emotional experience becomes "digested", which, in turn, enables him to begin re-building his world: "Dream thoughts allow us to feel (mentally) our bodily emotions, and thereby grow and evolve from our acceptance of them and the truth about ourselves which emotions carry as their ballast" (Grotstein, 2013, p. 119). And thus Darwish is able to tolerate the experience of absence as he begins to relinquish the object in the material world while simultaneously installing it in his inner world (Britton, 1992). He maintains his loved home within him as his unconscious phantasy liberates things from history, while also accepting that it no longer exists in the external world, as unconsciousness does not ascend. This is further echoed by his referral to his "first girlfriend", which could be inferred to represent Palestine. As he's asked to go to "their early days", one could further infer that this refers to his childhood. There is a sense of serenity evoked by this image, as Darwish re-finds his good internal objects that are assumed to have been established in his early childhood. His inner world is slowly being rebuilt, while also accepting that it no longer exists in the external world.

> then I awaken, and no city is in
> the city. No "here" except "there". And no there
>
> but here. If it weren't for the mirage
> I wouldn't have walked to the seven hills . . .
> If it weren't for the mirage!
>
> [Lines 20–26]

As Darwish reaches the end of the poem, he awakens from his dream-like state. At first a sense of sadness is evoked as the reality of the external world is faced, but there is also resistance within that sadness. Darwish is able to resist the "no city" because of the mirage that led him to the seven hills, a reference to Jerusalem. It is through the function of the mirage that Darwish is able to retain his loved city within him and thus re-build his inner world when faced with the pain of its ruins: "Without phantasies and without dreams you have not the means with which to think out your problem" (Bion, 1953). It also denotes how mourning for Darwish is as infinite as his exile. He remains in an inescapable cycle of mourning, and just as he finds his way through the ruins, the poem ends, and he returns back to the beginning: there is no ending to his exile. Exile has become his identity: "Exile is a part of my inner being. Exile exists not only in geographical terms. You can be an exile in your homeland, in your own house, in a room. Can I say I'm addicted to exile? Maybe" (Darwish, 2002, p. 77).

Conclusion

Undeniably, the "poetry of resistance" is more than just an expression of political discontent. It is the mode through which poets—and a result their readers—resist in the face of devastation. Through the poets' use of symbols and metaphors, their internal experience is transformed into external images. The readers experience this transformation in a contained form, and thus their own unmanageable emotions may be given meaning. Darwish's poem depicts this transformation, as well as how it is interlinked with mourning. Throughout the poem, Darwish conveys the harrowing experience of facing the ruins of his inner world. From this state of loss, his mirage led him through the ruins, and thus he began creating meaning out of his experience and, as a result, rebuilding his inner world. It becomes clear by the end of the poem that for Darwish this is an endless cycle of mourning, one that keeps him suspended between the ruins and the ideal home. Nonetheless, what is also clear is his ability to transform his pain into words contained within his poetry, which is what has sustained so many Palestinians. Even in his never-ending exile, he has provided a home for the homeless: "I built my homeland, I even established a state, in my language" (in Yeshurun, 2012, p. 52).

Notes

1 The war was fought between Israel and the Arab states of Syria, Egypt, and Jordan. Israel defeated the Arab states in a matter of six days, taking control of Gaza, the West Bank, and East Jerusalem, which were previously under the Arab states' rule.

2 The Oslo Accords are a set of agreements reached by the Israeli government and the Palestine Liberation Organization in 1993, which lead to the creation of a Palestinian Authority in parts of the West Bank and the Gaza Strip.

PART III

LITERATURE AND THE PERFORMING ARTS

Where the focus in Part II was on one specific genre, poetry, the scope of Part III is broader, containing chapters where the authors bring their psychoanalytic thinking to teaching on the Psychoanalytic Studies course to a play, an opera, and a novel.

In the first chapter, Michael Rustin, who teaches the Applications unit "Psychoanalysis, Drama and Society", describes the approach and the development of the unit that he ran jointly over a number of years, initially with Margaret Rustin and subsequently with other collaborators. He sets the work of the unit in the broader context of drama's traditional focus on family relationships, which have interested dramatists since the time of Aristotle, and he goes on to describe how the seminar leaders engaged students in thinking psychoanalytically about Shakespeare's plays.

Rustin encapsulates how he sees the relationship between psychoanalysis and Shakespeare's plays in the question, "What had Shakespeare understood, which centuries later has come to be of interest for psychoanalysts?" Like Edwards, he is clear that there is no hierarchical relationship between dramatists and psychoanalysis—both have a common interest in the complexities and dramas of the human mind and human relationships.

The cultural artefacts explored in chapters 10, 11, and 12—a play by Beckett, an opera by Puccini, and a novel by Ishiguro—might seem to be disparate; there is, however, a theme, introduced in Rustin's chapter, that draws them together: namely, the psychoanalytic concept of narcissism.

DOI: 10.4324/9781003564867-12

As outlined briefly in the Appendix ("6. Narcissism"), narcissism is a complex concept, and narcissistic states of mind (which are aligned more with the paranoid–schizoid than the depressive position) can be transient, as everyone fluctuates between the self-serving attitudes of the paranoid–schizoid position and the greater concern for the other inherent in the depressive position. However, in more severe psychopathology, narcissistic states can dominate the personality to the extent that they define what is described in psychoanalysis as a narcissistic character structure. Rustin cites Shakespeare's description of Richard in *Richard III* as representing a character type that shows a very close correspondence to the psychoanalyst Rosenfeld's (1971) definition of "destructive narcissism". Shakespeare expresses in the most poetic language his intuitive sense of the central features of this pathological personality structure within Richard—a hatred for any loving relationship, not only compulsive unconscious destructive and murderous phantasies but, in Richard's case, actual murderousness and an unconscious wish to exact revenge against the world as a result of being born deformed. As Rustin points out, in the scenario Shakespeare imagines, the playwright also understands that a psychopathology of this severity has its origins in the infant's earliest relationships. In the play, Shakespeare describes a meeting between Richard and his mother where she speaks to him in a way that reveals the degree to which she rejected him, hated him, and experienced him as her persecutor from the moment of his birth onwards. Thus, Shakespeare has captured something of the complexity of the conditions that might give rise to the development of such severe illness, a complexity that psychoanalysts struggle to make sense of in work with their patients.

Chapter 10, Maryam Ghasemi's essay, "*Rockaby*: Eros and Thanatos", introduces Freud's concepts of the two opposing forces within the human psyche: the life instinct (Eros) and the death instinct (Thanatos). Ghasemi notes that Beckett scholars have tended to focus on the deadened and deadening states of mind he portrays, which undoubtedly do infuse his writing to a great extent. However, she argues that in *Rockaby* the tension between the two psychic forces is more present than might first appear. She highlights how, as the protagonist, "a prematurely old woman", seems to be approaching death, there are suggestions that the life instinct in her comes to the fore momentarily but repeatedly as she asks for "more". Each section of the play begins with the woman waking after a period of withdrawal and saying one word, "more"—apparently meaning that she wants to hear more of the expressionless recorded story of her and her dead mother's lives, which forms the soundtrack of the play. The reader is invited by Ghasemi to consider whether that single word might also suggest the woman's libidinal wish for more life, more time in which to search for another—someone with whom there might be the possibility of a meaningful relationship. The scene has echoes of a dying person's clamour for water in a last attempt to hold on to life for just a little longer. The essence of the narcissistic state is an indifference to, or a withdrawal from, relationships and the external world, and, as Ghasemi points out, the woman's hope to find another, or at least to find one through a blind at a window, could be seen as the opposite of narcissistic indifference and, rather, as an expression of libidinal reaching out in the hope of a relationship.

As Ghasemi describes, Freud's concept of the death drive or death instinct was later developed by Klein, who saw the infant's attacks on the breast as a universal manifestation of the death instinct. This was the theoretical line that led to Rosenfeld's later more detailed formulations of narcissism. Ghasemi links her psychoanalytic perspective with relevant philosophical ideas, notably Badiou's notion of "Event", weaving them together into a multidisciplinary three-dimensional view of the play.

The chapter introduces the idea of Beckett's work as representative of traumatized minds, although it will always be unclear to what extent minds are traumatized as a result of external events, such as war, or whether the trauma might be intergenerational or developmental. The term "developmental trauma" is used to encompass the ongoing traumatic experience of the infant and young child born into a family where parental minds are disturbed, unpredictable, and unstable, or where hate and destructiveness dominate over love and generosity, making ordinary psychological development impossible.

Although Shakespeare's work suggests that he had an intuitive understanding of the relationship between early traumatic experience and the development of a character structure that later came to be described as "destructive narcissism", the originator of that term, Rosenfeld, developed his formulation from a different starting point.

In his seminal 1964 paper, "On the Psychopathology of Narcissism", Rosenfeld outlines two aspects of narcissism—libidinal and destructive—which he sees as always operating alongside each other. In his early papers he believes envy to be the main motivating force behind highly omnipotent identifications and the development of both aspects of narcissism; it is only later, in 1987, in *Impasse and Interpretation* (p. 87), that he refers more explicitly to the contribution of environmental factors, such as trauma and failure in containment, in the development of pathological narcissism (Spillius et al., 2011a).

Central in Rosenfeld's conceptualization of destructive narcissism is the idea of the internal gang, which continually works against any healthy part of the personality that moves towards a relationship with another. The possibility of a relationship that might involve an ordinary degree of dependency, leading to emotional growth, is consistently thwarted. Rosenfeld therefore describes destructive narcissism as achieved primarily at the expense of the dependent or libidinal self. As Tomaso Quaini describes in Chapter 11, "The Narcissistic World of Turandot", an understanding of this pathological character structure helps make sense of the ice-cold Princess Turandot's states of mind and behaviour, as they are communicated to the audience. The suggestion of intergenerational trauma is in the background here as we are told that one of Turandot's ancestors was raped by a Mogul prince, an external event in the past that might be one factor underlying her current cruelty to any potential suitor.

The two characters, Shakespeare's Richard III and Puccini's Turandot, are examples of the narcissistic character structure most often described in the psychoanalytic literature: destructive narcissism. Abnormal omnipotent projective identificatory processes are to the fore in these personalities, and, as described in the Appendix ("3. Projective identification"), projective identification is most usually discussed in terms of the expulsion of unwanted parts of the self into another. As Sagan (Chapter 5) describes, when working with very deprived populations, she was frequently left feeling wasted and unheard, and she understood her experience as her clients' unbearable feelings evacuated into her through projective identification.

However, in Chapter 12, "Identity, Identification, and Narcissistic Phantasy in the Novels of Kazuo Ishiguro", Diana Webster Thomas highlights another aspect of projective identification, which is predominantly acquisitive rather than expulsive. She explores the character and actions of the butler, Stevens, in *The Remains of the Day*, whom she describes as identifying "acquisitively and omnipotently with his own notion of greatness and dignity through his role as a great butler to a morally distinguished Lord of a Great House". She was interested to discover that Ishiguro uses his own term for what psychoanalysts would call projective identification. He referred to this process as "appropriation", and, as Thomas says, "He describes the inhering process of psychically taking for oneself another person to expel one's unbearable experiences and feelings attributively *into* or to extract the desirable *from*." In this and many other ways, Ishiguro demonstrates that artists are able to understand and describe the phenomena of unconscious mental life at least as well as are psychoanalysts.

The merging of personal boundaries with the aim of extracting desirable qualities from the other, and the associated distortion of reality that leads to these qualities being felt to be one's own, is a less frequently discussed use of projective identification. It has the libidinal quality Rosenfeld refers to, and this acquisitive process is based mainly on the idealization of the self. The self appropriates the object's desired qualities either by omnipotent introjective identification or forceful projective identification (Rosenfeld, 1964, p. 171). In contrast with destructive narcissism, where the cost is to the self, libidinal narcissism is achieved predominantly at the expense of the object (Spillius et al., 2011a). These processes could be viewed as a more extreme and pathological version of the passing identifications seen in ordinary development, such as the everyday example of a young girl who walks in her mother's shoes and perhaps briefly feels that she *is* her mother. The shoes are stepped into but then stepped out of as the child refinds her own self. This activity could be described as trying on another identity as part of an ordinary developmental process of finding one's own identity, which takes place during childhood and adolescence. To develop a strong sense of identity, the young person's identifications would need to be with parental qualities and capacities they have "taken in" through the process of ordinary introjection, rather than "taken on" through projective identification. However, Stevens' identifications lack this introjective quality. Thomas notes one point in the novel, where Stevens is planning to go travelling and tries to decide what to wear for his trip. He considers whether to put on one of Lord Darlington's old suits, which he has inherited, perhaps literally stepping into—and, as Thomas describes elsewhere, "inhabiting"—another person to the detriment of his own identity, which, she states, has become invisible as a result of his excessive use of projective identification. The reader never knows anything of Stevens' earliest life experiences and how he came to be the way he is, but it is noticeable that there is no mention of his mother anywhere in the book.

As in Austen's novel *Emma* and Eliot's *Middlemarch*, referred to in the Introduction, each of the main characters in the opera *Turandot* and the novel *The Remains of the Day* reaches a point at the culmination of the work where their narcissistic defensive structure and delusions of self-sufficiency begin to break down, and each becomes more in touch with reality and open to human warmth and relationships. Stevens begins to recognize, with feelings of disappointment and heartbreak, the time he has lost, as he always avoided any possibility of a relationship with the housekeeper, Miss Kenton, and instead gave his life and misplaced loyalty to his master, Lord Darlington. He is overwhelmed by a sense of inner desolation as he becomes aware of the depleted life he has been living. As Quaini describes, Turandot moves towards the depressive position as she gleans some understanding of her own inner world and the possibilities of love through what the slave girl, Liù, expresses. This is the beginning of the emergence of her own capacity to love.

It could be argued that it is the depth of understanding of states of mind and capacity of the authors of these works to convey unfolding processes of psychic change that give these and many other works of literature and the performing arts their emotional power and their ability to engage readers and audiences, including the authors of these chapters, over many centuries.

CHAPTER NINE

The teaching of drama, psychoanalysis, and society on the Psychoanalytic Studies course

Michael Rustin

From the beginning of the Psychoanalytic Studies course in 1993 until the present day, a one-term unit called "Psychoanalysis Drama and Society" has been offered as an element of its Applications strand. There were two principal reasons for this choice, in addition to the interests of the teachers themselves. The first of these was our understanding that the principal themes of classical European drama, and those of psychoanalysis, coincided in significant ways. Freud had, after all, named one of his most influential ideas, that of the Oedipus complex, after Sophocles' fifth-century BC tragedy, observing in the drama of Oedipus killing his father and marrying his mother the unconscious enactment of what Freud would come to see as a universal desire and fantasy. Freud also wrote of his deep respect for the writers and dramatists of classical literature, including the ancient Greeks, Goethe, and Shakespeare, declaring that their understandings of human nature had long anticipated and preceded those of psychoanalysis, even though they were articulated in a form different from that of Freud's aspiring new science. Freud (1916d) also wrote memorably about analogies he had seen between character-types that had been recognized and represented by the authors of great works of fiction (such as in *Macbeth*) and those that he had identified, as a psychoanalyst, as extreme or abnormal kinds of personality.

DOI: 10.4324/9781003564867-13

A book that Margaret Rustin and I found inspirational in thinking through the connections between the central themes of psychoanalysis and those of classical drama was *Tragic Drama and the Family* (1988) by the American psychoanalyst Bennett Simon. Simon pointed out the remarkable extent to which the tragedies of the ancient Greeks (and later classical plays such as those by Shakespeare, Eugene O'Neill, and Samuel Beckett), were focused on relationships within families, and the disasters to which these often gave rise. Examples are the tragedy of Oedipus and his family, Medea's murder of her own children, and Clytemnestra's murder of her husband Agamemnon, and her subsequent murder by her son Orestes, to name just three plays or dynastic sequences of plays by Sophocles and Euripides. Their tragic figures were invariably members of ruling dynasties, and through their individual fates the dramatists were able to represent those of the entire societies over which they ruled. Thus the tragedy of Oedipus came to light as a consequence of the plague that had cursed his city, Thebes, and had brought to everyone's awareness that something had gone seriously amiss in their world.

We came to recognize that it was not only ancient Greek tragedies that had focused their attention on the lives of families, but that this was also usually the case for most of the dramas of the modern Western tradition, from Shakespeare and the Jacobeans, through Restoration tragedy, on to the great revival of theatrical form accomplished by Ibsen and Chekhov, as well as, subsequently, in the work of great modern playwrights, such as Wilde, Miller, Pinter, and even Beckett—although in the work of these latter two writers it is often the absence or perversion of family relationships that is being explored. Examples are the parents abandoned in a pair of dustbins in Beckett's *Endgame* (1957), and a couple half buried in sand in *Happy Days* (1952a); Pinter's *The Birthday Party* (1960a) is scarcely a party, and *The Homecoming* (1965), in his play of that title, is to a home that is the location of memories of betrayal and the scene of their re-enactment. After studying examples of this great literature, we found we could ask our students whether they could name *any* plays in this tradition that did not have at their core relationships between family members, and, indeed, few good exceptions to the normal rule of this convention could be found.

It was not our belief that the *only* themes of the classical drama were those located in families. Rather, it was our understanding that it was through the close-up lens of family relationships that dramas explored the conditions of the larger societies to which their central characters belonged, in their representations on the stage and in their language. It could hardly be clearer that the classical dramatists such as the ancient Greeks and the Elizabethans were representing profound issues and conflicts within their own societies. Great modern dramatists—such as Ibsen, Chekhov, and Miller, or Beckett and Pinter—were in similar ways representing profound impasses and conflicts within the societies in which they lived and wrote, through their characters and their relationships with one another. A crucial modern development from Ibsen onwards was that the central characters of these plays ceased to be kings and aristocrats, whose fate determined that of the societies over which they ruled. As drama evolved, its heroes first became merely bourgeois citizens, as in Ibsen, or members of a decaying landed class, as in Chekhov, and then became more completely "democratized". Arthur Miller didactically insisted in his work that an ordinary man—Willy Loman in *Death of a Salesman* (1949)—could be as well depicted as a tragic hero as legendary Greek rulers had once been. Raymond Williams (1963) observed that in post-Second-World War theatre, characters were sometimes represented as entirely marginal to society—and even as vagrants, as in Beckett's *Waiting for Godot* (1952b) and in Pinter's *The Caretaker* (1960b). Williams' (1968) work enabled us to understand the significance of historical changes in the forms of dramatic representation. It was Aristotle's contention, in his *Poetics*, that tragedies conveyed universal truths or depictions of reality, through representations of particular individuals and their narratives. We believed that dramatists were discovering and expressing truths about the condition of the particular societies in which their characters and enactments were set.

We further believed that the innate connections between the dramatic representations of individuals and families, and their wider social contexts, might enable us to give psychoanalytic concepts and theories a more socially contextualized meaning than psychoanalysts had usually intended them to have. We had earlier, in our *Narratives of Love and Loss: Studies in Modern Children's Fiction* (M. E. Rustin & Rustin, 1987), developed an argument for such a social dimension of psychoanalytic ideas in a different genre of writing. Freud was always determined that his ambitious new science of psychoanalysis should be universal in its scope, discovering truths about *all* human lives that would not be confined in their relevance to any particular society. One can suggest that his adoption of a universalist world view came both from a commitment to the perspectives of the rational scientific Enlightenment and from his wish to avoid the identification of psychoanalysis as a "Jewish science" in the pervasively anti-Semitic culture in which he lived. We thought it was possible that the meaning of some key psychoanalytic ideas might be deepened, and given a more definite social location if they were seen through their embodiment in the characters and relationships of great plays.

A further reason for the choice of "Drama, Psychoanalysis and Society" as a unit of the course was related to how psychoanalytic ideas and methods could best be learned and taught. Essential to the conception of our Psychoanalytic Studies programme from its outset was that it should be "experience-rich", and especially rich in emotional experience, rather than merely didactic, cerebral, and theoretical in its approach to psychoanalysis. As discussed in Part I, it is for this reason that one of three strands of this course has always been devoted to infant observation and young child observation, its most distinctive feature. It has been hoped that students would learn about psychoanalytic ideas and ways of thinking through their experiences of observing young children and their families over nearly two years, and of reflecting on these in weekly seminars in groups of six or so fellow-students whose supervisors have always been child psychotherapists. The purpose of this work has been to expose students to experiences that have a central dimension of emotion. This is intended to enable psychoanalytic ideas to be learned about in a context where students are able to do "work" in interpreting what they are observing and feeling, in real life. Students in these observational settings are expected to be essentially inactive, although remaining sympathetic and friendly observers of children and their families, and to avoid taking any interpretive or quasi-therapeutic role. They thus gain some of the benefits of being exposed to the emotional lives of their subjects (not least its impact on themselves), while not incurring the responsibilities that are taken by therapists in such situations. We believed that this form of learning about psychoanalysis would add substantially to what can be learned through the study of psychoanalytic literature alone.

In introducing the study of drama as a unit in the programme, we set up a form of learning that was intended to have affinities with the observational strand of the course. (Incidentally, it has long been believed by some influential teachers of child psychotherapists that a prior training in literature can be of more value to students' learning than more scientific kinds of education in psychology, because of the empathetic understanding of human lives it encourages.[1]) One of the ideas that we developed from Bennett Simon's (1988) original insight supported our belief in the educational value of studying drama. We saw that audiences' experiences of theatre, the ancient location of Aristotle's experience of "catharsis" (audiences learning from their exposure to the action of dramatic tragedies) had parallels to the psychological functions of psychoanalysis in modern times. Just as the theatre (and cinema and television) create "symbolic spaces" in which audiences share intense experiences regarding human character and relationships, so the psychoanalytic setting constituted a parallel space for exploration. In the theatre, writers, directors, and actors create worlds of the imagination, with which audiences feel many kinds of identification. Audiences see aspects of themselves in those who are represented before them, and it is the gift of actors to be able to understand and perform such varied identities. In psychoanalysis it is the unconscious inner worlds of patients that find expression and recognition, in part through the transference relationship with the analyst. It is the relationship of such "inner worlds" to actual reality that is the primary work of analysis. The hope is that over time the experience of analysis may bring these inner and outer worlds into an alignment helpful to a patient's development. Joyce McDougall's (1986) metaphor for psychoanalysis was a "theatre of the mind", in which what was explored were "unconscious scripts" and their influence on personalities and behaviours. A psychoanalytically informed approach to drama can sometimes recognize the powerful presence of "unconscious scripts" in the characterization and action of great plays. Over the many years in which this unit has been offered, it has studied many dramas to which the relevance of psychoanalytic ideas can be seen.

There have been other units in the Applications strand of the course—for example those on poetry (the subject of Part II), on biographical narratives, on cinema and fine art—that have had purposes similar to those of "Drama, Psychoanalysis and Society", but these are not the topic of this chapter.

Development of the Drama course unit over 27 years

The Drama unit was taught for its first 18 years by two teachers, Margaret and Michael Rustin, who were together present for all the seminars. They had different capabilities relevant to the programme. Margaret Rustin is a child psychotherapist and brought her clinical sensitivity to the understanding of the plays being studied. Michael Rustin was (in the first instance) a teacher of sociology and brought a more theoretical and "sociological" orientation than Margaret's to the work. The early years of the course were a setting in which these two approaches were brought together in a focus on chosen plays, to see what could be learned from their conjunction. It was on the basis of their experience of teaching this course that Margaret and Michael Rustin wrote their book, *Mirror to Nature: Drama, Psychoanalysis, and Society* (2001).

In the early years, the two teachers' approach to the course was free-spirited, even improvisational. To explore the historical specificity of Western drama in its different phases, they presented plays (one per week!) from several of its major epochs. These were usually one or more Greek tragedies, Shakespeare plays, dramas from the period of nineteenth- and twentieth-century realism, and one or more "modern" post-Second-World-War plays. The teachers' approach would give an initial presentation of the play in question, selecting some key passages to study. The teachers and/or students would read aloud the chosen passages in as lively a way as they could. We would then offer some conjectures on possible psychoanalytic understandings of the plays and also some thoughts about their location in the societies for which they had been written and in which they were performed.

Looking back over 27 years, it seems absurdly over-ambitious to have hoped to do anything very useful in a ten-week sequence of 75-minute seminars, each devoted to a different play. But this was a new experience for everyone, and some powerful ideas were being explored, about the nature of the symbolic and emotional space provided by theatre and about the relevance of psychoanalytic ideas to the chosen plays. To further their own learning, and to keep the process fresh for themselves, the teachers often chose different plays for discussion in each year's sequence. The students were asked to undertake background reading, and the teachers circulated papers to them—sometimes their own. There was interest for students in being able to take part in lively and unscripted conversations between two staff members on plays that often had considerable impact on them. For some students, a "secondary" benefit of the programme was to be introduced to a field of great literature and performance of which some of them had little prior knowledge. In the early years, teachers and students went together to see some excellent productions of plays we were studying at fringe theatres. One overseas student, a psychiatrist from Taiwan, told us that the course had developed in him a passionate interest in Shakespeare, whose work he had not previously known.

The assessment arrangements for the course were extremely flexible. Students were required to write essays, and later a dissertation, on work from any element they chose from the various seminars devoted to Applications. There was thus no requirement for them to write about the Drama unit in particular. Students sometimes did good written work on drama and psychoanalysis, but they had the freedom to choose their own topic, and our Applications unit, like others, was free from the pressure of obligatory assessment. We were far in those early days from the prescriptive formulation of "learning objectives" and "learning outcomes" that has become customary in the academy—or, at least, from their enforcement.

After a decade or so we realized that our method of studying one play per week, drawn from the history of Western drama, had serious flaws, despite its exciting material. Our students were asking for a greater connectedness in the course. We decided to slow the pace, discussing around five or so plays in each term's sequence, instead of ten. A second change was to select plays that shared a principal common theme, of both sociological and psychoanalytic relevance. These themes were mostly related to stages of the life-cycle—for example, concerning relationships between siblings, within marriages, and between parents and children. We had one series on heroines. We chose plays that explored these different areas of experience. This clustering made it easier to compare the approaches taken within plays from different times, and to focus on selected psychoanalytic ideas in each sequence.

Another development took place in the middle years of the course, at the helpful suggestion of a student. She told us that her school library (she was a teacher) had a collection of video recordings of classical plays, from which it would be possible to borrow for the class. From this began the practice of screening selected extracts of productions of plays that we had chosen for discussion, as a way of giving the class an experience of a play that might be more intense and immediate than they might gain merely from reading or being read to. Outside the course, the lecturers found some enriching opportunities to explore some of the ideas of the course with actors and directors in relation to particular productions, and this experience informed their teaching.

In 2012 Margaret Rustin decided that her clinical work no longer allowed her time to teach the Drama unit. Since then, Michael Rustin has taught the course, although for three years, from 2014–5 to 2016–7, a former outstanding student of the course and its Drama unit, Jenny Abbott, (whose infant observation paper is included in Part I) was able to teach the course with him. As she discusses in her chapter in the first part of this book, she had formerly worked as a BBC documentary film-maker and was planning to train as a psychoanalyst. This was a successful arrangement, and it was hoped that this would lead to her taking on the full responsibility for the unit; unfortunately, this proved not to be possible for her.

It was at this time that a further significant change in the framing of the course took place. This was the decision to confine the syllabus wholly to plays by Shakespeare, which remains the current practice.

Teaching Shakespeare and psychoanalysis

One reason for confining the unit to the study of plays by Shakespeare was that from the perspective of exploring psychoanalytic ways of understanding drama in a social context, his work has an unequalled richness. It is also a field in which there is a substantial psychoanalytically oriented literature. With our earlier practice of selecting plays for study from different historical epochs, students were being asked to understand many social settings and theatrical genres within a very short time. We believed that a psychoanalytic attention to the plays, which was the main purpose of the course, would be helped if we focused only on Shakespeare.

A factor in supporting this choice was the increasing availability of high-quality film productions of many Shakespeare plays. Sometimes, as with Richard Loncraine's *Richard III* in 1995 and Rupert Goold's *Macbeth* in 2010, these had their origin in memorable stage productions. Sometimes they were originally conceived as films, as, for example, *Romeo + Juliet*, Baz Lurman's 1996 modern version of *Romeo and Juliet*, set in "Verona Beach", an imaginary location that evokes both U.S. and Latin American milieus. Many of these films brought more cinematic panache to dramatizing Shakespeare than did the BBC Television series made between 1978 and 1985, which filmed all of the plays and included some fine productions and performances. The quality of the directing, the acting, and the locations of some of these films—most of which were made as mainstream features—gave them a considerable impact on audiences, even where they retained most of Shakespeare's poetic texts. From the point of view of our unit, screening substantial extracts from such films overcame some limitations of accessibility for students unfamiliar with Shakespeare plays in the theatre. This was especially the case for the increasing proportion of students on the course for whom English was their second language.

There were, of course, discussions in class about the "authenticity" of such cinematic productions of these plays. Many of them involved major cuts in the spoken text (although Kenneth Branagh has said that his 1996 film of *Hamlet* is unique in having made no cuts at all to Shakespeare's text). By contrast, Olivier's classic 1955 film of *Richard III* transposed lines from *Henry VI*, another in the sequence of history plays. The quality of these films usually depends on their finding cinematic equivalents, in images, sounds, and locations, for what in the original texts is principally communicated through the dense and multivalent quality of poetic language. However, the seminar teachers argued that these texts had been written to be *performed* for audiences. We suggested that film-makers—many of whom had been leading figures in the theatre and had developed the essential conception of their films in their stage productions—were doing what Shakespeare had himself done in making use of the best performative means available to him. We noted also that in recent years the well-crafted real-time filming of stage productions (when they are screened in cinemas) has also been expanded in its expressive resources, thus creating another kind of hybrid performance, for both theatre and cinema audiences simultaneously. Actors' skill in front of a camera, through their capacities for expression and in the clarity in the enunciation of texts which close-ups can also augment, often adds considerably to the impact of a play. The active interaction with audiences in the exposure of the Globe Theatre in London can bring a loss of delicacy and subtlety, and sometimes even a pantomimic aspect. But there have been films of Globe productions that have captured extremely powerful and subtle performances—by Roger Allam in 2010 as Falstaff in the *Henry IV* plays, for example. British theatre, and the film-making that has developed from it, has in recent decades been strongly influenced by a tradition of respect for the close reading of texts, and especially of Shakespeare.

These debates on form and authenticity aside, we have been able to choose extracts, usually of 20 or 30 minutes each, from outstanding film versions of the chosen plays, for screening in classes. These have made available intense experiences of episodes, which could be considered in seminars. There are advantages in having speeches and exchanges between characters enunciated by great actors—such as Ben Kingsley or Nigel Hawthorne (in Trevor Nunn's 1996 film of *Twelfth Night*) or by Patrick Stewart and Kate Fleetwood (in Rupert Goold's *Macbeth,* in 2010), or by Ralph Fiennes' Coriolanus and Vanessa Redgrave's Volumnia (in Fiennes' *Coriolanus* in 2011)—if one wants students to be able to absorb their full meaning and impact. In assigning two weeks each to five plays over the ten weeks of each unit, we were able to make use of key scenes from film productions and thus provide focal points for learning about the plays from a psychoanalytic perspective.

A question that we thought it essential to ask for each of the plays we had chosen was, what had *Shakespeare* understood that has now, centuries later, come to be of interest for psychoanalysts? We wished to challenge any incipient belief that a student might have that the deepest forms of understanding a work of drama or fiction comes from a knowledge of psychoanalysis and its theories, with plays and their characters cast as if they were objects whose depths of meaning it requires a psychoanalytic critic to disclose. We took a quite different view of where understanding was to be found. We believed that it was to be gained from the study of the texts of the plays themselves, and from their interpretations by directors, actors, and designers. The understanding of human nature and character, of course, has a different form when it is represented and conveyed to audiences in dramas about imagined lives from that derived from psychoanalytic consulting rooms or formulated as theories of personality development or psychopathology. These understandings are in a relation of being different and parallel to one another, and not one of a hierarchy or relative depth of knowledge. But all of these provide insights of their own kind. One aim of our course was to show how much Shakespeare knew and understood four centuries before psychoanalysis was even thought of, and to think about these different forms of understanding in their relation to one another.

Psychoanalysts, following Freud himself and including, among others, in Britain, Ernest Jones (1949), Ella Freeman Sharpe (1950), Donald Meltzer and Meg Harris Williams (1988b), Harris Williams and Margot Waddell (1991), James Fisher (1999), and Ignes Sodré (2014), have long found Shakespeare's work to be extraordinary in its insights into unconscious mental life, anticipating their own psychoanalytic perceptions. Contemporary productions of plays sometimes reflect the depth of Shakespeare's understanding and of its particular relevance to the world of today. Sometimes this relevance is established by transposing the imagined worlds that Shakespeare created to settings or "structures of feeling" (Williams, 1977, pp. 128–135) that are resonant for modern audiences. Olivier's portrayal of Henry V as a British warrior hero at the time of the Second World War, and the transcription of *Romeo and Juliet* into *West Side Story*,[2] a 1957 musical about American adolescent gangs in the 1950s, are examples. We shall suggest more modern instances below. Sometimes new productions of plays seem to reflect, in their perceptions and emphases, ways of thinking that have only recently emerged in psychoanalytic writing.

One can recognize that what modern producers of plays or films do when they "update" the setting of a play has its parallel in Shakespeare's own practice as a dramatist. His work displays a complex relationship to historical time. The plays are set in many historical and geographical locations, real and imagined. These include ancient Rome (*Julius Caesar, Antony and Cleopatra*) mythical ancient Greece (*Troilus and Cressida*), medieval England (the history plays), and Renaissance Italy, which was more or less Shakespeare's own time (*The Merchant of Venice, Two Gentlemen of Verona, Othello*). Some plays (*A Midsummer Night's Dream, The Tempest*) have the quality more of fantasy, although these, too, are shown to have some anchorage in the relationships of power of that time. Shakespeare often shows in these plays an astonishing understanding of historical contexts remote from his own, and was surely finding meanings in dramatic actions in these imagined settings that were relevant to audiences in his own society. For example, the issues of royal succession and its dangerous uncertainties, which are central to many of his plays, surely reflect the preoccupations of late Elizabethan England. Elizabeth I is said to have observed, when she saw *Richard II* (which is set in 1398) performed in 1601: "I am Richard II. Know you not that?" The Earl of Essex had been executed for treason in the same year for having plotted against her.

We recognize that the areas of life Shakespeare was exploring correspond to many phenomena that are equally significant to our own lives, many of which have been fields for psychoanalytic inquiry. These include, for example, oedipal jealousy, sibling enmity, adolescent disturbance, marital discord, ageing and the loss of potency, dictatorship and tyranny, and patriarchal oppression, which is, in his plays, often exercised over young women who lack the protective figure of a mother. (Perhaps their vulnerability reflects not so much the literal absence of mothers as their lack of power in Shakespeare's world.) *The Merchant of Venice*, for example, is a profound exploration of prejudice against Jews, even though practising Jews were excluded from England between 1290 (when they had been expelled) and 1660. The portrayal of Caliban, shown as Prospero's slave in *The Tempest*, seems to be an early representation of the social relations of colonialism, whose beginnings lie in Shakespeare's time. It is because Shakespeare's plays help us to better understand ourselves that they remain such a central presence in our culture.

Theoretical preoccupations in psychoanalysis have influenced the ways in which psychoanalysts have thought about particular plays. Ernest Jones (1949), for example, focused on the Oedipus complex in his writing about *Hamlet* in 1949.

Some of the ways in which consideration of particular plays in this course, and the insights that they embody, have been informed by recent psychoanalytic thinking. The first of these is *Romeo and Juliet*. This was the topic of a valuable paper by the child psychotherapist Beta Copley (1993), which drew on the understanding of adolescent states of mind, which she had developed in her work as a psychotherapist in the Tavistock's

Adolescent Department. The present writer developed a view of the play that was deeply influenced by the ideas of Wilfred Bion (M. J. Rustin, 1991). One of Bion's great contributions to psychoanalysis has been his understanding of the importance of thinking, of the need for space for reflection, in human development.[3] For Bion, this begins with the function of mothers in "containing" the anxieties of their babies and, through absorbing their impact and processing them mentally, being able to render them bearable by the infant. "Thinking in Romeo and Juliet" (M. J. Rustin, 1991) took note of the repeated attacks on space for thinking that are portrayed in the play, and the catastrophe to which these give rise. The invasions to which thought is subjected have different sources, both internal and external, and their consequence is usually a resort to precipitate action. One source is the anxiety that arises from the fragility of political authority in the Verona of the play's setting and from the dangers this may give rise to for the rival Capulets and Montagues if they antagonize Verona's Duke. So Capulet demands that his daughter marry Paris, the Duke's kinsman, within days of her cousin Tybalt's death, and he refuses to listen to her when she pleads with him not to insist on this. Romeo and Juliet are each so overwhelmed by their passion for each other that they feel compelled to take extreme risks, whatever the consequences, resorting to the magical solution of drugs to escape from their impossible situation. Throughout the play, the natural order of time is disrupted, everything taking place in a frantic rush in which reflection is made impossible. The Nurse and the Friar have the role of mediators between the young people and their respective families—they have the role of surrogate parents—but their position is so vulnerable that they cannot slow down the disastrous rush of events. The argument of this interpretation is, of course, what Shakespeare represented in the detailed action of the play. What a psychoanalytic account contributes is a theoretical conceptualization of what is happening, which enables one to recognize aspects of character and action that have many applications beyond the particulars of the play itself.

Our second example is *Macbeth* (M. E. Rustin & Rustin, 2002b). Here our particular interest was in the processes of projective identification between Macbeth and Lady Macbeth, as they jointly undertake their terrible crime of murdering Duncan, their king, and seizing his throne. Our love of this play arises from its representation of the Macbeths as the forerunners of a modern marriage, in which they are deeply involved with and dependent on each other (until Macbeth abandons his wife and returns to the delusional witches)—although, of course, in disastrously destructive terms. We have written about this play as a "matrimonial tragedy". The play continually presents an idea of a good family as a kind of negative of the Macbeths' actual lives. Banquo observes the "temple-haunting martlets" in the battlements of Macbeth's castle, which will prove to be a misleading image of benign fertility; there are the children we learn the Macbeths do not have and, by contrast, Banquo's loving relationship with his son, Fleance; Lady Macbeth plays the gracious hostess to the guests she intended to murder. She recognizes, when the deed is done, that Duncan was a good man, who reminds her of her own father. So while Macbeth is causing the destruction of the actual families that, he believes, threaten him—a mother and her children among them—we have been put in mind of what might have been. We have been pleased when our students have shared the sadness that one can feel for both Macbeth and Lady Macbeth at the play's end—a response evoked in Rupert Goold's 2010 film version of the play.[4] We were influenced in our understanding of both *Macbeth* and *Romeo and Juliet* by the historian Lawrence Stone's (1977) writing about the origins of modern "companionate marriage" in the sixteenth century. We understand both *Romeo and Juliet* and *Macbeth* as representations of emerging forms of life. Both of these two examples end in tragedy and disaster, the specific causes of which are illuminated in the plays, but which are, perhaps, in a broader historical sense, the consequence of their "prematurity".

A third example is *Coriolanus*, through which Jenny Abbott and I examined another kind of projective process, deeply understood by Shakespeare and represented though his principal characters. This was the projection, or projective identification, by a powerful, narcissistic mother (Volumnia) into her son (Coriolanus), and the development in Coriolanus of a "false self" and a virtual possession of his identity by his mother from which he was not able to escape. The loss and absence of a husband for Volumnia and of a father for Coriolanus seem to explain the role of manly omnipotence which Coriolanus was pressed to adopt by his mother's intrusive projection. This was of a warrior identity that was unavailable to a woman but which she unconsciously desired for herself. The nature of projective identification, and the way it has trapped its object, could hardly be more completely represented than in this play. One of the sequelae of this development is Coriolanus's indifference to the tender and affectionate qualities of his wife, Virgilia, who is trapped in the emotional ambience of her mother-in-law's household, and the location of his strongest passions in a homosexual attachment to Tullus Aufidius, the military leader of the Volscians, the enemies of Rome. The fighting between them is erotic in its intensity. *Coriolanus* also explores the powerful projections into political figures that take place in situations of intense anxiety, which subject Coriolanus to great pressures, overwhelming his judgement.

The fourth play, *Richard III,* is an example of a remarkable correspondence between the representation of a character by Shakespeare and a description of such a "character type" (recalling Freud 1916d) by a psychoanalyst. Richard is an almost perfect representation of the character structure defined by Herbert Rosenfeld (1971) as "destructive narcissism". Its essential qualities, and their perverse capacity to seduce, are articulated in speeches and asides by the character himself.

Here is Richard:

> . . . But I, that am not shaped for sportive tricks,
> Nor made to court an amorous looking-glass;
> I, that am rudely stamp'd, and want love's majesty
> To strut before a wanton ambling nymph;
> I, that am curtail'd of this fair proportion,
> Cheated of feature by dissembling nature,
> Deformed, unfinish'd, sent before my time
> Into this breathing world, scarce half made up,
> And that so lamely and unfashionable
> That dogs bark at me as I halt by them;
> Why, I, in this weak piping time of peace,
> Have no delight to pass away the time,
> Unless to spy my shadow in the sun
> And descant on mine own deformity:
> And therefore, since I cannot prove a lover,
> To entertain these fair well-spoken days,
> I am determined to prove a villain
> And hate the idle pleasures of these days.
> Plots have I laid, inductions dangerous,
> By drunken prophecies, libels and dreams,
> To set my brother Clarence and the king
> In deadly hate the one against the other:
>
> [Act I, scene I, lines 14–35][5]

Shakespeare provides us with an account of the childhood experiences that have given rise to Richard's hatred for any relationships of love that he comes in contact with. He seduces, marries, and brings to her death the widow of the man he has recently killed. He has his unsuspecting brother Clarence murdered. He orders the death of the two princes in the Tower, the two sons of his elder brother, Edward, the King, as well as Rivers, his brother-in-law, the Mayor of London, and Buckingham his former ally. From the instrumental point of view of Richard's all-consuming desire for power, all these characters in one way or another stand between Richard and the Crown he craves to have and keep. But Shakespeare is also representing in Richard's actions and character a compulsive, unconscious drive to destroy and to avenge the injury that he feels has been done to him since his misshapen birth. Lest there be any doubt about the origins of Richard's perverted character, Shakespeare has him meet his mother, on the eve of his final battle. She tells him, and the audience, the story of his early life, and of her rejection of him:

> *Richard*: "And cam'st I not at last to comfort you?"
>
> *Duchess of York*: "No, by the Holy Rood, thou know'st it well
> Thou camest on earth to make the earth my hell.
> A grievous burthen was thy birth to me;
> Tetchy and wayward was thy infancy;
> Thy school-days frightful, desp'rate, wild, and furious,
> Thy prime of manhood daring, bold, and venturous;
> Thy age confirm'd, proud, subtle, sly, and bloody,
> More mild, but yet more harmful, kind in hatred.
> What comfortable hour canst thou name,
> That ever graced me in thy company?"
>
> [Act IV, scene iv, lines 165–175]

In the light of Rosenfeld's ideas, we can see this as a story that describes a pure case of destructive narcissism and its imagined origins.

The final example of a connection between Shakespearean drama and psychoanalysis is a particular production of *Twelfth Night,* made first for the stage and then as a feature film in 1996 by Trevor Nunn. My point of reference here is the film. It seems that central to Nunn's particular reading of this play is an insight that relates closely to one of the most important advances in modern psychoanalytic thinking—namely, Bion's conception of the importance of containment through the process of thinking. One wonders how this conjunction comes about, what subtle links there may sometimes be between psychoanalytic thinking and the wider culture, including that of the theatre.[6]

Feste the Clown is in one way marginal to the society of the play (Malvolio almost has him cast out of Olivia's household at its beginning), yet he has access to every part of it. We (the audience) observe him observing the action and learn what is happening through his desire to understand it. He "contains" the action of the play, the misrecognitions and distresses that pervade it, through his comprehension of its action, as it takes place, in which he is both participant and observer. The audience is invited to see the play through his observant eyes. Nunn, and the beautiful performance by Ben Kingsley, gives his presence a reparative quality, just as the "containing" process has in Klein and Bion's psychoanalytic perspective. Early in the play, Feste's reminding Olivia of his past connection with her father, and thus with her as a child, enables her to trust him and to emerge from her melancholia following her father's and brother's deaths. At the end of the film, Feste bestows a kind of blessing on Viola. Now that she is reunited with her brother, whom she had believed to be dead, she can recover her female identity, and the barriers of misrecognition between herself and Orsino are resolved. At this moment of discovery, Feste places around Viola's neck the gold necklace that she had abandoned on the beach where she came ashore after her shipwreck, and which he has retrieved, to her amazement. His gesture, as this climactic moment of the play, makes clear that she has been held in his mind throughout, as the troubled action has unfolded.

At the end of the play, when, according to the dramatic conventions of comedy, three marriages are to take place, Feste takes his leave, following his admission of his role in the harsh humiliation of Malvolio. ("And thus the whirligig of time brings in his revenges.") But he speaks the epilogue for the play. He is now the voice of the dramatist who has created this world and given it meaning. We imagine that Feste's own capacity to contain and understand, through poetry and music, will enable him to bear being alone, as he walks away from the households to which he has been attached, as they embark on a new phase of life.

> But that's all one, our play is done.
> And we'll strive to please you every day.
> For the rain it raineth every day.

I hope that these examples—there could have been others—demonstrate the way in which in this course we have been able to show the depth of Shakespeare's understanding of many aspects of human experience through the form of inquiry represented by poetic drama—but also how psychoanalysis has been able to achieve its own different form of understanding of these same experiences. What is central to our approach is the belief that these perspectives can be complementary, each able to inform the other.

Notes

1 We take the view, however, set out most fully by M. J. Rustin (2019c), that psychoanalysis is itself in important aspects a science with its own unique object of investigation—unconscious mental life—the attributes of which give rise to its specific methods of research.

2 *West Side Story* was filmed for the second time by Stephen Spielberg in 2021, with music by Leonard Bernstein and Stephen Sondheim.
3 A fine, accessible account of Bion's theory of thinking, and of its relevance to clinical practice, is to be found in O'Shaughnessy (1981).
4 There are, of course, other ways of interpreting and responding to this play and to its principal characters.
5 The quotation is from the 1981 Arden edition of the play, edited by Antony Hammond.
6 Productions of Shakespeare have often explored contemporary political resonances (Kott, 1967), although it is psychoanalytic /psychological connections that are our focus in this article. The Loncraine/McKellen film of *Richard III*, for example, is set in the upper-class circles of pre-War London and imagines a potential British Fascism of that time.

CHAPTER TEN

Rockaby: Eros and Thanatos

Maryam Ghasemi

Samuel Beckett is often regarded as an absurdist and pessimist author whose work represents the existential deprivation of the human being. Seen like this, his protagonists communicate an experience of a paralysing narrative of birth, repetition, and death. This is clearly depicted in his 35-second-long play *Breath* (1969, p. 369): faint light, a stage littered with rubbish, a faint brief cry, a second cry identical to the first, and then silence. Life in this sense is a short breath that expires in death.

It seems that Beckett's work is playing in a register that is not far from what Sigmund Freud (1920g) theorized as "death instinct",[1] which came, later, to be called "Thanatos".[2,3] For Freud, the founder of psychoanalysis, literature was an important site of knowledge for postulating and advancing his theories. In this chapter I contemplate one of Beckett's short plays, *Rockaby* (1980), through the medium of Freud's theory of Eros and death drive.

Having seen the play a few times in various countries, acted by different actresses, performed to socioculturally different audiences, I am well aware that it will not be possible to do justice to the play without seeing it in its dimensionality—that is, the dialectical or, rather, "trialectical" relationship between plot, character, and audience. Any analysis of any of these components in isolation would inevitably risk reductionism and incomprehension if we think of a play not as a text but as a social relation played out in a specific relational space between plot, actor, and audience.

DOI: 10.4324/9781003564867-14

The particular context in which the story is shown and how it is perceived by the members of this particular audience makes the play a constant act of construction of meaning.

Bearing this in mind, it would also be impossible to explore these interwoven aspects of the play without simplifying the complexities in this short chapter. Hence, I focus on just one aspect of the play and analyse it as a text. I first introduce Freud's theory of Eros and death drive and its reception among his successors. Then I contextualize Beckett's work within historical and philosophical traditions. Thinking through the reception of his work among different scholars and thinkers, I consider the dichotomy of life and death in *Rockaby* in the light of Freud's concepts of Eros and death drive and Alain Badiou's notion of "Event" (2005).

Eros and Thanatos

In *Beyond the Pleasure Principle* (1920g) Freud took a controversial step beyond his attempt to provide scientific evidence and grounds for his metapsychological theories. In a highly speculative (and one could argue courageous but uncomfortable) shift, he introduced the existence of a different characteristic of the drives, which contradicted his earlier discovery of the pleasure-seeking nature of the drives. In "Formulations on the Two Principles of Mental Functioning" (1911b), Freud argued that the course taken by mental events follows the pleasure principle. This implies that when unpleasurable tensions are presented in mental life, an automatic regulatory function, characterized by its pleasure-seeking tendency, is set into motion to avoid or lower the tension and produce pleasure as the final outcome of mental activities.

However, in his clinical work and observations he encountered a phenomenon that could not easily be explained by the theory of the pleasure principle. The event that caught his interest and later led him to the revision of his theory was the repetitive reliving of trauma by war veterans and patients suffering from traumatic neurosis. This would occur in the form of the return of the repressed memory of the original scene of trauma in the patients' dreams, symptom formations, or the patients acting out their traumatic experiences in the transference. He also noticed this in children's repetitive play of losing and finding an object (*fort–da*) as an attempt at the mastery of an undesirable situation. All these indicated the existence of an unconscious drive that does not obey the neutralizing function of the psyche under the commands of the pleasure principle or, rather, derives *pleasure* from the repetitive re-enactment of the traumatic event. The repetition is an unconscious automatic movement as a result of the traumatic event escaping the channels of remembering and becoming a memory (Freud, 1914g) or, in Bion's language, escaping the thinking apparatus that can cope with thoughts (Bion, 1962b). Hence the outcome is not in the service of deriving pleasure: it presents itself as a destructive act and pure pain.

The observation of this phenomenon raised many questions and difficulties concerning the ever-pleasure-seeking nature of the drives—whether the repetition compulsion could be explained according to the pleasure principle or whether this is a rupture from it, which necessitates a revision of the earlier hypothesis. This predicament paved the way for speculation about the existence of a different characteristic of the drives, separate from or even in opposition to that described in "Two Principles of Mental Functioning". Freud (1920g) attributed the clinical phenomenon of compulsion to repeat to the characteristic of a drive he called "death instinct", sometimes referred to as "Thanatos".

This is arguably one of the most significant concepts developed over the course of the evolution of psychoanalysis, which gained fundamental clinical importance in the work of some later psychoanalysts. It is the hypothesis that life in the living substance is preserved by a drive that brings it together as a unity. Freud (1920g) called it Eros or "life instinct" and argued that it derives its energy and power from "libido", which, in turn, is a manifestation of the sexual instinct (p. 60, footnote). In opposition to Eros, Thanatos seeks to break down the unity of the living being. This drive addresses an obscure realm in the function of the psyche that cannot be fully comprehended by the observational method. It cannot be demonstrated and proved by empirical and conventional scientific approaches, and its existence cannot be attributed to the organic lesions of the nervous system. It is the speculation that the deepest and most obscure territory of the psyche, namely the unconscious, bears in itself a trace of the inorganic origin of the living organic, the inanimate state of the *matter* before coming to life. Freud argues that "as the inanimate things existed before living ones", there is a tendency in all living organisms to seek to restore the inanimate state. As he put it: "the aim of all life is death" (p. 38).

There has been no unanimous agreement regarding the existence of the death drive, and it continued and still continues to create much controversy in psychoanalytic communities. Some of Freud's disciples discredited it as being merely a speculative hypothesis and an imaginative artefact of the destructiveness of the First World War. For these critics, there is no proof for the existence of a drive inside the living organism directed towards self-annihilation. Jones (1961, p. 405) dismissed it as a

"Schopenhauerian position".[4] Otto Fenichel (1935) viewed the inherent impetus towards death as an idealistic deviation biologizing the neuroses. Theodor Reik (1941) associated the death drive with masochistic suffering and argued that masochism is, in its essence, a search for pleasure, like the urge for sacrifice in Christian martyrdom for final victory. Thus, death drive is not a primary drive, as suggested by Freud, but, rather, a secondary formation.

Melanie Klein (1932) was among Freud's successors who embraced the concept as a useful instrument to support her own theory of the formation of a harsh superego at a much earlier stage than had been proposed by Freud. Rather than being a biological entity with no representation in the unconscious, the death drive was, for her, a psychic perception present in primitive unconscious phantasies from the beginning of life. The anxiety experienced by the infant is an effect of the fear of hostile and persecutory forces, activated by the death drive. Relying on her observations and the various manifestations of destructiveness she encountered in the clinic, she came to believe in the existence of a primary unconscious self-destructive force operating intra-psychically as well as inter-subjectively by being projected outside to the Object. For her, the representation of the death drive in the new-born's psyche was the aggressive and cannibalistic phantasies of devouring and being devoured by the *breast*. To protect itself from this fear, the infant introjects a good and nurturing breast, which allows it to survive the perception of a bad and withholding breast.

The French psychoanalyst Jacques Lacan not only reaffirmed the concept of death drive but also treated it as central to psychoanalysis. In his Seminar 11, *The Four Fundamental Concepts of Psycho-Analysis* (1977), Lacan presented the death drive as one of the four major concepts, together with the unconscious, repetition, and transference. He, too, opposed Freud's notion of death drive as biological drive (Lacan, 1960b). The notion, however, had different theorizations at various periods of his psychoanalytic work. In his early work, alluding to Melanie Klein's development of the concept, he conceptualized death drive as "the nostalgia for wholeness" (Lacan, 1938, p. 23), a yearning for the pre-oedipal union with the mother's womb and breast. In this vein, death drive is linked with the painful experience of birth and weaning (p. 20), which leaves a permanent trace in the child's psyche, a longing for a lost pre-birth paradise and "the most obscure aspiration for death" (p. 23). According to this formula, death drive is linked with the maternal imago, in that the longing for the maternal imago can become a longing for the pre-birth state, the union once experienced in utero. Later, Lacan (1977) postulated death drive as the repetitive tendency of drives to transgress the limits of the *pleasure principle*. As Evens observes, for Lacan:

> The purpose of the drive [*Triebziel*] is not to reach a *goal* (a final destination) but to follow its *aim* (the way itself), which is to circle round the object. Thus, the real purpose of the drive is not some mythical goal of full satisfaction, but to return to its circular path, and the real source of enjoyment is the repetitive movement of this closed circuit.
>
> [Evens, 1996, p. 47]

And, finally, Lacan argued that the death drive is not separate from and opposed to the sexual drive—a duality Freud had established in his conceptualization of sexual drive (Eros) and death drive—but, in his view, it is, rather, an aspect of sexual drive. In a radical twist to the concept, he went on to claim that "every drive is virtually a death drive" (1960a, p. 719) in the sense that every drive seeks its own extinction, involves repetition, and attempts to surpass the *pleasure principle* into the realm of excess enjoyment, where pleasure is experienced as pain.

It could, however, be argued that even though Freud used the concepts Eros and death drive in a biological sense, at times these notions do not have exactly the same connotations as drives in the biological meaning of the terms. In *Beyond the Pleasure Principle* he uses death drive to refer to the living organism's inclination towards death, whereas in *Civilizations and Its Discontents* (1930a) he refers to these concepts not only as drives directing the organism towards life or death, but also to mark a *desire* for life (and relationship) or the withdrawal of this desire in human beings, that is more in the realm of the symbolic and culture rather than nature. Hence, for Freud, the war he had witnessed before postulating his theory of the death drive could itself be regarded as a testimony of the existence of a drive in human beings, with the destructive tendency finding an outward expression in the symbolism of war. He believed (1930a) that civilization and its cultural achievements worked in the service of Eros by gathering together individuals and building a multitude of human beings in one great unit of humanity. In the same vein, one could argue that the war he found himself engulfed by represented a death cult—a pull toward disunity, division, and evidence for humans' aggressive and destructive tendencies.

Despite his dualistic model, describing Eros and the death drive as two *things* and setting them in opposition to one another, one could also infer from his theorization of the concepts that Freud was aware of the complex nature of death drive and the impossibility of separating it from life itself. He noted that these two primal drives—Eros and death drive—which are "the essential content of all life" (1930a, p. 75) seldom appear in isolation. Rather, they rule the world jointly, albeit in an antagonistic relation and in highly varying proportions. As Rosenfeld (1971/1988, p. 2) points out, the constant interplay between these concurrent drives, which makes them unrecognizable to our judgement, explains "the rich multiplicity of the phenomenon of life".

Philosophical and historical context of Beckett's work

Beckett's work has been analysed by a wide range of scholars from different traditions and disciplines. He lived in France for most of his adult life and rose to fame in Parisian circles during an active period in existential philosophy, and so one of the main approaches often taken to his works is to categorize them as existentialist literature. George Bataille (1951) and Maurice Blanchot (1953), among others, focused on the harsh facts of the human situation, the utter darkness, despair, and crawl towards death, at the heart of Beckett's work. For them, the derelict and transient figures in his trilogy, *Molloy* (1951b), *Malone Dies* (1951a), and *The Unnamable* (1953), incarnate the essence of being. They are the real anguish of a real existence—all around us, in fact, they are the reality in its purest form. In his essay "The Theatre of the Absurd" (1960), Martin Esslin, using the definition given by Ionesco (1957) in a note on Kafka, considers Beckett as one of the defining playwrights of the Theatre of the Absurd movement in that it "has no purpose, or goal, or objective" (Esslin, 1960, p. 4). The "special type of absurdity" in Beckett "is melancholic, coloured by a feeling of futility born from the disillusionment of old age and chronic hopelessness" (p. 4).

Seen through this lens, Beckett's writings encapsulate the spirit of a modern post-theological world in which, as the German philosopher, Friedrich Nietzsche announced, "God is dead" (1882, p. 109). In this world, forsaken by God, the divine compass pointing towards *meaning* has collapsed, and human-beings are left on their own to create their own meanings and essences. Existentialist philosophy was born out of this world view. Its premise is the primacy of existence to essence—that is to say, there is no mode of being predefined and no path predetermined; rather, it is to be created once *one* is in the world. This philosophy has the *being* itself as its ontological standpoint. The duty of human beings is not dictated by any metaphysical guidelines, there is no Messiah to redeem and save, but human beings are responsible for their own actions and for creating their own meanings for life. This is precisely what can be called freedom in an otherwise deterministic existence, according to the French existentialist philosopher, Jean-Paul Sartre (1943).

Waiting for Godot (1952b) can be seen as one of Beckett's earliest and most significant attempts to represent a post-messianic world, where the era of theological imagination has come to an end, and in which no rescuer enters the scene. The world in this two-act play is matterless; it consists only of a road and a bare tree; and two anxiously waiting tramps in the middle of nowhere. The plot is centred on the theme of waiting and the human predicament. The absent figure of Godot, whose coming will redeem and rule the destiny of the characters, invokes God or the Messiah. Act 2 of the play is a repetition of Act 1, with slight difference: "nothing happens, twice" (Mercier, 1956, p. 6). Godot never arrives.

In his essay, "Trying to Understand *Endgame*" (1961), the German philosopher Theodor W. Adorno interprets Beckett's oeuvre as a debate on *meaning* itself. He argues that the absurd is diluted to an idea in the Existentialist literature. He states that for Existentialists, such as Sartre, the absurd is a content represented within a traditional form and its "comprehensibility of presentation" (Adorno, 1961, p. 237), whereas, for Beckett the crisis and decay of sense is not only at the level of idea and content, but the form itself: "the form overtakes what is expressed and changes it. The impulses are raised to the level of the most advanced artistic techniques" (p. 237). For Existentialists, the absurd remains a theme outside the human subject, implying that there is an unmediated subject that is *a priori*.

Existentialists, then, go as far as freeing the subject from meaning in order to then burden them with the responsibility of creating their own sense. This, for Adorno, is an ideological position, which renders human subject ahistorical and metaphysical. However, the absurd, in Beckett work, is not what one is confronted with, but the decay of meaning necessarily creates a crisis of expression on a formal level. In this respect, the absurd is not an existential situation. Adorno argues that the destruction of meaning is a given presupposition in Beckett's work and the existence of the free unified subject, who, according to the Existentialist philosophy, in the absence of metaphysical meaning, creates its own meaning, is an illusion. Hence understanding the meaning of *Endgame* "can mean only understanding its unintelligibility, concretely reconstructing the meaning of the fact that it has no meaning" (p. 238).

In his attempt to understand *Endgame*, Adorno (1961, p. 241) makes references to the unfolding historical events in relation to the destruction of meaning in Beckett and argues that *Endgame* depicts the ruined landscape after the Second World War, where everything, including nature, is destroyed:

Hamm: Did your seeds come up?
Cloy: No.

Hamm: Did you scratch round them to see if they had sprouted?
Cloy: They haven't sprouted.
Hamm: Perhaps it's still too early.
Cloy: If they were going to sprout they would have sprouted. [Violently] They'll never sprout!

[Beckett, 1953]

Approaching Beckett's works through the mediation of history, one can also argue that they are representations of a traumatized mind. Although there is no explicit reference to any particular time period or event, as one would find in post-war literature in the traditional aesthetic of realism, Beckett's writings correspond to the brutal reality of the world surrounding him: "humankind continues to vegetate, creeping along after events that even the survivors cannot really survive, on a rubbish heap that has made even reflection on one's own damaged state useless" (Adorno, 1961, p. 240). As argued by some commentators,[5] it is important to contextualize Beckett's work in the post–Second-World-War era. As someone who joined a resistance cell in France to fight against the German occupation and later witnessed the colonial atrocities committed by France in the Algerian War of Independence,[6] Beckett was an eyewitness of the disaster and horror that were part of his everyday landscape in Paris. Thus, his plays do not only transcend the historical and the geographical to address existential human deprivation, but they also depict the despair and horror in the external world, which have found their way into his characters' psyche. His protagonists represent the death of imagination, a deprived internal world where thinking fails repeatedly. They try to give representation to a catastrophe about which they cannot gain any understanding. Like the *loss* in the melancholic, the awareness of the disaster has been withdrawn from the consciousness of Beckettian subjects.

As the extent of the horror of the war was becoming known, Beckett's work became a hallucinatory repetition of movements and words heading towards annihilation. The dialogues regress to silence, sentences become words, words become speechless acts, and actions cease. He did to literature and drama what, in 1915, the Russian artist, Kazmir Malevich, did to the history of painting in *Black Square,* his iconic solid-black canvas. *Black Square* established the zero point of painting—it was difficult to see where art could proceed from there. One may also argue that Beckett's plays are the theatrical representation of what Adorno famously pronounced: "To write poetry after Auschwitz is barbaric. And this corrodes even the knowledge of why it has become impossible to write poetry today" (1955, p. 34). Language is sterilized, and the subjects "can't go on". In a dialogue with the French writer and art critic Georges Duthuit, although commenting on a painting by Pierre Tal Coat, Beckett also seems to speak about his own struggle with aesthetic practice and expression.[7] He tells Duthuit that Coat's revolutionary work is disturbing only "a certain order on the plane of the feasible" (Beckett & Duthuit, 1949, p. 103), whereas for him the expression should be "that there is nothing to express, nothing from which to express, nothing with which to express, no power to express, no desire to express, together with the obligation to express" (p. 103).

Event

Despite the psychic horror and *nothingness* that run through Beckett's work, he has also inspired some thinkers as an author whose work is an affirmation of meaning and hope. In his polemical interpretation of Beckett's literary and stage works, the French philosopher, Alain Badiou (2003) decisively calls Beckett's lesson a lesson of courage and hope. Unlike—or, rather, opposite to—the nihilistic and existentialist reception of his thinking among the majority of Beckett's scholars, for Badiou his work harbours love and optimism. But how is this Beckett possible?

Badiou argues that traditionally Beckett's critics have considered him as an absurdist and a pessimist, who moves towards a "nihilistic destitution" (2003, p. 55)—towards a "radical opacity of significations" (p. 55). For Badiou, on the other hand, there is evidence of desire and a relentless effort in Beckett, implying that there is a possibility of a happening and hope: "Little by little—and not without hesitations and regrets—the work of Beckett will open itself up to chance, to accidents, to sudden modifications of the given, and thereby to the idea of happiness" (p. 55).

Badiou argues that although one can find a trajectory of a belief in predestination in Beckett, he does not remain in this deterministic cycle; rather, his work moves to the exploration of the potential and the possible. In Badiou's (2005) philosophy as a whole, the existence of possibility amid all the deadly repetitions is called the "event". This notion points to an unforeseen encounter with the figure of an other, creating a rupture in history and within the subject itself and opens up spaces of possibilities. It is precisely the possibility of an encounter in Beckett's work that makes a hopeful and affirmative reading of him possible. The *chance* of an event is Beckett's way out of what Badiou (2003) calls the "Cartesian terrorism" of alternation of "being" and "vain reflection" (p. 55). "Event", characterized here as meeting an other, is a "third term" that fractures this dualism and interrupts the "grey black of being" (p. 15). As Badiou puts it:

> it was necessary to find some third terms, neither reducible to the place of being nor identical to the repetitions of the voice. It was important

> that the subject be opened up to an alterity and cease being *folded* upon itself in an interminable and torturous speech.
>
> [p. 55]

Here is where, for Badiou, hope and freedom can be found in Beckett: the possibility of the encounter with an other and the possibilities that come with this. Hence, the very act of searching for an other and the chance of meeting an other is affirmation of life. For Badiou, the encounter, being Two, is the moment of construction of the social, the collective subjectivity, and a rupture in the predetermined human condition and existential deprivation. The event of encounter in Beckett is so powerful that it exceeds the feeling and the desiring body: as one of his characters in his novel, *Murphy* (1938), says: "And to meet . . . in my sense exceeds the power of feeling, however tender, and of bodily motions, however expert" (quoted in Badiou, 2003, p. 28).

It is worth noting that for Badiou the encounter, becoming *two*, is an experience that is not an inevitable but, rather, contingent. It *might* happen. Hence, he calls it a "chance" (p. 17), an "event-incident" (p. 21). And if it happens at all, and if the subject is open to this possibility, it will bring forth the *two* out of singularities and solitudes and generate love and happiness:

> The Two of love introduces a new opening onto the sensible world, away from the endless circuits of language. Love permits beauty, nuance, '*colour*'. It also permits—in fact, it is the only event to do so—happiness.
>
> [Badiou, 2003, p. xvi]

One can find a similar description when Freud defines the core of Eros as search for another. He writes: "In no other case does Eros so clearly reveal what is at the core of its being, the aim of making one out of more than one . . ." (1930a, p. 45).[8]

Rockaby: Eros and Thanatos

Rockaby is a play about a "prematurely old" (Beckett, 1980, p. 433) woman sitting in her dead mother's rocking chair and rocking to and fro. She is dressed in a glittering black evening gown, with unkempt grey hair and huge eyes in a pale face, increasingly closed throughout the play. A gradually fading bleak light is on her face and chair, and the rest of the stage is in complete darkness.

A recorded voice is telling the story of her and her dead mother's lives while she is rocking and listening to it. The story is told in a shattered, expressionless, minimalistic (or, rather, poetic) repetition. The distance of the voice, the automatic rocking of the chair, and the absence of any emotion make it clear that the *story-telling* is not a remembering of the past by the woman but a repetitive enactment of a vague attempt, ending in a deadlock.

The voice summarizes the woman's life in four phases. At the beginning, she is out "going to and fro", searching for another soul like herself:

> all eyes / all sides / high and low / for another / another like herself.
> [Beckett, 1980, p. 435]

Then she retreats home, sits at her window, draws the blind up, and continues her search from there:

> quiet at her window / only window / facing other windows / only other windows / all eyes / all sides / high and low / for another / at her window / another like herself / a little like / a living soul / high and low/to and fro/at her window/to see/be seen.
> [p. 438]

But her "famished eyes" are stopped from searching for an other by the closed blinds of other windows:

> all blinds down / never one up / hers alone up.

She retreats even more and limits the scope of her search for only one blind up,

> one blind up / no more / never mind a face.
> [p. 439]

When this attempt, too, fails, she pulls the blind down and walks down the "steep stairs" to the basement, where her mother had rocked herself to death:

> till her end came . . . dead one day / no / night / dead one night/ in the rocker / in her best black / head fallen / and the rocker rocking / rocking away.
> [p. 441]

The woman stops her search, sits in her mother's rocking chair, and closes her eyes:

> right down / into the old rocker / those arms at last / and rocked / rocked / with closed eyes / closing eyes / she so long all eyes / famished eyes/all sides.
> [p. 441]

Each section of the play ends with the voice, chair, and the light slowly coming to rest; after a long pause, the next section starts, with the woman suddenly opening her eyes, looking at the deep dark in front of her, and asking for *more*. Then, the chair starts rocking again, and the recorded voice goes on with telling the story. She asks for *more* four times, each time more softly than the previous time, until she stops asking for it, and this is when the chair stops rocking, and the voice stops talking, and her head sinks. The light fades out slowly.

Rockaby is a play in dying. Through repetitive movements, words, and silence it gradually deprives itself of all the elements that bring it into life: plot, light, woman, voice, eyes, chair, rocking, all move towards zero point, an inanimate and static state. If one takes it too literally, *Rockaby* is then a play about a tragic death of a joyless life. However, despite what might appear, death is not a welcomed bliss for the protagonist. She fractures the predestined universe of life and death by striving for love, by carrying on searching, and, in Badiou's term, by inviting "possibility" and "chance", despite the knowledge of her mortality. By being open to alterity and searching actively for an other, the woman is prolonging life and deferring the end. Even though this unremitting labour of love, looking "all eyes . . . all sides . . . high and low. . ." stops, and the woman's head falls on her shoulder, there are many resistances and obstacles put in the way by Eros. By asking for *more,* the woman interrupts the play/search for love from coming to an end and keeps the story going. So even though her existence consists of constant repetitive movements, there are momentary ruptures of the circular movements and postponements of the end.

The hope to find an other, or at least see "a blind up", can also be seen as the opposite of narcissistic indifference towards external objects and the world. Rosenfeld (1971) argues that in the destructive narcissistic state, due to self-idealization, the individual perceives the external objects as parts of the self. Hence, the phantasmatic desire of reuniting with the mother is the expression of the death drive, as previously argued by Lacan. The denial of separateness enables an avoidance of the traumatic encounter with the otherness of the mother and dependency and need associated with separateness. Rosenfeld saw an obvious relation between narcissistic withdrawal and Freud's theory of the death drive. In the destructive narcissistic state, the idealized self avoids encounter, any positive libidinal object relationship or love relationship with the external world and, by extension, the construction of the "collective subjectivity". It also avoids the libidinal part of the self that depends on others, as everything is seen as an extension of the self, a regressive atomized state of returning to the mother's uterus.

In *Rockaby,* however, the repetition of movement and stillness is not without tension, brought about by a desiring subject. She is looking out, searching, hoping to find. Not only is alterity acknowledged in *Rockaby,* but it is also desired. There is a longing for "another", for love's "twoness", which is the opposite of the fusion of two identical entities. Even though the desire is not fulfilled and the encounter with an other never occurs in the play, the libidinal drive goes on searching for an object. The object is not found, but the longing for a "living soul" continues in a repetitive movement until the desire is withdrawn from the external world and ceases to go on. At this point the woman walks down to the basement, where there is "no window facing other windows", sits in her mother's rocking chair, and dies her mother's death.

The retreat from being out to the basement, from going "to and fro" to rocking in her dead mother's chair, from looking out through the window to sitting with closed eyes, and from searching for an other to listening to her own recorded voice is the moment when Eros gives up. The woman is turned inward, folded upon herself, in solipsistic seclusion, and life, the search for an other, has given in to the hidden aggression of a desireless and motionless existence. The woman does not ask for *more* any longer and the recorded voice goes on with its torturous repetition,

> and rocked / rocked / saying to herself / no / done with that / the rocker / saying to the rocker / rock her off / stop her eyes / fuck life.
> [1980, p. 442]

. . . until the chair stops completely.

Concluding remarks

The antagonism of life and death, argued by Freud as the essence of all life, finds its theatrical representation in Beckett's *Rockaby* in the form of *being out* and searching for an other and *stepping down* to the basement, where the character is caught in a repetitive act, until she reaches the exit of death. However, the triumph of isolation and death over life is not the conclusion to be drawn from the play. What takes the play beyond a nihilistic and absurdist reading is the resistance of the character to the eventless repetition. Her call for "more" ruptures the smooth decline of her being and searching for an other. But it seems paradoxical that, on the one hand, Beckett radically subtracts his character from any ornamentations, material attributes, and even pretentious language, and, on the other hand, his characters ask for "more". To think with Badiou (2003), one could interpret the dispossession not as a sign of existential poverty and human deprivation, but a success. The peripheral possessions must be lost so that the "essence of generic humanity" (p. 3), the elementary skeleton of existence, can be subtracted. Seen like this, neither is losing a destitution nor is asking for "more" a desire to repossess what is lost. "More" is then the name of life itself, the woman's desire to go on, to search, and possibly reach. This implies a "possibility" of an "event" within and beyond the given condition, and the meaning of life is to strive to actualize this.

The possibility of an "event" runs through Beckett's writings as a subtle gesture of life amid the deadliness of his works. In one of his other short plays, called, *Not I* (1972), the moment the mouth, the only "protagonist" in the play, turns away from searching for a divine source or meaning for her condition, she realizes that there is no predefined meaning in her suffering and in life itself. This realization enables her to find meaning in the very act of *going on*, when she says ". . . no matter . . . keep on . . ." (p. 383). In *Waiting for Godot,* when Estragon, tired of waiting, tells Vladimir that he "can't go on like this", Vladimir replies: "That's what you think" (1952b, pp. 87–88).

It brings a new perspective to the understanding of *Rockaby* when one shifts one's attention to Beckett's own personal experience and his relationship with his mother. It can be argued that *Rockaby* is a play that encapsulates Beckett's personal life and his life in writing (if one could ever distinguish between them). His childhood friend, Geoffrey Thompson, said in an interview that understanding the nature of relationship Beckett had with his mother is essential to understanding his personality (Miller, 2013)—and, one could argue, essential to understanding his work. According to Alvarez (1992), there is only one plot in Beckett, and his various writings are different expressions of this single theme, which is Beckett's own depression. As a young man, he suffered from panic attacks, an arrhythmic heart, and night sweats, which took him to psychoanalysis. He underwent intensive analysis for more than two years with Wilfred Bion at the Tavistock Clinic. He also embarked on an extensive study of psychoanalytic texts and was particularly interested in Otto Rank's *Trauma of Birth* (1924) and the two primal traumata of birth and weaning. He also attended lectures delivered by Carl Jung at the Institute of Psychological Medicine at the Tavistock Clinic where he listened to the story of a young female patient recounted by Jung as someone who "had never really been born!" Beckett's own anguish stemmed from his suffocating relationship with his mother and her "savage loving", as he put it in a letter to the Irish poet, Thomas MacGreevy (Kim, 2010). He gave an account of his psychoanalysis to James Knowlson in 1989, when he mentioned recalling "intrauterine memories" of being trapped in his mother's womb, unable to escape, being in pain and crying to be let out, but no one was listening (Knowlson, 1996, p. 177). It is not hard to identify the representation of Beckett's maternal imago in his work and characters. However, unlike his character in *Rockaby*, who identifies with her dead mother and walks down the steep stair to die in her mother's fashion, he chose a different fate. He wrote. Writing was his way of transcending the suffocation and longing. It was his desire for "more", the Eros amid all the paralyzing meaninglessness of dwelling in a mortal world, and his novelty amid all the deadly repetitiveness of life. However, alienated from his critics, audience, and journalists, he wrote in order to relate to these very people and to life itself. He had an obligation to *go on;* this was a fate he shared with his immobile protagonist, in his novel, *The Unnamable* (1953), when the protagonist ends his disjointed monologue with this sentence: "you must go on, I can't go on, I'll go on" (p. 407).

Notes

1 Strachey's translation of the Freudian *Trieb* as "instinct" has been criticised by many for being a biologizing notion that refers to innate animal responses, with no psychological representation of stimuli originated within the organism. Lacan (1960b, p. 680), for instance, proposes "drive" rather than "instinct" as a more accurate translation of *Trieb*. Here instinct is used only when the quote is directly from the *Standard Edition*.

2 Freud never used the term "Thanatos" in his writing. According to Jones (1961), it was Wilhelm Stekel who, in 1909, used the term to signify the death wish.

3 It is important to note that before Freud's conceptualization, the hypothesis of the existence of "death drive" had already been introduced by the Viennese psychoanalyst Sabina Spielrein, in her paper "Destruction as a Cause of Coming into Being". In this essay, published in 1912, she argues that the most powerful drive, namely sexual drive, harbours, in addition to positive feelings, negative feelings such as anxiety, resistance, and disgust. These negative feelings correspond to the "destructive component of the sexual instincts", which she later formulates as "death instinct within the sexual instinct". It has been argued by some psychoanalytic scholars that this essay anticipated the hypothesis of the existence of "death drive" put forward by Freud in 1920 (see, for example, Carotenuto, 1980, and Britton, 2003).

4 The notion of death is central to Arthur Schopenhauer's philosophy. He argues that existence is a constant dying, and he interprets death as the aim and purpose of life. He maintains that the streaming of time, in which the individual is caught up, is constantly turning the present into the past, and so the past is the repository of death—of no longer existing events. In other words, existence is a constant process of dying (Janaway, 1999).

5 See, for instance, Rustin & Rustin, 2002a, and Boulter, 2008.
6 See Morin, 2017.
7 In the *Three Dialogues,* Duthuit tells Beckett that his views on the painters under discussion are "violently extreme and personal point of view", and that he should try to remember that the subject under discussion is not himself.
8 It is important to note that for Badiou & Troung (2012) love is always between *two* and this becoming *two* does not lead to *oneness,* whereas Freud's notion of love implies fusion and *oneness* of two people (1930).

CHAPTER ELEVEN

The narcissistic world of Turandot

Tomaso Quaini

This chapter is an attempt to bring the reader into the experience of watching and listening to the Italian opera *Turandot*, an opera by Giacomo Puccini, posthumously completed by Franco Alfano in 1926 and set to a libretto in Italian by Giuseppe Adami and Renato Simoni. I focus particularly on a passage of the opera in which the princess Turandot's narcissistic world starts to waver under what I argue to be the pressure of internal integration. I dissect this passage and analyse it from three different perspectives: the plot, the theatrical display, and the music, which, as Sterba (1965) and, more recently, Nagel (2010) describe, has the power to capture the unconscious. Nagel draws on the well-known Freudian percept of the interpretation of dreams, with their visual content and verbal analysis as the "royal road to a knowledge of the unconscious activities of the mind" (Freud, 1900a, p. 608), a road she refers to as the "Royal *Oral* Road"; she semantically expands the idea, suggesting that music travels the "Royal *Aural* Road" to the unconscious.

I consider the emotional impact of the opera on the spectator, who finds him/herself drawn into what is described by some authors as a powerful regressive mother–infant experience: the theatre often being compared to the maternal womb with its containing function. As Brigid Brophy points out, the theatre places the audience in the position of the infant, and in so doing, "the audience renounces the power of speech in

DOI: 10.4324/9781003564867-15

favour of the persons on the stage and signifies its own feelings only by the infantile methods of inarticulate cries and hand-clapping" (Brophy, 1988, p. 40). Specifically in relation to being in the audience of an opera, Rustin and Rustin argue that the intensity of the emotional involvement that an opera calls for through its great displays of light, movements, vast range of sounds, and colour "evoke the impact of maternal care and behaviour on young babies" (M. E. Rustin & Rustin, 2006, p. 2).

With this in mind, allow me now to enter the theatre, listen to the vast range of sound, and "bathe myself in the emotion" of the beginning of *Turandot*.

The beginning of the opera

Here I am sitting in the theatre surrounded by the continuous chatter of elegant people, which gradually fades as the lights go down. The orchestra leader makes his entrance, and I suddenly find myself a member of a huge audience that applauds him as the light switches from us to him. The usually dreaded dark becomes, for once, my silent companion and triggers in me an unexpected and exciting anonymity that passes through my body as a little electric discharge. A sense of safety wraps my soul, but the illusion that whatever I am going to see will not affect me at all breaks at the very first notes of *Turandot*.

The fortississimo unison accented chords in the woodwind, brass, and strings (Bar 1, Ricordi), which begin the opera, instantly sets up a menacing atmosphere. Through the use of unison and the dissonant interval of a tritone (the interval of an augmented fourth or three full tones) between the second and third chords, Puccini creates a sense of tonal ambiguity in the first two bars. The interval of the tritone is known as the *diabolus in musica*, or the devil in music. It demands resolution and is typically used to portray conflict and unease. This, plus the overall tonal ambiguity, generates a wariness and uncertainty in the listener. A sense of rejection and of being unwelcome spreads around the theatre as the audience finds itself in a scene set in front of the wall of Peking: the set design mirrored on the stage by the curtain still being closed and in the music through aurally aggressive dissonance, harsh orchestral timbres, and loud dynamics.

After only a few seconds, a strong sense of tension and suspense follows in the music, skilfully underlined by Puccini through repeated monotone notes. A sinister atmosphere announces the subsequent speech by a Mandarin, a solemn and threatening baritone who, appearing on the stage with the curtains still closed, seems to be speaking directly to the audience, giving them the following warning:

> People of Peking!
> This is the law:
> Turandot, the Pure, will be bride
> Of the man, of royal blood,
> Who solves the three enigmas
> That she will ask him.
> But whoever faces the trial
> And is defeated,
> Must bow to the axe
> His haughty head!
>
> [Act 1, lines 1–10][1]

According to Rusbridger (2008), the music helps the audience to identify immediately with individual characters' states of mind, but here, on the contrary, I think that the audience is warned from the beginning *not* to enter the stage and not to identify with one of those men who want to win the love of Turandot, since the threat, a castration threat, is to be beheaded—a fate that befalls the Prince of Persia at the beginning of the opera. Consciously or not, the audience starts to have the feeling of being part of (or looking at) an over-controlled world. "Listeners in the theatre . . . are challenged to take part in the very process of 'working through' the artistic message" (Noy, 2009, p. 4, quoted in Nagel, 2010). To borrow a Freudian expression, is the shadow of a cold object (Turandot) already falling upon the audience's ego? Being aware of the intensity of this "overture", I need now to step outside the theatre for a moment to give myself and the reader some time to recover before carrying on with the analysis. Taking advantage of this respite, I give some background information about the opera.

Background to the opera

The Italian composer Giacomo Puccini wrote *Turandot* in 1924, when Western culture in Europe was particularly interested in what was thought of then as the exotic and the oriental. It is, in fact, in the faraway kingdom of Peking that the opera takes place. Its music subtly contributes to the oriental character of the opera by use of the pentatonic (five-note) scale, which, together with Chinese-sounding ornamentation, creates an oriental atmosphere in this faraway world. This is a world still populated and dominated by gods and deities, one of which the Princess Turandot herself embodies.

Yet prior to this particular opera, the composer's artistic output was under the influence of *Verismo* (internationally known as Realism), which was oriented towards demythologizing the gods and myths. Puccini's best-known opera, *La Bohème,* sits firmly within this tradition. As a result of this and in contrast to *Turandot*, the characters of his previous works were prevented from claiming any operatic grandeur (Conrad, 1948).

However, according to Conrad (1948), if the realism of Puccini's previous creations was intended to dismantle the gods, myths, and religious mystery that were so characteristic of the "classic opera", with *Turandot* (and *Il Trittico*) the Italian composer returns to where he believes opera belongs, in the realm of myth. Greenfield, in a similar vein, describes *Turandot* in his book *Puccini: A Biography* in the following way: "Its heroine was diametrically opposed to the typical Puccini heroine. Far from sweet or pathetic, she was a cruel, heartless tyrant, who scorned love and fought against it" (Greenfield, 1980, p. 257).

I believe that a psychoanalytic exploration of the opera can lead us to a slightly different conclusion from the one proposed by Greenfeld and Conrad, in which Turandot's godlike aura seems to obscure values like sweetness and simplicity. Does this opera belong entirely to the realm of myth, "abandoning" the values of Realism?

Here I raise this, and the following question: "What states of mind does the opera convey that can be further elucidated through a psychoanalytic lens?"

I try to answer these questions throughout the chapter by focusing my analysis on three characters in the opera: Turandot, a beautiful and cold princess who reigns over a faraway Chinese Kingdom; the Unknown Prince alias Calaf—son of Timur; and Liù, Timur's slave, who is secretly in love with the Unknown Prince.

Brief summary of the opera

At the beginning of the opera a Prince of Persia is to be executed, as he has just failed to solve the three riddles that Turandot poses to any suitor of noble blood who wants to marry her. The people await the beheading, but, as the Prince of Persia enters, the crowd is suddenly moved and pleads with the Princess to pardon him. However, Turandot confirms the Prince's sentence.

Among the crowd is the Unknown Prince, who, entranced by Turandot's beauty, immediately falls in love with her. Liù, who also happens to be there with Timur, tries to convince him to change his mind, but blinded by this sudden love, the Prince challenges for Turandot's hand.

During the second act, the audience comes to know a terrible truth about the Princess: one of her ancestors was raped by a Mongol Prince. It is for this reason that Turandot wants to retaliate against anyone who asks for her hand.

However, the Unknown Prince is eventually able to solve the riddles, and an exchange of roles between him and Turandot takes place. The Unknown Prince, in fact, witnessing the reluctance of the Princess to love him back (as the law requires her to do if someone is able to solve the enigmas) will pose her one riddle: should she learn his name before dawn, he will die and relieve her of her duty. A furious Turandot orders that everyone in Peking who might know his name must be tortured. Among these, only Timur and Liù know the Prince's name.

It will be Liù who, by declaring that only she knows the name, will save Timur from torture, and, by refusing to disclose it, will face the Princess and play a pivotal role in ultimately making her falling in love with the Unknown Prince.

Turandot's complex

Turandot is described in the opera as a cold and beautiful deity, often compared with the Moon, therefore distant from embodying any values of realism. She is defined by Conrad as ". . . less a character than a complex: a vagina dentate" (1948, p. 200). This is a strong and powerful image of what could otherwise be described in psychoanalytic terms as a deeply narcissistic character.

The whole opera is, in fact, a magnificent depiction of a narcissistic world, with its contrasting coexistence of omnipotent power and submissive fragility in which any "other" represents a threat that has to be got rid of. It is a tale of resistances and defences against integration and change, where Turandot's narcissistic kingdom strives to remain unchanged.

Rosenfeld, drawing from his clinical experience, talks about destructive narcissism, and, focusing particularly on the destructive parts of the self says,

> They are directed both against any positive libidinal object relationship and any libidinal part of the self which experiences need for an object and the desire to depend on it. The destructive omnipotent parts of the self often remained disguised or they may be silent and split off, which obscures their existence and gives the impression that they have no relationship to the external world. In fact they have a very powerful

> effect in preventing dependent object relations and in keeping external objects permanently devalued
>
> [Rosenfeld, 1971/1988, p. 246]

I find this quotation particularly important in the context of the opera, as it summarizes several aspects contained within it. With this formulation of destructive narcissism in mind, I first address the question of whether the Unknown Prince can perhaps be considered the external object or the "positive libidinal object" that seeks love, and whether Liù might represent the part of Turandot's self that needs an object to depend on. The Unknown Prince plays a pivotal part in the resolution of Turandot's narcissistic world, but here I focus mainly on the role of Liù.

Who, then, is Liù?

I believe Liù embodies a denied split-off part of Turandot that seeks love for, and dependence on, an object. In the opera she is a slave who is literally tied to the Unknown Prince's father, Timur, on the stage and is deeply in love with the Unknown Prince.

In performance, her depressive figure stands out timidly and yet powerfully among the other characters and retains, in my view, beauty and dignity as her voice has the power to slow down for a moment the impetuousness of the Unknown Prince's sudden love for Turandot.

Liù's aria, "My lord, listen, ah! Listen!" towards the end of the first act is full of love and compassion as she desperately tries to stop the Unknown Prince putting his life at risk as he declares his love for Turandot and his intention to solve the riddles. It is an unexpected and desperate caress in the face not only of the Prince, but also of the audience, who, still shaken by the chilly overture, finds its original and primordial need to be held satisfied in her voice. Hence Liù's song brings a sense of something maternal: a cohesion and fluency to the rhythm of the opera.

It is important to note an interesting aspect of the opera. While it is, indeed, named after Turandot's character, Turandot herself is on the stage for no longer than Liù or any of the other characters. On the contrary, she remains "disguised and silent" for most of the time, particularly in the first act. Yet Turandot is *actively against*—to use Rosenfeld's words (1971—any "positive libidinal object relationship and any libidinal part of the self which experiences need for an object and the desire to depend on it" (1971/1988, p. 246). How, then, can her narcissism be actively displayed when she is not present on the stage?

This is where I think the chorus plays a central role.

The role of the chorus

Greenfield describes *Turandot* in the following way: "a pageant, a spectacle. It called for huge crowd scenes and large choruses, neither of which had been a part of any of the composer's previous, more intimate operas" (1980, p. 257).

At the beginning of the opera, and particularly during the first 20 minutes, the audience loses itself in this overwhelming "spectacle" of voices and masks displayed in "huge crowd scenes and large choruses". Turandot's narcissistic shadow spreads in the theatre, and with that the spectator's identity experiences a sense of threat. Similarly, when stepping into the realm of the unknown, Kohut says that on hearing a piece of music for the first time, the ego experiences it as "a chaotic, threatening experience that cannot be mastered" (Kohut, 1950).

It is difficult for the audience to have a clear idea of what is going on at the beginning of the opera. All the main characters make their entrance in the first act: the Unknown Prince, his father Timur, Liù, and Turandot herself, although she doesn't speak at all in the first act. However, I don't think this means that she is not already communicating through the voice of the chorus.

It is, in fact, as underlined by Greenfield (1980), the chorus that is the protagonist of the first act, enchanting the audience's confused ego and leading it to admire the interplay of different voices that are able to communicate a range of emotions at an unconscious level through the music. We come to know who Turandot is also through the eyes and voices of the people in the crowd, whose feelings are at her mercy.

I now raise another question: is the cold Princess controlling them, psychoanalytically speaking, by projective identification?

Rosenfeld (1971), analysing the aggressive aspects of the narcissism of certain patients, describes them as

> often highly organized as if one were dealing with a powerful gang dominated by a leader who controls all the members of the gang to see that they support one another in making the criminal destructive work more effective and powerful. . . .
>
> The main aim seems . . . to control the members of the gang so that they will not desert the destructive organization and join the positive parts of the self or betray the secrets of the gang to the police.
>
> [Rosenfeld, 1971/1988, p. 249]

Do we see the crowd acting in a gang-like way when, at the beginning of the first act, the chorus incites Turandot's guards to murder the Persian Prince, who, as we come to know, had failed to solve the enigmas, embodying in this way her sadistic desire for revenge? Might we understand that the people become the victim of Turandot's power, as the chorus begs for pity (in the music, with almost damned voices) when it is roughly dispersed by the guards? At one point we experience the crowd calling for Turandot with distant, melancholic, beautiful voices, idealizing her as a divine figure and begging her Moon-like presence to appear from the stairs of the palace. The chorus calls, with seductive voices, for other people to come "where Turandot reigns! Sweet lovers, come forwards, come!" (Act 1, lines 16, 17) attracting in this way new victims for Turandot and so guaranteeing for her—using Freud's terminology when he describes some aspects of melancholia (1917e [1915], p. 251)—the continuous operation of abuse, causing suffering and deriving sadistic satisfaction from the constant presence of a victim-object that cannot be given up.

In her paper, "Projective Identification: Clinical Aspects" (1988), in which she discusses projective identification from a Kleinian perspective, Betty Joseph identifies various aims of this primitive defence mechanism. One aim could be to project the self, or part of it, into the object to dominate and to control it. In this opera, something is projected into the crowd, but I wonder whether through the performance something is projected into the audience too. Another aim of projective identification can be to maintain an omnipotent narcissistic balance: in the background of Turandot's ancestor's trauma of rape, the crowd is invested to constantly attract new "sweet lovers" who, by being sacrificed and tortured one by one, become in this way the victim-objects that can guarantee an abusive retaliatory circle.

Is this what is happening in this faraway Chinese Kingdom? Is this what the crowd is caught up in, and what is conveyed at an unconscious level to the audience's ears?

Bion (1962a) recognizes that projective identification can also be used as a method of communication. Are the crowd's voices in the music—at times damned, at times melancholic, other times glacial, but also, and predominantly, beautiful—the mirror of Turandot's narcissistic image and hidden feelings? I wonder whether, in fact, the fear, withdrawal, solitude, and sense of rejection that are falling on the ears (and in the ego) of the audience are the shadow of Turandot's narcissistic world.

The beginning of the narcissistic resolution in the third act

We are now in the middle of the night, and a chorus of male and female voices sings an obsessive thought whispered by, in Rosenfeld's terms, the "mafia-like" chorus that, with distant catatonic voices, keeps repeating the same thing, giving voice to Turandot's command:

> No one must sleep!
> No one must sleep!
> The name of the stranger
> must be revealed before morning!
>
> [Act 3, Scene 1, Lines 4–8]

In the meantime the princess has withdrawn into her "cold room" as the Unknown Prince himself, echoing the chorus, describes it: "No one must sleep and you too Princess, in your cold room . . ." (Act 3, Scene 1, Lines 16, 17). The image of the cold room, brings to my mind Steiner's concept of "psychic retreat":

> A psychic retreat provides the patient with an area of relative peace and protection from strain when meaningful contact with the analyst is experienced as threatening . . . they retreat behind a powerful system of defences which serve as a protective armour or hiding place.
>
> [Steiner, 1993, p. 1]

In this sense, one is tempted to allocate to the Unknown Prince the role of the analyst who was, in the first place, by solving the riddles, able in the second act to make "meaningful contact" with the princess. Perhaps Turandot experiences this contact as a threat, and she retreats from it, defending herself against the warmth of true love.

Who can help her step out from this room and not be afraid to know true love?

Here lies the importance of Liù's contribution both in the opera and in Turandot's internal resolution.

Liù and Turandot's scene

It is only towards the end of the opera, when Turandot is desperate to know the Unknown Prince's name, that, Turandot and Liù "speak" to each other for the first time.

Here I give the reader the actual words sung by the two women. I then analyse the exchange from three different angles: that of the plot, the acting, and the music.

Turandot: "Speak!"
Liù: "I'd rather die!"

Turandot: "Who gave your heart such strength?"
Liù: "Love, Princess!"
Turandot: "Love?"
Liù: "Such love, secret and unconfessed
so great that these torments are sweet for me,
because I make a gift of them for my lord . . .
because keeping silent I give him
your love . . .
I give you him, Princess,
And I lose everything!"
. . .
"Bind me! Torture me!
give me torments and pain!
as supreme gifts
of my love!"

[Act 3, Scene 1, Lines 157–173]

a. *The plot*

Betty Joseph, discussing perverse relationships, describes how one of her patients

> was dominated by an aggressive part of himself that not only attempted to control and destroy her work but that was actively sadistic towards other parts of the self which would be more available for help were they not masochistically caught up in the perversion.
>
> [Joseph, 1982, quoted in Steiner, 1993, p. 52]

If, in the second act, the Unknown Prince was acting like an analyst whose work is under attack through the Princess's attempt to get rid of him, Liù, representing the more available part of Turandot's self, seems instead to be caught up in a somewhat sadomasochistic relationship with the Princess when she sings:

> "Bind me! Torture me!
> Give me torments and pain!
> as supreme gifts
> Of my love!"

But if I may digress briefly, I would like to draw a parallel between the opera *Turandot* and George Orwell's 1949 novel, *Nineteen Eighty-Four,* to underline that within this perverse relationship it is Turandot and not Liù who is the fearful one.

Whereas in the famous Room 101 Orwell's protagonist, who dared to have a forbidden love relationship, shows his weakness by betraying his partner, in Puccini's opera Liù, in contrast, shows her bravery, keeping secret the Unknown Prince's name and revealing to the Princess that what gives her the strength to resist the torture is love—the same love that Turandot, after the solution of the riddles, is required to give to Calaf and of which the Princess is terribly afraid.

But why is Turandot so fearful of loving the Unknown Prince?

Both the world of *Nineteen Eighty-Four* and the world of Turandot, I think, represent the love that, as an emotional internal life (or the Freudian life instinct) and symbol of freedom, poses a threat that must be destroyed in order to preserve the tyrannical narcissistic balance of an over-controlled, singular world. Perhaps it is a love that could also represent fear of dependency and involvement, with the consequent risk of being hurt or betrayed.

Let me quote here what Segal and Bell say about narcissistic patients: "There are many patients who experience love as a threat, fearing that it will deplete them . . . they fear they do lose part of themselves through projective identification" (Segal & Bell, 1991, p. 163).

I think that this "depletion" (similar to the Freudian "impoverishment of the ego", as mentioned previously) is what Turandot (and not Liù) is afraid to face in her (cold) Room 101. Her deepest fear is perhaps lodged and projected into Liù, who says: "Because keeping silent I give him your love, I give you him, Princess, and I lose everything." Might this be a fear, then, of *losing everything* and of losing control of her kingdom as the consequence of the duty to love the Prince?

b. Theatrical display

The opera is not only about its plot but also, as importantly, it is about how the story is conveyed in the particular context of the theatre through inventive instrumental and vocal music, through the dramatic action and the staging. As Rustin and Rustin say, "The multi-dimensionality of opera is its most striking characteristic. It is not only orchestral and vocal music with the impact of the libretto on a vast scale, but also sumptuous theatrical display" (M. E. Rustin & Rustin, 2006, p. 2).

It is interesting to note how this highly emotional and meaningful musical scene, when Liù and Turandot come to "talk" to each other, is preceded in the opera by moments of almost erratic acting, displayed in many movements on the stage on the part of the crowd, the ministers, the Unknown Prince, Liù, and Timur. They all participate in creating confusion, like the wind and rain that precede a storm.

In the meantime Liù has, as we have seen, been literally tied with a rope to her master Timur for the whole duration of the opera.

It is in the background of this tumultuous scene in which Turandot's guards and ministers desperately try to make someone give them the name of the Unknown Prince that Liù, representing, in Rosenfeld's terminology, "the dependent sane part of the self . . . trapped . . . inside the psychotic narcissistic structure" (1971/1988, p. 251), bravely comes out into the light on the stage and, as she stands up, distancing herself from Timur, speaks directly to Turandot. Puccini succeeds, I think, in creating a powerful emotional impact on the grateful audience, which, still at the mercy of the fragmentation of several voices, suddenly finds much-needed containment in Liù's voice.

She first claims that she is the only one who knows the Unknown Prince's name ("The name you seek, only I know"), in this way saving Timur from torture. She then also claims that she will never say that name, thus saving the Unknown Prince from his death.

An incredulous Turandot, witnessing this gesture of bravery, asks Liù who gives her "such strength", and, as we have seen, Liù's answer is "love".

It is particularly interesting to observe Turandot's acting on stage at this moment in the performance.[2] As Turandot hears and comes to realize that Liù's driving force and courage derive from the purest form of love, she literally turns around and takes a few steps back. It is not a turning away, though. Rather, I think, it is a turning inwards, as she appears touched by Liù's confession—her reaction is to retreat, perhaps to digest what she has just learned from Liù.

Her stepping backward in this way not only creates an internal space for her to receive Liù's words, but it also allows the audience to come emotionally closer to Liù, to feel her pain and empathize with her unconditional love. It creates an unexpected emotional movement, whereas previously there had been rigidity and only space for Turandot's self.

It could be said that here the audience, as we shall see also towards the end of the chapter, unconsciously acts as a third and participates in the narcissistic resolution of the opera.

Hindle (2000) analyses an opera by Ravel, *L'Enfant et les sortilèges,* in which the little protagonist, a rather spoiled and defiant child who, in consequence of being told off by his mother for not having studied, frees himself from her binding love and gives himself over to the power of hatred. His aggression comes to the fore in beating and wounding objects and animals around him once he is left alone. However, as he observes the animals crying lovingly and supporting each other in response to his attacks, something changes within him. Hindle points out this moment in the opera and, describing it as the protagonist's developmental change, says,

> His awareness of their capacity to mourn appears to set in motion a retreat from his infantile grandiosity and a move towards an awareness of his helplessness and need. Rather than 'premature guilt', the child is faced with having to bear guilt for damage that is irreparable.
> [Hindle, 2000, p. 1191]

It seems to me that both in Ravel's and in Puccini's operas, in order for the protagonists to move on from an omnipotent and destructive narcissistic stance, they first take a step backwards into themselves, into what could otherwise be described as a move towards or into the depressive position.

The beginning of the integration between Liù and Turandot seems finally to take place as the princess witnesses Liù's ability to give voice to her feelings, something that again can be compared to Ravel's opera, as Hindle says, "Only when the animals voice their thoughts and feelings is the child able to glean an understanding of their inner worlds hitherto unavailable to him" (2000, p. 1193). It can also be added that only when the audience feels what Liù is giving voice to that Turandot is able to glean an understanding of her inner world, hitherto unavailable to her.

By stepping backwards, Turandot also gives me now the space to analyse what is conveyed in Liù's voice and her interaction with the princess in the music, as it is in the music rather than in the lyrics that the audience can feel a moment of unexpected harmony and union between the two protagonists—another sign, perhaps, of the beginning of Turandot's internal integration.

c. The music

Liù is seized by her torturers and falls to her knees. The crowd commands her to speak, and so does Turandot who, witnessing her unfailing resistance, asks her with surprise:

> "Who gave your heart
> Such strength?"

Liù replies:

> "Princess, love!"

Turandot, somewhat confused, asks again:

> "Love?"

It is in some ways a pity to have already reported and analysed the actual words of the two women. Analysis of words, as suggested by Nagel, "can obscure the capacity of music to evoke and convey multiple meanings not related directly to verbal narrative" (Nagel, 2010). It is a pity because, listening to the music, which seems suddenly to become an untouchable essence, I find myself enchanted by the lightness of this quick and intense "talk" between Turandot and Liù, where the latter, a slave, gives to the former, a princess, the secret of her strength (and weakness?), love.

It is as if we are now in the eye of the storm, where there is a sudden and almost unreal calm, and if I pretended for a moment not to have the plot in front of me, I would find myself pleasantly confused by their talk. The words are, in fact, difficult to grasp and slip away from any cognitive effort to be understood. The lens of rationality is blurred, and one has something of the feeling of being cradled in this fused and confused alternation of who is speaking to whom. The emotional wave emanating from the music is such that the audience almost forgets that one is a princess and the other a slave, although on the stage Turandot is still physically on a higher level than Liù.

This exchange between Turandot and Liù is a rare moment of harmonic clarity in the opera (6 bars before figure 24; Puccini, 1926, p. 378). Chromatically uncoloured chords of C major, F major, D minor, and A minor are played at a high tessitura (pitch level) in the upper strings, which are divisi (divided), with fewer instruments on each part allowing for an extremely quiet and ethereal accompanimental dynamic, thus highlighting the duet of voices.

Turandot and Liù sing at a similar tessitura, and their respective melodies follow on immediately from each other, so that there is no perceived gap in their conversation, nor is there overlap between their statements. This results in the impression of one voice singing one long phrase. This merging of Turandot's and Liù's voices in the music could also perhaps signify a merging/coming together of Turandot's inner world, which has thus far been fragmented. This coming together is, however, in contrast with what is conveyed in the plot and in the acting, where Turandot literally steps away from Liù on the stage.

An unexpected natural harmony between the two women's voices is created, and this has the power to invite the audience to regress to a very early stage in life. As Hindle and Godsil describe so well when talking about the experience of listening to the mother's voice:

> Consciously, the memory of one's mother's voice elicits many thoughts and feelings. Unconsciously, it may open the door to a deeper

> longing—a wish to return to a state of unconditional love, being held in mother's arms and ultimately the womb.
>
> [Hindle & Godsil, 2006]

This fusion and con-fusion of the two women reminds me of Freud's description of Leonardo da Vinci's painting, *St. Anne with the Madonna and Child*. In a footnote added in 1919 Freud, trying to interpret the particular configuration of the two female figures in the painting and drawing a parallel with those of the artist's childhood, writes,

> . . . one is inclined to say that they are fused with each other like a badly condensed dream figure, so that in some places it is hard to say where Anne ends and Mary begins . . . it seems for the artist the two mothers of his childhood were melted into a single form.
>
> [Freud, 1910c, p. 114]

The spectator, too—as if driven, in a "cathartic experience" (Kohut, 1950), suddenly back into childhood by the rarefied sound of the violins—is made to believe that he is facing what could be described as two "goodly (well) condensed" mother figures.

To summarize my argument, it is, I think, in the unconscious layer of the music that the dyadic "perverse" relationship of perpetrator and slave, as personified by Turandot and Liù, qualitatively changes in the two following and interconnected ways. First, in a dream-like moment Liù appears to become Turandot's mother. Does Turandot's deepest fear find for a moment in Liù the containment she was seeking? In Bion's terms (1962a) it seems to me that Turandot's "nameless dread" (a psychoanalytic expression that I find strikingly similar to the Unknown Prince's name itself), her beta elements, are first, as we have seen, projected onto Liù (who in fact earlier in the opera said: "I know his name. . . . My supreme pleasure is to keep it secret and to have it for myself alone!" Carrying on with Bion's terminology, Liù, through reverie, appears to be able to receive these projections and then modify them, so that Turandot can introject the fear but in a "detoxified" form—in the music in an almost untouchable form—love. In relation to this, Waddell (1998b) in a chapter titled "Late Adolescence", writes,

> Maturity is slowly acquired through the experience of having the more infantile and insistent projections received and rendered both bearable and meaningful. . . . A coming-out-of-projective-identification then becomes possible, the foundation, as we have seen, for adult identity and for intimacy.
>
> [Waddell, 1998b, p. 190]

At the end of the opera the cold (and perhaps rather adolescent) princess appears not to fear saying the Unknown Prince's name any more when she sings, joyfully,

> "August father . . . I know the name of the stranger!
> His name is love!"

Second, as suggested by Freud's interpretation of the painting, like the child in relation to Mary and St. Anne and Leonardo in relation to his childhood, the spectator, too, in an unexpected oedipal triangulation, becomes a child cradled by the voices of the two mother figures "who melt into a single form" in the scene.

In Rosenfeld's words, it seems to me that in this speech the defused instincts of love (Liù) and hate (Turandot), to simplify it to the bare minimum, merge together in a wonderful and touching moment of high melody.

For the first time in the opera Turandot is able to lower her narcissistic defences and open herself to an internal dialogue with the denied and feared part of herself, signalling in this way the dawn of her integration, which will, sadly, culminate in Liù's death.

Liù's death

In a letter Puccini wrote to his librettist Adami in early 1922, two years before his death, he didn't hide his wish to make the conclusion of his opera a great duet finale between Calaf and Turandot: ". . . this must reach the greatest possible heights of fantasy. . . . In this great duet, Turandot's ice gradually melts away. . . ." In the same letter he also talked about Liù, saying, "I think Liù must be sacrificed through suffering . . . and why not? This death can be an element in the softening of the Princess' heart" (in Greenfield, 1980, p. 268).

It was central henceforward in the Maestro's thoughts that Liù's death should be strongly connected with the resolution of Turandot's narcissistic defences.

But what is the significance of Liù's sacrifice, then, from a psychoanalytic point of view? Is the implicit idea that emotional growth in the end depends on maternal sacrifice if Liù has the role unconsciously of a maternal object?

Odgen, in his paper "The Music of What Happens", reports a session in which a patient, Ms S, speaks about her anxiety of finding herself perhaps less dependent on him and more able to have a mind of her own. He writes,

> I spoke with Ms S at the end of the meeting about her fear that having a mind and a voice and a life of her own would result in an end to the

> relationship with me that would feel so absolute as to feel like one or the other of us had died.
>
> [Ogden, 1999, p. 988]

It is interesting that in this session the patient brought a dream in which, as absurd as only a dream might be, her ability to swim in an ice-covered lake was contrasted with an image of a grass-covered statue of a woman who is able to cook. Odgen understood the grass-covered "cooking" statue as a sign of her increased capacity to be creative and independent, as opposed to the narcissistic icy state she had previously been "swimming in".

But whereas Ms S had the opportunity in her analysis to think through with her analyst about moving on in her life, with its correlated anxieties of losing the very person who was able to make her more independent, in Puccini's mind, on the other hand, Turandot's internal integration must come, instead, at the cost of the person who helped her in "softening her ice", as he so openly confessed to Adami.

In the opera the prince turns quickly from feeling sorrow about Liù's death back to his courtship of Turandot, who appears, once more, impenetrable to the emotional consequences of the death of her maternal object (Liù) and limits herself to playing the same reluctant adolescent role until the end, when she finally gives her love back to Calaf.

Margot Waddell, in the chapter cited above, speaks about the process of becoming an adult and recognizes that at the bottom of this experience lies the challenges of the depressive position:

> . . . the realistic estimation of the actual qualities of the other . . . the capacity to bear the loss of the external presence, but nonetheless to retain that presence internally in the face of absence . . ."
>
> [Waddell, 1998b, p. 192]

In the absence of a real protagonist, a third, who could mourn Liù's departure, I am left wondering whether it is the audience's tears, my tears, that are flowing while listening to Liù's heart-breaking final words—the only emotional space for mourning the loss of the princess's (and the audience's) maternal object.

> "Yes, Princess, listen to me!
> You, who are enclosed in ice,
> Conquered by such flame,
> You will love him, too!
> Before the dawn,
> I will wearily close my eyes,
> So He can win again.
> And I'll never see him more!"
>
> [Act 3, Scene 1, Lines 184–191]

. . . and as soon as she has said this, she suddenly seizes a dagger from a soldier and stabs herself to death.

Conclusion

To return to a question I raised at the beginning of the chapter, and in the light of my exploration of the opera, I find it highly arguable whether Puccini actually renounced *"in toto"* values belonging to the Verismo, such as sweetness and humility in *Turandot's* heroines, unless one discounts Liù as one of the main protagonists of the opera. I wonder whether the authors Greenfield and Conrad, who claimed such a thesis, were somehow blinded by Turandot's powerful use of projective identification and splitting off defences, which resulted in them not being able to value, in Waddell's words (1998b), "the realistic estimation of the actual qualities of the other", the other, in this context, being Liù.

It is known that Puccini composed the opera up to the point of Liù's death, after which, in some kind of symbiotic emotional resonance, his own health gradually deteriorated until, before long, he died. The task of finishing the opera was passed to Alfano, who carefully followed the maestro's original sketches and completed the opera in the form it is generally performed today (Greenfield, 1980). This has put many directors in the position of having to choose: should the opera end where Puccini stopped writing, or continue with Alfano's ending?

Within the context of this chapter, I have personally opted to end my analysis exactly where the maestro left it, leaving me with some questions about my reasons for doing so. By stopping with Liù's death, am I reluctant to describe a somewhat adolescent love, the one between Calaf and Turandot at the end of the story, which is seemingly capable of denying the loss of the maternal object that enabled them to fall in love?

Or did I want to give dignity to Liù's version of love, which, instead, celebrates values like dependence and sacrifice—antidotes to Turandot's narcissistic poison?

Or, alternatively, by having chosen not to continue with the analysis, am I finding it difficult to indulge in further thinking and move on from both Liù's and the composer's deaths, which, seeing them as a parental couple, would leave me with no other task other than to separate from them and become independent?

I started this journey of analysing *Turandot* by stepping inside the womb of the theatrical performance and losing myself in a child-like position in face of the extraordinary performances of the male, female, and choral voices. Rustin and Rustin, referring to an observation made by Esther Bick on infants in interaction with their mothers, describe the audience sitting immobile in a theatre as an experience in which "we too may feel rather baby-like in our anticipation of what will come our way, waiting for a degree of tension and longing of the excitement of the song and dance which will unfold" (M. E. Rustin & Rustin, 2006, p. 2).

As I now step outside the theatre, I know I won't be "waiting for a degree of tension and longing of the excitement of the song to unfold" any longer.

I know there won't be the "vast range of sound" to listen to and to lose myself in, nor "displays of light, movement and colour" to admire and be amazed by (M. E. Rustin & Rustin, 2006, p. 2). I know, instead, that once the stage curtain is closed and the lights are switched off, I will now have to face what comes next: the echo of the silence and the void of the empty theatre . . . and, as I am now touching on them, I have the impression, but it is just an impression, of glimpsing once again Liù's feeble halo reverberating in the dark.

Acknowledgement

I would like to thank Anna Lush who advised on the musical elements.

Notes

1 https://www.murashev.com/opera/Turandot_libretto_English_Italian
2 Wiener Staatsoper, directed by Lorin Maazel, 1983, with Eva Marton (Turandot), Jose Carreras (The Unknown Prince), and Katia Ricciarelli (Liù) (https://www.youtube.com/watch?v=jkPuXzjpL-g&t=20s).

CHAPTER TWELVE

Identity, identification and narcissistic phantasy in the Novels of Kazuo Ishiguro

Diana Webster Thomas

Ishiguro, trauma, and history

Kazuo Ishiguro, born in Nagasaki in 1954, came to Britain in 1960, aged 5. His books are best sellers and have won many prizes, and three have been adapted for films,[1] with his work translated currently into some 36 languages. This chapter about his novels begins with some reflections on their distinctive qualities, and on how a psychoanalytic perspective, and especially one drawing on post-Kleinian ideas and their focus on narcissism, can be illuminating in understanding them.

Ishiguro's narratives intersect with troubled times in history: times of war or social upheaval, and the weakening of some of the stable institutions that provided authority and containment. Ishiguro has commented that he is not primarily "interested in the solid facts [of history]". Instead, "the focus . . . is elsewhere, in the emotional upheaval" (Ishiguro, quoted in Mason, 1986). What drew me to his novels, and arrested me on reading each one, was the gap between the trauma and emotional pain suffered in childhood in such turbid times and the calm, deliberate tone of the texts. Salman Rushdie (1989) captures this quality in his observation on *The Remains of the Day*: "Just below the understatement of the novel's surface is a turbulence as immense as it is slow."

Many of Ishiguro's characterizations, often via protagonists' first-person narrations, show us enacted psychological defences of which the narrators

DOI: 10.4324/9781003564867-16

are largely unaware as they struggle to preserve their sense of dignity and self-worth. Pathos lies in the dramatic irony that they do not know the true nature of their actions and cannot know that they do not. Ishiguro's ways of managing psychic pain in the texts link in many aspects to those behaviours and attitudes explored within the psychoanalytic study of narcissism.

Critics of Ishiguro mention the "psychology", the "interiority", the "internal", and "identity" in his novels, and several have made pertinent links with Freud. But it is the Object Relations psychoanalytic theory of narcissism, with its solid body of research and clinical experience, that provided the tool with which I could best explore the states of mind and behaviours of Ishiguro's narrators. The post-Kleinians, in particular, address the extremes of painful emotional upheaval and catastrophic change, such as those traumas of war and social upheaval in the novels, and they theorize the defences that are activated to protect the subject from psychic disintegration.

Ishiguro produces responses for readers through the way he evokes the extreme states of mind and feeling of ordinary people and their need for self-respect and dignity. He explores, especially, their hopes and expectations in love and work, and the pain that comes of disappointment (if it is recognized), the sense of partly wasted lives, and of time as finite. His writing can also offer the pleasures of irony, word-play, imagery, inter-textual allusion, subversion of genre, and the humour of incongruity. With both pathos and detachment for the reader, the huge response to his work suggests that it penetrates a substantial area of contemporary psychological experience.

Within each novel, Ishiguro describes or alludes to the narrator's childhood trauma and failures of dependency, and in so doing points to the emotional origin of the psychic defences. He shows the psychic mechanisms that produce their defensive psychic structures, and the ensuing behaviours, idiom, and personal relationships peculiar to each narrator. As a way of understanding this writing, I propose the psychoanalytic dynamic of trauma, identity, identification, and narcissistic phantasy, arguing that the authentic self (ego) becomes invisible through excessive projective identification and the re-introjection of a distorted self. I also show how Ishiguro figuratively represents such states of mind, using the aesthetic resources of language, and "expands" the conventions of the novel to embody his themes. It was illuminating later to find that Ishiguro, in interviews (for example, Krider,1998/2008, pp. 132–133), had coined his own term for the psychoanalytic process of projective identification: "appropriation". He describes the inhering process of psychically taking for oneself another person to expel one's unbearable experiences and feelings attributively *into* or to acquire or extract the desirable *from*.

A framework for reading

The question of a critical template for my work was a challenge, in view of I. A. Richards' tenet that criticism requires both an account of value and an account of communication (Richards, 1924, p. 25). Hitherto, most psychoanalytic literary critics have focused on the values in the content of the work as suited their interests.[2] However, as Ishiguro is a considerable stylist and embodies narcissistic states of mind in the forms of his prose, I resolved to include the dimensions both of values and of literary techniques in this study.

It was necessary to briefly identify the humanism with which the historical continuities of the English novel and its concerns with reality, self-knowledge, and moral and psychological consciousness were consistent with the psychoanalytic approaches of Klein—approaches rooted in, but developing from, Freud. This, then, linked to those of post-Kleinian development, but focusing on severe trauma and borderline cases. These preoccupations complement Ishiguro's own psychological and ethical interests, along with his writing methods, which he views as simply *expanding* the territory from a late twentieth-/twenty-first-century perspective.

Ishiguro, in his interviews, sees himself as using an "in-between" version of the traditional humanist model by adopting some deconstructive tactics in his writing. Eagleton (1983, pp. 133–134) points out that deconstructive approaches to language allow for the fact that "one term of an antithesis secretly inheres with the other" and that words might be defined in terms of their opposites and derivations. The idea of such porous boundaries in language struck me as a relevant literary analogue here of the narcissist's dissolution of personal boundaries of the "other", by regarding him as an extension of the self through projective identification. Sodré's (2004) clinical commentary, entitled "Who's Who? Notes on Pathological Identifications", illustrates this action of the mind. Ishiguro frequently uses words of "merging", such as foggy and floating, also to suggest this. His expressions of fluidity and drifting, likewise embody the way the memory slides in and out of time past and present, often distorting events and relationships in the process.

Ishiguro, with the post-Kleinians, also perceives that with trauma, there is a loss of affect, and since *meaning* is rooted in feelings and inter-subjectivity, a diminished capacity for symbolization, and therefore thinking, results. His narrators speak in subtly limited idioms. He ironically subverts the humanist, realist novel—the novel of consciousness and progress to self-knowledge—showing it in its *failed* form. I call this, here, "the deficit model" and have devised a critical framework for discussing the novels derived from three complementary sources. It allows critical reading to hold in tension:

1. a humanist model
2. a post-modernist-ironic/deconstructive model
3. a Kleinian-post-Kleinian account of human behaviour and experience

Ishiguro holds these within ethical and reality constants, producing a realist surface and the slow turbulence that Rushdie describes. The tensions are vivid. The self-knowledge and resolution, typical of the traditional-humanist plot outcome, for example, is undercut by protagonists' weak self-knowledge and in the indeterminacies of the later deconstructive turn, likewise rendered in terms of inviting the Kleinian visions of fragmented-dissociative experience.

I offer this critical framework, suggesting it is responsive to the central theme of my study—Ishiguro's "emotional upheaval"—that is, the defensive mind in action as it deals with trauma. The novels demand such a critical framework that draws together three strands of knowledge: an implied background of the values and writing conventions of the novel in the traditional humanist tradition; a subtle subversion of this model in its ironic, post-modernist register by the judicious use of some deconstructive narrative tactics—my "deficit" model—to convey the emotional depletions of narcissism; and, third, a coherent, psychoanalytic theory, rooted in clinical work—post-Kleinian object relations theory. The Kleinian ethical and reality-seeking imperatives and the notion of countertransference are retained, but the focus is on catastrophic change, trauma, borderline states of mind, and narcissism. These dynamics and themes characterize all of Ishiguro's novels in various and evolving ways. Through his explorations of post-apocalyptic trauma in *A Pale View of Hills* (1982) and the vicissitudes of narcissism and creativity in *Artist of the Floating World* (1986) and *The Unconsoled* (1995), Ishiguro's novels support an attentiveness informed by the post-Kleinian theoretical approach and the broader framework set out.[3]

The Remains of the Day

I want now to further explore the value of this approach via a close reading of just one of Ishiguro's novels—perhaps his best-known work, *The Remains of the Day* (ROTD). Ishiguro explores a fractured period: England before and after the Second World War, and the impoverished emotional life of the butler-narrator, Stevens, in service at Darlington Hall, and its aristocratic owner, Lord Darlington. The novel is a firm reminder that while Ishiguro is certainly a psychologically attuned writer, evoking elusive states of mind, his novels also subtly envelop powerful social and historical themes.

The Remains of the Day (1989) is often known via James Ivory's 1993 film version, in which many will remember the performances in the principal roles of Anthony Hopkins and Emma Thompson. Partly because of such adaptations, Ishiguro enjoys enormous reach, with a readership both sophisticated and popular. He says: "I don't share the cynicism about the dumbed-down audience. There's an audience out there that's literate in many kinds of way . . . hungry for new adventures" (quoted in Groes, 2011, p. 261).

In *The Remains of the Day,* Ishiguro subverts the genre of English country house novel concerning the personal lives of the aristocratic families, with the minor, servant, characters from "downstairs" used as comic foils or confidantes, P. G. Wodehouse's Jeeves (1916) being the most notable example. This novel can also be seen as a critique of the English novels in which the house represents the moral values of the householder, such as Jane Austen's *Mansfield Park,* E. M. Forster's, *Howards End,* or Evelyn Waugh's *Brideshead Revisited.*

Identity, dignity, and crisis

Across his work, Ishiguro finds numerous ways to explore the question of identity, often linked to the sense of dignity and self-worth, whether by the clones in *Never Let Me Go* (2005) or in the musings of artists in *Artist of the Floating World* or *The Unconsoled. The Remains of the Day* provides an extended narrative frame within which to witness such explorations, often specifically in term of *dignity.* Stevens, the country house butler, is prone to extend reflections on matters of identity and worth.

> [P]rofessional prestige lay . . . in the moral worth of one's employer. . . . [T]he world was a wheel . . . with these great houses at the hub . . . each of us harboured a desire to make our small contribution to the creation of a better world . . . [and] serve the great gentlemen of our times in whose hands civilisation had been entrusted.
>
> [Ishiguro, 1989, pp. 115–116]

Stevens again:

> [T]oo many people believe themselves capable of working at these higher levels without having the least idea of the exacting demands involved. It is certainly not suited to just anybody.
>
> [p. 172]

Ishiguro articulates here an interest in the human need to be not "just anybody" or a nobody, but to have a place, an identity, moral worth, self-respect, and the respect of others. Kleinian language might further suggest a good object at the core of one's emotional being.

Stevens, adrift in the rupturing sociocultural climate of the mid-twentieth century, has believed in good faith, but misguidedly, that impeccable work and unswerving loyalty to Lord Darlington, to the exclusion of all else, was the route to a fulfilled and morally estimable life.

In this novel, the central character's narcissism is dominated by acquisitive projective identification—*I am you*—and a delusory grasp of reality. Stevens, in late middle age, reaches a painful awakening to his wasted hopes for love and for dignity in work.

The historical context is important in view of the way Stevens' memories reach back to the fragmenting earlier half of the twentieth century from the vantage point of the 1950s and the sale of Darlington Hall. This was the time of the collapsing Empire, the recent humiliation of the Suez Crisis, and a weakened Great Britain. Stevens has suffered a loss of identity with the break-up of the culture of large aristocratic houses and the slow fracture of the social class system. Stevens, now an ageing servant, has endured cumulative social and private trauma.

In a meticulous account, no mention is ever made of a mother. The primary, core object is either absent or dead; there is the loss of his older brother, Leonard, killed in the Boer War in a very "un-British" (dishonourable) attack on a village, and an elderly father, who has had to be taken in as "staff" and has died on the job, at the age of 72. He has endured the humiliation of knowing that his Lord Darlington, with whom he has identified and idealized, had been publicly shamed, among others, as a Nazi sympathizer before and during the Second World War.

Darlington Hall has been a self-enclosed community with the owner–Lord as the head of household and including the servants. By mid-century, many such houses had been sold off to affluent Americans, who pursued their own versions of English living. In this case, the new American owner, Mr Farraday, has included Stevens, the genuine English butler, in his purchase as part of the package.

The title, *The Remains of the Day*, suggests the routine clearing of guests' leftovers: the dregs of time that remain after a lifetime's service, and the decline of all hopes and expectations;[4] and a further level, Freud's "day's residues" or "*Tagesrestes*" (Freud, 1900a), which surface in dreams or in re-enactions in the external world. Such fragments represent wish-fulfilment, internal conflict, or "split off", intolerable experience akin to Stevens' half-buried memories, emerging as he motors towards the West Country to meet Miss Kenton, the housekeeper at Darlington Hall twenty years earlier, apparently to replenish his staff plan. Time, in Stevens' emotional world, has barely moved, as he recalls himself and Miss Kenton in the 1920s, when they were both young, at the top of their professions, and the mainstays of one of the most prestigious English country houses.

The plot is minimal. It is 1956; Lord Darlington has been dead three years; the House, now owned by the American, Mr Farraday, is half-empty, covered in dust sheets, and to be unoccupied for five weeks. Stevens is now older and making errors and needs to add to his staff. At the surface level, the question, Stevens believes, is a professional one. As he had received a brief, friendly letter from Miss Kenton, the former Housekeeper (who has been Mrs Benn for twenty years); he has construed, in phantasy, that because she has briefly left her husband three times and is currently staying with a friend, her marriage must be over, and she must want a home and her old position back. As part of a short motoring holiday in the West Country, with petrol paid for, he will make up his new staff plan by bringing back Miss Kenton.

At an unconscious level, the plot question is whether or not this journey—his first away from Darlington Hall—is a quest for love and companionship. He might, in post-Kleinian terms, be object-seeking, retrieving a relationship that had been previously psychically "split off" as unacceptable. Had he been impervious to her affection because of a lifetime's misplaced loyalty to his late master, Lord Darlington? Stevens is socially and relationally adrift. His is a journey towards self-knowledge, albeit with a tentative ending.

Structurally, the outside frame story is Stevens' six-day solitary car journey to the West Country, and, in counterpoint, the inner story is his selective, self-idealizing journey through memories of his life during the past decades at Darlington Hall. They focus on the climax of his career, the 1923 secret international conference, with Miss Kenton as housekeeper, in Darlington Hall. It is circular—almost a round trip, but with some important geographic and psychic detours on the way.

In this novel, the short car journey focuses firmly on the nature and quality of Stevens' relationships: I therefore explore Stevens' behaviour in relation to his three significant figures, Lord Darlington, his father, Stevens Senior, and Miss Kenton/Mrs Benn, the housekeeper. I comment on the states of mind Ishiguro devises, narcissistic forms of omnipotent thinking and action, namely: denial, control, grandiosity, triumph, smugness, and disparagement. I discuss the metaphors of landscape and architecture to do with perspective, especially on the presence or absence of "view" and windows, as ways of seeing reality.

Stevens: identity and identification

The important theme of losing identity emerges as Stevens, self-idealizing, identifies acquisitively and omnipotently with his own notion of greatness and dignity through his role as a great butler to a morally distinguished Lord of a great house. He also identifies with the English landscape in a way comparable with the "undifferentiated identification" of Rosenfeld (1964, p. 172),[5] claiming it to be:

> "the most deeply satisfying in the world . . . best summed up in the word, 'greatness'. . . I distinctly felt that rare and unmistakable feeling . . . that one is in the presence of 'greatness' . . . we call our country Great Britain . . . the landscape of our country alone would justify the use of this lofty adjective. . . . I would say that it is the very lack of obvious drama or spectacle that sets the beauty of our land apart . . . the calmness of that beauty, its *sense of restraint*."
>
> [1989, pp. 28–29, emphasis added]

The reader, however, begins to perceive a poignant irony in that Stevens is a limited, uneducated, un-travelled man, who has already stated: "It has been my privilege to see the best of England, sir, within these very walls [Darlington Hall]" (p. 4). He has known the English countryside only vicariously, from reading Mrs Jane Symons's out-of-date guide book, *The Wonder of England*, yet he positions himself as "any objective observer" (p. 28).

Stevens believes that his aim in life is to achieve "that balance between attentiveness and the illusion of absence that is essential to good waiting" (p. 72). He is concerned with his performance for others, rather than the idea of being himself. He is immersed in self-idealizing within a myth of Englishness, claiming that,

> "[B]utlers only truly exist in England . . . other countries have only man servants", declaring that, "Continentals . . . and Celts are as a breed incapable of the emotional restraint required . . . dignity is beyond such persons. . . . as with] the great butler . . . it is with the English landscape, . . . one simply *knows* one is in the presence of greatness."
>
> [pp. 43–44, original emphasis]

Stevens conflates role with identity when he says, of dignity:

> "[A] butler must not abandon the professional being he *inhabits* . . .great butlers are great by virtue of their ability to *inhabit* their professional role and *inhabit* it to the utmost . . .they wear their professionalism as a decent gentleman will wear his suit."
>
> [pp. 42–43, emphasis added]

A butler of any quality, he declares, must be seen to *inhabit his role utterly*. He cannot just don it when it suits him, like a "pantomime costume", or drop it like a "façade", to reveal the actor beneath.

But the role inhabits *him* to the exclusion of any personality derived from inter-subjective exchanges and the "sense of oneself as a creator of meanings" (Ogden, 1986, p. 217). Stevens adds, more tellingly, that role can only be relinquished when one is "entirely alone" (1989, p. 169), for in his view, personal relationships are a distraction. At this stage, the notions of relating naturally to others in a spirit of mutuality, and of the value of relationships per se in giving meaning to life, are entirely outside his consciousness.

Stevens' preoccupation with clothing shows how he both disguises and reveals his need for professional cover to cloak his emotional life. In the prologue, planning his trip, he considers his "costume": either a new travelling outfit or one of Lord Darlington's old suits, old-fashioned and formal, which he has inherited. But, then, as he sees himself as a special kind of son and heir, these suits seem appropriate.

Similarly, Stevens, as the first-person narrator, is given an idiom that obscures the self and conveys his emotional dissociation. In object-relations terms, his mode of symbolization, like his clothing, is designed to mask the self and exclude emotion. The code of "butler-speak" is formal, formulaic, functional, emotionless and distancing, derivative, and circumlocutory, with double negatives and balanced syntax.

Interpersonal dialogue, elegant or otherwise, he never engages in, as spontaneous, natural exchanges are not seemly. He often refers to himself via the depersonalized "one" or "one's person", and houseguests as "distinguished personages". Such language is inappropriate in crucial emotional situations, such as Miss Kenton's bereavement or his father's dying. His own feelings of grief and disappointment are disguised by "a laugh" or said to be "strange". When Miss Kenton seeks permission to close his dead father's eyes, he can say only:

> "Please don't think me unduly improper in not ascending the stairs to see my father in his deceased condition just at the moment. . . . I know my father would have wished me to carry on just now. . . . To do otherwise, I feel, would be to let him down."
>
> [p. 196]

It is possible that the "him" is Lord Darlington, his psychically adopted father, with whom he identifies (Segal, 1983, p. 270).[6]

Lord Darlington

Stevens' relationship with Lord Darlington is the significant one of his life. By 1923, Lord Darlington has become Stevens' replacement, class-father through the process of acquisitive projective identification, intensified by moral narcissism and his phantasy of himself as the indispensable facilitator in their "joint" efforts at the *hub* of international diplomacy for peace. This was not an unreasonable aim, after the recent horrors of the First World War.

Stevens believes he has found both moral worth and a landed aristocratic family in the single and childless Lord Darlington.

For Stevens, the central question is the "great" butler and who ranks within that exclusive elite? (pp. 29–33) He implies that *he* is it, despite his self-deprecation. Professional prestige, he claims, lies in the moral worth of one's employer, "who needs to be an enlightened force for good . . . furthering the progress of humanity" (p. 114). Stevens re-internalizes aspects of Darlington, casting himself as a top professional (acquisitive projective identification), *morally* superior, and contributing towards a better world. His destiny is to enable, to facilitate, those "in whose hands civilisation has been entrusted" (p. 116): aristocrats and members of the Foreign Office in high social and political circles. This is a distorted self-view.

Stevens sees the world as a wheel at the hub of which are the great houses where the real political debates and key decisions are held in privacy and calm. He, himself, is at the hub of Darlington Hall, masterminding the privacy and calm, much as a General masterminds manoeuvres on the battlefield, for "History could well be made under this roof" (p. 77). Without him, the top-secret conferences cannot effectively take place, nor the mighty, international decisions made.

Stevens' narcissistic identification with Darlington defends him from, for example, the humiliating interrogations by two guests who, late one night, quiz him in order to ridicule his lack of knowledge of world affairs (pp. 194–196). It is poignant to see that Stevens is out of his depth, explaining that such things are out of his "realm", unaware that Lord Darlington, too, is out of his depth in believing that democracy is outmoded and that countries should be run by strong (fascist) leaders, as in Germany and Italy (p. 198).

The last word of the chapter in which Stevens sums up the secret international conference, is "triumph" (p. 110), signifying that narcissistic defence with an element of sadistic gratification over the "other". And he is triumphant. Stevens' self-deprecation, with his sententious "my humble standards" and "I do not delude myself", show his pride in the compliments and a real need for some narcissistic self-congratulation.

Lord Darlington belongs to the network of European aristocrats and gentlemen whose narrow code of honour includes being sporting to past enemies. He *is* uncritical, self-focused, and amateur. Ishiguro implies that his efforts might even have been driven by personal homo-erotic motives, to do with his very dear German officer friend, Herr Bremann, who visited Darlington Hall in officer's uniform just after the First World War and returned at regular intervals. It was a "close" friendship; Darlington spoke of him "with intensity" and visited Berlin several times in 1920 (p. 71).

Given Stevens' unthinking, acquisitive loyalty, he embraces Lord Darlington's anti-Semitism (pp. 146–147), sacking the two Jewish maids without a qualm, despite Miss Kenton's outrage (pp. 148–149). Later, in a spirit of narcissistic triumph, he taunts her by asking why she has not already left the house since she had been so shocked. She admits that she has nowhere to go. She, however, uses her mind independently, while Stevens evades thought, regarding politics as "out of my realm". Towards the end (pp. 224–225), Stevens recalls Mr Cardinal's exasperation with him:

> "Are you not at least *curious* about what I am saying?"

His own typical reply is,

> "I have every trust in his lordship's good judgement."
>
> [p. 225]

He has to hear out Cardinal's ruthless exposé of how Darlington, his godfather, had been Hitler's most instrumental pawn, but Stevens refuses to see himself as a pawn of the pawn.

By 1956, Stevens' ego has been so depleted in projection that he has a deficit of "observation and judgement". Stevens has no independent voice and so far does not want one, but during his disturbing journey west in Mr Farraday's Ford, he re-delivers his views on greatness in the unfamiliar territory of Moscombe, a small village in Devon where he gets lost in every sense.

After the hillside view of the "perfect" English pastoral landscape near Salisbury, Stevens encounters a more disturbing view from the twisting lane on the hill in Devon, where he breaks down. He is no longer self-sufficient, having run out of petrol and radiator water, nor is he entirely protected from other views of Englishness. Trampling through the pastureland to get help, he finds the turn-ups of his "aristocratic suit" soiled and his fixed attitudes disturbed.

Mr Harry Smith, an ordinary middle-class Englishman, argues the case for democracy, declaring that whatever your social level, you have the right to express your opinion freely: it is "what we fought Hitler for—otherwise we'd just be slaves now" (p. 186).

In Moscombe, however, with Mr Farraday's car and Lord Darlington's old suit, Stevens is unwittingly in "role" and mistaken for a Lord himself. He is reckoned to speak almost like a gentleman, but if the locals are deceived, the doctor is not, tactfully asking if he were some sort of *manservant*. Stevens accepts the term with some relief, although in his prime he had held it in utter contempt.

In retrospect, Stevens rejects "mindless loyalty", judging his to have been trustingly and "*intelligently* bestowed" (200, original emphasis); that the likes of him can never be in full possession of the facts and have to trust. He adds, defiantly,

> "It is hardly my fault if his lordship's life and work have turned out today to look, at best, a sad waste—and it is quite illogical that I should feel any regret or shame on my own account."
>
> [p. 201]

Father

Throughout the journey, memories of Stevens' butler-father rise to the surface, although none recalls a loving, containing parent. By the end, at Darlington Hall, they speak with mutual embarrassment (p. 64). Stevens identifies with him as a butler rather than a father, retaining this as a shadowy ego-ideal. He allows that his father *was* a dignified butler, despite no command of language, a poor accent, and no general knowledge. His recollections are not personal but reside only in some defining set-piece anecdotes, the most vivid of which recalls his father's gifts as a raconteur and as judge of professional qualities.

He tells of his father's tale of another admirable butler in India, who failed to panic on discovering a tiger under the dining room table, shot it with the twelve-bore gun prior to a grand dinner party, and announced:

> "Dinner will be served at the usual time and I am pleased to say that there will be *no discernible traces left*."
>
> [p. 36, emphasis added]

Stevens senior, like his son, found dignity in the impression of "absence" with no "discernible traces" left—but only up to a point.

When the elderly father arrives at Darlington Hall in 1922, having neither home nor savings after a lifetime in service, the power relations between father and son are reversed. Father enters the story as an under-butler, although Stevens, out of the respect owed to himself, insists that he retain some status and be called Stevens Senior, not simply William. In any case, this father has long been replaced by the admired father-mentor, Lord Darlington.

Either out of staff protocol or an oedipal need to control (if not kill) the father, Stevens does not make father's room comfortable, nor communicate with him except as staff. During this time, Stevens denies the fact of his father's failing powers, which have to be pointed out repeatedly to him by Miss Kenton. These he dismisses with contemptuous irritation: the dustpan and brush unattended in the entrance hall, the china statues displaced, the dripping nose while serving at table, or a silver fork, found with traces of polish on it. Then, finally, one day, walking up to the summer house, Stevens senior trips, falls over in front of everyone, and drops a loaded tea-tray. Eventually, Lord Darlington himself remarks, "these errors are trivial in themselves: but you must yourself realise their larger significance" (p. 59). Stevens agrees that they could undermine the secret international meeting, so dear to them both.

The professional end of Father, the second fall, is devastating in its narcissistic inhumanity. Stevens, unfamiliar with his father's bleak quarters, is surprised how high up some rickety stairs the room is, how like a prison cell, and that there is no "view" apart from roof-tiles. Father has been up three hours already, and is in uniform. He is addressed by his son in the third-person passive voice, as if he were an abstract entity. The harsh early morning light enhances the harsh rigour of their conversation. The father is contemptuous and humiliates the son; the son is omnipotent and depersonalizes father.

> "I have come here to relate something to you, Father."
>
> "Then relate it briefly and concisely. I haven't all morning to listen to you chatter. . . ."
>
> "Father has become increasingly infirm. . . . His Lordship is of the view as indeed, I am myself, that while Father is allowed to continue with his present round of duties, he represents an ever-present threat to the smooth running of this household, and in particular, to next week's important international gathering. . . . It has been felt that Father should no longer be asked to wait at table, whether or not guests are present."
>
> [pp. 64–65]

The climax to Stevens' professional career is the unofficial international conference of 1923, and present are the German ambassador, Ribbentrop, selected American and French diplomats, and English Nazi sympathizers. But Ishiguro has Stevens senior collapse over his cleaning trolley in a grotesquely comic attitude of obeisance. Father is taken up to his room. He is 72, and has had a stroke.

During the following conference day, Stevens, on his father's instructions, is summoned upstairs but feels that he cannot be spared and eventually attends briefly. He appears oblivious to the significance of the situation: clearly, his father is dying, and equally clearly, Stevens presents himself as unaware that Father is trying to say goodbye.

> "My father opened his eyes and turned his head a little upon the pillow and looked at me."
>
> "I hope Father is feeling better now", I said. . . ."
>
> "Everything in hand downstairs?"
>
> "The situation is rather volatile . . ."
>
> "An impatient look crossed my father's face. 'But is everything in hand?' he said again."
>
> "Yes, I dare say you can rest assured on that. I'm very glad Father is feeling better."

Stevens' evasion of intimacy continues,

> "He went on looking at his hands for a moment. Then he said slowly: 'I hope I've been a good father to you.' "
>
> "I laughed a little and said: 'I'm so glad you're feeling better now.' "
>
> "I'm proud of you. A good son. I hope I've been a good father to you. I suppose I haven't. . . ."
>
> " 'I'm so glad you're feeling better now, . . .' and took my leave."
>
> [p. 97]

Stevens remembers the banqueting hall, the delegates, and the conflicting pressures in immense detail, as opposed to the bleak account of his dying father. Miss Kenton has called a doctor, who is waylaid by the French delegate for his blisters, while Stevens maintains the conviviality of the conference with port, denying any feelings of irretrievable loss.

Miss Kenton/Mrs Benn

As Stevens drives westward, expecting to recruit "Miss Kenton" for Darlington Hall, he considers his relationship with someone who has been Mrs Benn for 20 years. He omnipotently overrides the reality of the boundaries of time, oblivious to two decades' worth of enormous change. Consciously, he believes that his past connections with Miss Kenton were professional, with him always in control.

Alone, off-duty in his pantry, Stevens would often read romances, experiencing love vicariously. He was appalled when the real Miss Kenton once came in, making playful comments about his reading and teasing him about some pretty maids. His pantry—the box-like, viewless, "prison cell" room—is, metaphorically, a "psychic retreat" (Steiner, 1993, p. xi). It is a refuge or sanctuary in which Stevens remains stuck, denying flexible thought and strong feelings such as love and compassion.

As he drives, Stevens's mind uncovers "turning points" in their relationship. When he claims that he, too, was distressed by the sacking of the Jewish maids, Miss Kenton is exasperated, saying, "Why, Mr Stevens, why, why, why do you always have to *pretend?*" (p. 153). Just to share his feelings at that moment would have helped her to feel less alone in Darlington Hall. When Miss Kenton's aunt, her only "mother", died, Stevens was glad that she remained composed and felt only a "strange" sense that behind her closed door, she was weeping. He hovered for a while, but instead of offering sympathy or comfort or even being aware of the sadistic edge to his behaviour, he narcissistically denigrated her work by criticizing her new maids.

When Kenton had carefully trained a new employee to be a good housekeeper, perhaps as a replacement if she, Kenton, were to marry, she asked him if, at the top of his career, he might wish for something more. He remained impervious to her meaning, declaring undying loyalty to Lord Darlington until his destiny in history should be completed. He was faintly contemptuous of her intention to marry a butler gone into business in the neighbouring village. He twice offered perfunctory congratulations, then smugly added, "there are matters of global significance taking place upstairs and I must return to my post" (p. 219).

As he drives closer to their meeting, a faint memory of her weeping behind her door resurfaces. Stevens has stood outside many doors as an over-hearer, an on-looker, detached, dissociated, and living vicariously. Miss Kenton's letter had mentioned one happy time of their enjoying a view *together,* which Stevens recalls with something like yearning.

Now, late in the narrative, Stevens seems to be thinking of it in connection with his broadening perspective, his own lost time, and potential closeness with Miss Kenton (pp. 67, 180). He knows that Kenton is spirited, independent and has true dignity, having sometimes challenged his intransigence in her own critical voice. And she has empathy for others, having watched over his dying father, closing his eyes in death.

Lord Darlington has been dead three years, and Stevens is struggling with the new freedom that Mr Farraday offers him. He re-reads Miss Kenton's letter. It is sad and nostalgic, but she does not ask to return to Darlington Hall. His first response to it is one of extended narcissistic condescension, in which he projects his own emptiness attributively into her.

> ". . . It is of course tragic that her marriage is now ending in failure. . .no doubt she is pondering with regret decisions that have left her, deep in middle age, so alone and desolate . . . of course, Miss Kenton cannot hope . . . ever to retrieve these lost years. . . ."
>
> [p. 48]

As Stevens approaches Cornwall, he re-reads the letter more realistically and concedes that it expresses no clear desire to return and that it may have been his own professional wishful thinking, given the errors he has been making now that he is older (p. 140). On the day before they meet, he checks the letter again, thinking that he may have read more into her lines than was wise. He retreats into denial, becomes emotionally disengaged, and says of their approaching interview, "aside from a few informal exchanges, it will be essentially a professional one", still assuming that her marriage has broken down and she is without a home (p. 180).

The day before he is to arrive at Little Compton, he again recalls his past failure to console her in her grief and begins to recognize time lost. He uses the depersonalizing pronoun "one" but cannot minimize the enormity of his failures to respond to a possible life companion by referring to their disagreements as "small incidents" and mere "misunderstandings", and hopes that are "forever irredeemable". He concludes,

> "[I]t was as though one had available a never-ending number of days, months, years in which to sort out the vagaries of one's relationship with Miss Kenton; an infinite number of further opportunities in which to remedy the effect of this or that misunderstanding. There was surely nothing to indicate at the time that such evidently small incidents would render whole dreams forever irredeemable."
>
> [p. 179]

Two days after their meeting, Stevens sits alone on a bench on the pier in Weymouth, an isolate, but with his feet on the ground. Now, he can *view* the end of his hopes with the "sun setting over the sea" but is waiting for the lights to come on. He has reached the turning point of his internal and external journeys. He now has a perspective on the "evening" of his life. He has met with Mrs Benn and seen reality for what it is.

Recalling their recent tea together, Stevens has noticed her graceful ageing and her pleasant defiance. Mrs Benn is still the person, he realizes, "who *inhabited* my memory over these years" (p. 232), recognizing in one of his favourite words, the existence of feelings (p. 236). He has had the shaming tale to tell of Lord Darlington's national disgrace and last empty years as an invalid. Mrs Benn assured Stevens that she certainly did *not* think that she had written of her life as stretching out like emptiness before her. Despite some periods of discontent, she will again return to her husband; she has a daughter and a grandchild coming.

Stevens' rigid, narcissistic psychic structure is liquefying as they wait at her bus stop in the drizzle, with the view of empty fields, intensifying Stevens's own emptiness. Only then does he ask her if she was unhappy, since she has left her husband three times. Mrs Benn had grown to love him, but she had sometimes wondered what life she might have had with him, Stevens. Her eyes fill with tears: it is too late for Stevens to reciprocate. All he can do is smile.

Only later, on the bench in Weymouth, does he allow a stranger beside him to know that "... at that moment, my heart was breaking" (p. 239). And only when envying the happy groups and couples on the pier can he tell this stranger: "It's no use. I've given what I had to give. I gave it all to Lord Darlington" (p. 243).

His own tears now flow for his disappointment at the loss of Miss Kenton, his misplaced identification with Lord Darlington, and his inner desolation. Ishiguro builds into the text many images of the hard, brittle psychic structures of defensive narcissism fragmenting and *dissolving* with the steady rain, the drizzle, a puddle, her tears, his tears, and his heart breaking.

The shame of recognition bursts out in his lament of narcissistic rage and disappointment as happens "when ... grandiose aspirations are found to be discrepant with reality, and this discrepancy is apparent to others" (Mollon, 2002, p. 34).

> "At least he [Darlington] had the privilege of being able to say at the end of his life that he made his own mistakes. ... He chose a certain path in life, it proved to be a misguided one, but there, he chose it, he can say that at least. As for myself, I cannot even claim that."
>
> [Ishiguro, 1989, p. 243]

As Stevens struggles to give meaning to a depleted life, he begins to perceive that ordinary people, "the likes of you and I ... try to make our small contribution count for something true and worthy." If you do make sacrifices to this end, "that is ... in itself, cause for pride and contentment" (p. 244). He observes those around him without trying to control them, noticing them *exchanging* (pp. 13, 245, emphasis added) one bantering remark after another and decides that the secret of human warmth resides in banter. Banter might be the start of the two-way, reciprocal exchanges that are part of containment and object relations.

Life in 1956 with his new American owner is disorientating. Mr Farraday does not worry about the silver, makes saucy jokes, gives him holidays, use of a car, and freedom. The ageing Stevens, who has neither friends nor family and a tendency to errors like his father, does not see any option other than returning to Darlington Hall, although other butlers in the story have retired or gone into business. He will relate to Mr Farraday and his "strange" American ways through "banter".

Bantering, as Stevens recalls near the beginning, might be a skill for which he has some flair (pp. 16–17), for although his joke fell flat, he knows the reason. Practising three witticisms a day (pp. 130–131) does not sound too promising, but with his awakening to human warmth and object relationships, Stevens might find a more solid personal identity and contentment in the evening of his days.

Stevens' psychic organization is now more flexible: not the earlier, rigid one of a butler whose behaviour was grandiose, denying, controlling, and disparaging. He is now a man capable of self-recognition, insight, and the acceptance of reality. While Stevens has made a circular external and an unexpected internal journey, there have been important detours in which he has psychically changed. Although he is left with only "remains" as internal objects, he is planning exchanges of human warmth in a changing national culture, from which he need not be dissociated.

Dedication

The thesis on which this article is based is dedicated to the memory of Jorge E. Thomas.

Notes

This chapter, which is drawn from its author's larger doctoral thesis, has been edited for publication in this book by Iain MacRury and Michael Rustin, who were her PhD supervisors.

1 At the time of writing.
2 Post-Kleinian psychoanalytic literary criticism has usually focused on the psychological thematic material in works of literature and bypassed matters of communication. Psychoanalytic critics, such as D. Bell, R. Britton, A. Hyatt-Williams, L. Miller, M. E. Rustin, M. J. Rustin, H. Segal, I. Sodré, J. Steiner, and M. Waddell, for example, are part of this tradition, using theory developed by Bion and Rosenfeld in the 1960s up to the present day. There is a significant literature relating earlier Kleinian psychoanalytic ideas to fiction, some of it contemporary with Kleinian development—for example, L. Stonebridge (1998, 2007), who writes on anxiety in mid-twentieth-century British fiction.

3 In the thesis-length account (Thomas, 2013), looking at all his works, I explore more fully the conventions of the novel form and the narrative strategies that embody Ishiguro's themes of fragmentation, expectation, and disappointment. Given the childhood traumas of his narrators, how does Ishiguro shape, in words, their states of mind, personal relationships, and plot trajectories, their language idioms and enactments? How are these rendered in the elliptical style of his prose?
4 The Earl of Halifax's autobiography, *Fullness of Days* (1957), sits ironically in this context of emotional emptiness. In the novel he is a real person who praises the silver at the Hall as a contributory factor in the apparent success of the 1923 secret international conference.
5 The separate identities of patient and analyst are not differentiated, as in Freud's "oceanic feeling".
6 Segal writes of the permanent narcissistic personality structure built up by the "re-internalization of the projectively possessed object".

PART IV

CONTEMPORARY LIFE

The premise underlying the Psychoanalytic Studies course is that any activity humans are involved in can be usefully thought about from a psychoanalytic perspective. This includes their relationship with the natural environment, as well as individual, group, and societal processes. Sometimes these explorations can lead to greater understanding of human behaviour on a deep level; at other times they can do little more than raise questions about possible unconscious processes and underlying motivations.

Given the freedom to write their Masters dissertation on whatever subject captures their imagination, students have chosen a huge range of topics over the years. Among many others, titles have included "The Greek Riots: A Psychosocial Approach"; "Is Homelessness a Choice? A Psychosocial Exploration of Rough Sleeping in the UK"; "To Tweet or Not to Tweet? A Psychosocial Exploration of Human Relationships on Twitter"; "Celebrity: Why Are We a Nation Obsessed?"; "Drowning or Waving? An Exploration of Fears and Fantasies Evoked by Swimming and Being in Water"; "Fascism and the Body–Mind Relationship"; "Latin American Migrant Women in the United Kingdom: A Psychoanalytic Perspective", and "Street Children: A Study of Some Psychoanalytic Aspects of Their Lives".

The titles above are not included here, but something of this diversity is represented in this fourth and final part under the broad heading, "Contemporary Life".

DOI: 10.4324/9781003564867-17

The first two chapters in Part IV (Chapters 13 and 14) were written some time ago. Yong Suk Lee's chapter on the Korean pop song, Psy's "Gentleman", was written not long after the song and music video became a worldwide hit, following its release in 2012; Gabrielle Smith's exploration of the sport of BASE jumping dates from around the same time. Although these essays date from a particular moment in time, the themes in each have a timeless quality—the unconscious dynamics revealed and the questions raised are as relevant now as they were at the time of writing.

The final two chapters (chapters 15 and 16) were written much more recently, during or soon after the 2020/21 Covid 19 pandemic period, and it is clear how influential the particular circumstances brought about by the pandemic have been on the authors, albeit in different ways.

Chapter 13, "Psy's 'Gentleman'—Between the Ugly and the Beautiful", explores the viewer's aesthetic response to the song and music video. Highlighting the polyphonic nature of the course's interdisciplinary approach and themes running through the present book, this chapter could equally well have found a home in one of the other parts: there is an implicit link with earlier chapters as Lee notes that, with its obscure lyrics but strong beat and rhythms, the emphasis in the brief video is on pre-verbal sound rather than verbal meaning. He quotes Hannah Segal (1991, p. 62), who states that "art embodies and symbolizes and evokes in the recipient a certain kind of archaic emotion of a preverbal kind", and, with the emphasis on pre-verbal emotion and nonverbal communication, we are again firmly grounded in the world of the infant and infantile states of mind, which were the focus of Part I and which form the bedrock of psychic life.

Lee explores the unconscious elements suggested in the song and video, and although oedipal dynamics are hinted at, he believes the main underlying processes are those of primary importance in Kleinian theory: destructiveness and repair. The psychological process of moving from destructiveness and ugliness to repair and beauty suggested in the brief video is compared to similar movements that unfold over much longer time frames in two substantial artistic works, one from Western and one from Eastern culture. Each of these has stood the test of time and become a classic. Lee raises interesting questions about whether music videos that are only a few minutes long can bring an aesthetic experience to the viewer, and, if so, what sort of aesthetic experience that might be. He questions whether there is something vital in the development from destructiveness to repair (the move from the paranoid–schizoid to the depressive position) that is captured in the longer works but missing in the brief video. He asks what might contribute to the greater emotional depth and the audience's deeper feeling of pain in relation to the opera and story he explores compared to their experience of the music video, which, despite its brevity, seems nonetheless to have captured something universal.

Reflecting the range of subject matter in this part, we then take a leap into Chapter 14, an ambitious investigation into BASE Jumping where Smith explores what motivates participants to take part in such a dangerous sport and what the implications might be when they live the dream of flying, rather than just dreaming it. She makes extensive use of BASE jumpers' own words as they paint a vivid picture of various aspects of their experience. Each individual will have their own relationship with the sport, influenced by their internal world and predominant states of mind, but what comes through strongly in Smith's chapter is the difficulty of making sense of the sport, as there are so many contradictory ways of understanding possible underlying motivations. As she says, "For every possibility there was an equal and opposite alternative". Important questions come to the fore—to what extent might participation in BASE jumping be motivated by the life instinct or the death instinct, or is it, as one jumper notes, the space between life and death that is important here? Is the sport deadly or life affirming, frontier-pushing or omnipotent and narcissistic? How might we understand the intrinsic balance between danger and reward? Does the strong group of BASE jumpers provide a healthy, supportive group structure, or might it act as a mafia-like gang, supporting group members to maintain a lack of contact with reality? Smith describes a sport filled with the tension of contradictory forces, fear versus a wish to fly, and of living on the edge. As one writer, Stephen Lyng, describes, it involves "negotiating the boundary between life and death, consciousness and unconsciousness, and sanity and insanity."

In this final part, which has the inherent quality of something coming to an end, all the chapters bring to mind "relationships to time" of one sort or another. The timespan of artistic structures, a particular moment in time for humanity, the passage of time, including looking back to the beginning of the Psychoanalytic Studies course and looking forward to the future, are all overtly addressed or present in the background. Contemplation of one's place in time and awareness of time past, present, and future necessitate being in touch with reality, but a different relationship with time seems to underlie some of the BASE jumpers' descriptions of a particular moment in their experience. One comments that when they step off the object, "What has happened has happened, what will happen will happen, and there's nothing I can do about either. I exist in that moment . . .". Another muses, ". . . when pushing off to jump, I never think about what's coming next. The past doesn't exist. The future doesn't exist. There's only now." The jumper takes responsibility for his survival through meticulous preparation and accumulated technical skill but with each jump, that begins with this moment of peace, there is still much that is unpredictable.

This leads us into the following chapter (Chapter 15), where we come firmly back down to earth, and themes of corporate and individual agency and responsibility are discussed. Leila Taheri explores how and why the Welsh Harp Nature Reserve in North London quickly deteriorated from a world-class wetland to a litter-strewn, unsightly dumping ground and how she and a group of volunteers were instrumental in returning it to a more pleasant and uplifting environment for wildlife and local people. She sets the study in the broader context of the worldwide plastics crisis, and she examines the intersection of individuals, society, and culture to understand the conditions that facilitate care for the environment. Thinking psychoanalytically about how individuals' inner lives interact with the outside world, she draws on relevant theories, including Meltzer's (1967) idea of the "toilet–breast mother". As a development of this idea, she introduces her own interesting concept of the "placenta womb–mother", which she sees as a more accurate description of a littering individual's phantasy relationship with the environment.

Taheri puts forward a convincing argument about the detrimental effects of the "culture of uncare" (Weintrobe, 2018), which, Weintrobe believes, activates the uncaring parts of the self, and Taheri describes her central role in engendering a culture of greater care towards the nature reserve within the responsible organizations and local population. In contrast to a culture of uncare, she describes a culture of care as one that "faces reality, recognizes the staggering scale of issues, and apologizes for past neglect"; she goes on to say, "Such a culture successfully mourns the fact that the earth is not a toilet–breast mother and has limitations".

This reality-based relationship to humankind's present and past misuse of the earth's resources, based in a depressive state of mind and a capacity to mourn, leads to a wish to make reparation, perhaps with the hope of leaving something better for those who come after us.

Part IV concludes with Clare Parkinson's "Beyond Competence in Social Work: Where Are We Now?" (Chapter 16). As well as again reflecting something of the range of subject matter that students engage with, this chapter links with the other strand of the book, which could be described as "thinking psychoanalytically about pedagogy". Here Parkinson looks back to her Masters dissertation, written more than 20 years ago, on the teaching of social work, and she revisits the content, considering to what extent there has or has not been progress since that time. She explores how social workers learn to practice, and whether there are opportunities for them to really learn from experience in their training in the way

Bion understood it. She explains Bion's "Theory of Thinking" (1962b) and makes use of this to consider whether and how professional bodies can help create conditions conducive to thinking, or perhaps do the opposite. She discusses Bion's view of omniscience as a substitute for thinking, and she suggests some of the dangers of an omniscient state of mind, such as the tendency towards a certainty that we can see prejudice in others rather than allow the challenge to our own sense of identity when we need to recognize it in ourselves.

Parkinson tracks developments over the last two decades, and she raises questions about what gets lost when the measure of trainee social workers' capabilities is based on whether or not they have met a particular competency in an individual area. What happens in those circumstances to reflective practice and the capacity to engage with complexity? Thoughts about the impact of the Black Lives Matter movement and recent greater recognition of the need to "decolonize" the social work curriculum are woven into the chapter, as they are becoming integrated into recent social work learning and practice. Parkinson notes the sobering reality that "the corrosive impact of racism in contemporary life is indeed an obstacle to thinking and learning".

Having described the tension between an apparently wide recognition that relationship-based practice is important and the pull towards attainment being measured by competencies, Parkinson concludes on an optimistic note, as she sees psychoanalytically informed social work research becoming well established and productive.

At the time of writing, optimism in the world is in short supply, as fighting has once again broken out in the Middle East and war continues to rage in Ukraine. The world seems a long way from being able to come together to tackle climate change with the urgency needed. However, perhaps there can still be hope for the future when Taheri and Parkinson's chapters show what can be achieved when one person or a small group brings thoughtful attention and in-depth understanding to the status quo. The transformation of a large open space started with Taheri as a lone litter picker; the psychodynamic approach to social work training is being maintained and promoted by a small but dedicated group, with Parkinson at the forefront.

This book has been about looking beneath the surface and trying to understand, through reflection and psychoanalytic thinking. The writing, covering many different subjects, suggests that these processes can, in small ways, lead to constructive ways forward based on the necessary engagement with reality, despite the many challenges the world currently faces.

CHAPTER THIRTEEN

Psy's "Gentleman"—between the ugly and the beautiful

Yong Suk Lee

The term "popular culture" usually refers to trends in fields of art and in the expressions of groups of people. In popular culture, a certain value and expression is shared (Matsumoto & Juang, 2013, p. 21), and popular culture can "provide helpful ways of managing internal anxieties and conflicts from which we all suffer" (Richards, 1994, p. 5). Thus, by investigating popular culture from a psychoanalytic perspective, we can understand the interaction between popular culture and our unconscious mind. Furthermore, a study of this kind will provide a useful opportunity to understand the universal processes of the mind if we were to examine pop culture beyond the locality of national culture.

The second worldwide hit song, "Gentleman", by Korean singer Psy, has become popular but is also controversial. In 2012, Psy's "Gangnam Style" was a chart-topping success, both in South Korea but also across the world, and the song became YouTube's most-watched video of all time (BBC, 2012). Psy's follow-up single, "Gentleman", has emulated the success of "Gangnam Style", at the time of its release being viewed over 412 million times on YouTube (YouTube, 2013) and becoming his second top ten hit in many countries, including the UK and USA. The music video of this song, which includes scenes of a male figure teasing a woman sexually, has, however, caused some controversy since its release. The song's chorus sounds like the obscenity "motherfucker".[1] In Korea, which still has a culture of a strong Confucian tradition, this evokes sensitivities. On

DOI: 10.4324/9781003564867-18

19 April 2013, an influential newspaper in Korea, Munhwa.com (2013), reported on the controversy surrounding this song. According to this newspaper, there were two issues with the song in South Korea. First, the song violates both moral and family values, and, second, the video's lasciviousness led to it being viewed by some people as pornography. In this context, Korean Public Broadcasting (KBS) banned the Psy's "Gentleman" video from being broadcast.

If so many have criticized the production as being merely sleazy pornography, then why has it become a worldwide hit song, topping the iTunes Chart in over 40 countries? In my opinion the song and video could not be loved throughout the world if it were just an expression of sadism. I therefore consider whether there is some kind of aesthetic experience between "Gentleman" and its viewers that has led to this song becoming a megahit beyond national barriers and across languages.

Consideration

In order to explore "Gentleman" from a psychoanalytic perspective, it is important to consider that although Freud wrote articles on Jensen, Leonardo, and Michelangelo, as he was interested in the artists and their works, he also noted that the application of psychoanalysis to the cultural community beyond the consulting room should proceed with caution (1930a, p. 144). Since Baudry's 1984 classification of a psychoanalytic exploration into four main approaches, which he used to examine a literary text (see Introduction), there has been a shift in psychoanalysis, and, rather than analysing the unconscious mind of a patient, the unconscious interactions between two parties are emphasized. A similar shift has occurred in the application of psychoanalysis to art. Nowadays, the aesthetic reaction between artists and viewers is the primary focus of interest, as in Baudry's fourth method. Hanna Segal's theory of art can be seen to be typical of this approach. In her paper "A Psycho-Analytical Approach to Aesthetics", in contrast to Freud, Segal focuses on "why we should derive such pleasure from listening to the day-dreams of a poet" (1952, p. 196). Her argument could be briefly summarized as follows: after the artist experiences the destruction of his world, he tries to recover and repair it through his art. We, the viewers or spectators re-experience the same and "share experience where the chaotic world is turned into the unified and harmonized world by his re-creation in his art" (p. 204).

This essay examines "Gentleman" through the concept of the viewer's aesthetic reaction, principally focusing on the fourth method noted by Baudry, which he described as "The aesthetic response of the reader".

The reasons for doing so are the following. First, the subjects in the song and music video are not real people, as they are within a case history, and the content of a music video is usually relatively superficial in comparison with that of most novels and plays. Second, there is limited information about the writers or directors of the song and the music video. Moreover, these artworks are the result of a co-creation. Therefore, the main focus of this chapter is to explore the aesthetic response of listeners and spectators to the song and music video.

A question that needs to be considered is whether the audience of Psy's "Gentleman" is typical? It could be argued that listeners to pop music usually communicate with singers and their songs in relatively passive ways. If an artist releases a new song via CD, iTunes, or a concert, audiences generally tend to buy or download it and enjoy it privately. They seldom show their response publicly, except by attending concerts. However, in the case of Psy's songs, many fans have actively uploaded their reactions to the videos to YouTube, capturing themselves by webcam, dancing, singing, laughing, or talking. This would suggest that the videos of the music have as much importance as the songs, and the audience enjoys Psy's aesthetic experiences through identification with "Gentleman" and the world portrayed in the video. But with whom, why, and how do they identify? This essay explores this process in an examination of the form of the song's lyrics and the contents of the music video.

Lyrics of "Gentleman"

The form of the song's lyrics is considered in relation to both preverbal and verbal meaning. My opinion is that the song's lyrics encourage preverbal communication, for two reasons. One, the song is formed from both the Korean and English language, so its comprehension is difficult, except for a small number of people who are fluent in both languages. The other is the vagueness of its content. What is the meaning of its refrain? Obscure lyrics are loaded onto beats and rhythm, thus being sound, rather than story. In other words, their importance is as preverbal sound rather than verbal meaning. Segal (1991) remarked that in musical, visual, or verbal art, the form can bring us into deep unconsciousness, the reason for this being that the form is the embodiment of an unconscious meaning. For her, "art embodies and symbolizes and evokes in the recipient a certain kind of archaic emotion of a preverbal kind" (p.62).

The refrain of the song is also very peculiar with respect to any verbal meaning. For example, the refrain implying "motherfucker" is not well matched with other lyrics. These repetitive lines remind viewers/listeners of the fundamental object relations between a mother and a father, already complicated by the suggestion of oedipal stirrings. It could be considered that "Gentleman" stimulates a preverbal and archaic interaction in the unconsciousness of the listener through its vague lyrics and two distinct languages.

Music video of "Gentleman"

In reviewing the contents of the music video, I focus on the stream of dances. In my opinion, the dances within the music video are the key to understanding the aesthetic response. Segal differentiated between plastic arts and performance arts (Quinodoz, 2008, pp. 39–40). The latter focuses on the role of the body. In performance arts, the aim is to have complete control over one's body, although this is never actually attained. I think the dances in Psy's video are a kind of performance art that attempts to control chaos and transmute mess into rhythm. According to the stream of dances, "Gentleman" could be divided into three phases—an early phase, a middle one, and a final phase.

The early phase: indifferent and narcissistic dances combined with harassments

In the first scene, a male figure in a tuxedo—"the gentleman"—kicks a traffic cone, a symbol of law and order. He then dances alone in a boutique, where old men are seen behind him showing little response to him. Similarly, in the next scene, when a woman is seen dancing alone behind him, he sits with some older men and doesn't show any signs of a response to her. Then he and another man dance separately and indifferently in the playground. Later, the main character is seen to be harassing both women and men; he or someone other than himself, always dances alone, indifferently and grotesquely. In the first part, there is one scene of a group dance. However, the male figure and women dance back-to-back; and there are many perverse and aggressive behaviours on the part of the male character.

The middle phase: the gentleman meets the woman and persists in perverse dance

The male figure meets the woman in a gym. He takes off his jacket, throws it at her, and subsequently she follows him. Abruptly the beats and sound become fast and intense. The woman unexpectedly kicks the man's seat as he attempts to sit down at a bar. He falls down. Inversely, she now teases him. Now he responds to her provocation through deviant acts—namely, he performs a perverse dance in front of her. The camera focuses on a woman's face, waist, buttocks, and legs, following the gentleman's gaze. In the same manner, viewers who identify with him can share his voyeuristic gaze. Notably, the woman sucks a fishcake on a stick, and its mayonnaise trickles out around her mouth, suggesting an association with fellatio. In this phase aggressive and perverse dances mirror scenes that are full of equivalent acts.

The final phase: a harmonized group dance

In the cross-cutting between the gentleman and the woman, the eating scenes metaphorically suggest sexual intercourse. Later, the gentleman holds the woman's hands, and the couple dance in the forefront, while other dancers, including those teased by him earlier in the video, dance together behind the two of them. They dance rhythmically and harmoniously to the music. Interestingly, the rest of the group no longer dance back-to-back but facing each other.

Throughout the early and middle phases, the male figure is seen to perform many perverse acts. His behaviours can be seen to be fetishistic (grabbing the breast of a female mannequin), voyeuristic (undoing the strap of a bikini and staring at the woman's body parts) and anal sadistic (expelling wind into a girl's face). These acts could invoke in the viewer a feeling of ugliness. Why do people clearly enjoy these scenes, despite the invoked feeling of ugliness? Here, there is a basic question. Is this ugliness the opposite of beautiful? In my opinion, Segal's theory could provide an answer to this question and could help to explain the success of "Gentleman". Segal divides aesthetic experience into two categories, "ugly" and "beautiful", and remarks that the contrary concept of the former is not the latter but, rather, the unaesthetic, or the indifferent or dull (Segal, 1952, p. 205). In her book, *Dream, Phantasy and Art*, Segal (1991, p. 91) suggests that the content of art symbolizes aggression and internal disaster while the form itself reconstructs a harmonious world. For her, the "ugly" deconstructs the form, but through its restoration, the beautiful is made.

It could be construed that the perverse and aggressive contents in "Gentleman", are the "ugly", which destruct and break up the internal world. Simultaneously, this ugliness could be the driving force for repair to reconstruct the ugly into a new form. In my opinion, the dances and beats that form the base of this music video are the driving force for the subsequent reparation and reconstruction. In the stream of dances and beats, destructive interaction caused by the Gentleman's perverse and aggressive acts is repaired. If we look closely at the three phases, we can see that the dances change according to this process.

In the early phase, the solitary dances are indifferent, chaotic, and narcissistic. Even where the group members dance together, they dance back-to-back. There is neither interaction between group members nor echoes between the dances. Dances in this phase reflect exactly the style in which the gentleman teases people: therefore, audiences watching this phase could feel just ugly. In the middle phase, however, we can find a sign of transformation, suggested by an abrupt change in the beat and noise. The forms change when the woman appears, although the gentleman still gazes at her perversely and dances in a perverse manner. Interestingly, the woman teases the gentleman too, unexpectedly kicking his seat from him so that he should fall down. In other words, she attacks him. At the beginning of the final scene, the eating scene can be seen to suggest, by way of the cross-cutting between the man and woman and the intense beats and rhythm, metaphorical intercourse. After this, the couple begins to dance, and then everything changes. Following them, everyone, including the man's earlier victims, dance together rhythmically. In this process, spectators can identify with the gentleman in the music video and feel that all the chaos and ugliness has been transformed into harmoniousness and beauty with streams of dances and beats.

In summary, the gentleman's perverse and aggressive behaviours throughout the video have a destructive intent. Because of this, the woman attacks him. The beat and dances that form the basis of the video change, and, finally, the destructive interaction is repaired. Following this, spectators identify with the gentleman and feel the ugliness to have been transformed into beauty.

Two traditional examples of aesthetic experiences of the ugly and the beautiful

Ravel's Opera: traditional Western culture

These aesthetic experiences of the ugly and the beautiful relating to the process of reparation within the audience can be found in the arts and their appreciation, regardless of locality or time. Two traditional examples, Western and Eastern, can be used as evidence of this.

Ravel's opera, *L'Enfant et les sortilèges: Fantaisie lyrique en deux parties*, is a good illustration. This work is discussed in an essay by Melanie Klein (1929), who associated artistic creativity with "reparation", although she didn't explicitly use this term as she only began to use it after this article had been published. Later, Segal (1952) drew on Klein's ideas about reparation in her paper.

Ravel's opera has the same structure as the "Gentleman" music video. It is made up of three phases: the early phase, where a boy has a temper tantrum after he is scolded by his mother for breaking a teapot and a cup, trying to stab a squirrel with his pen and tearing the wallpaper; the middle phase, where the things he has abused come to life and attack him; and the final phase, which begins with a scene in which the squirrel is hurt. The boy bandages its paw and whispers, "Mama!" Klein explains that the boy's cruelty toward things and animals resulted in their attacking him. Conversely, after he cares for the wounded squirrel, they help him.

If we watch this opera (YouTube, 2011), we can see a process similar to that in Psy's music video unfolding. As with the dances and beats in "Gentleman", here opera music is the driving force behind the reparation and reconstruction of destructive interaction. In the early phase, a naughty boy destroys his surrounding world, so spectators feel ugliness. However, in the middle phase, with the change of music—namely, the change of forms—things that were abused by the boy attack him. In the final phase, after the boy has treated the squirrel, the animals stop hitting him and sing together. In this process, viewers can identify with the boy and feel that everything damaged is repaired. In other words, in their minds, all the chaos and ugliness of the earlier phases is transformed into harmoniousness and beauty by the operatic music.

Song of Heungbu: traditional Eastern culture

Another example can be found in traditional Korean music, in a musical story called "Heungbuga" (Song of Heungbu), which is performed by a singer and a drummer. Its story is as follows (Yang, 2008): Long, long ago, there were two brothers, Heungbu and Nolbu. Nolbu, the older, was wicked and greedy, whereas Heungbu, the younger, was kind-hearted and empathetic. Nolbu had an organ called, "Simsulbo" protruding from his left ribs, which caused him to behave maliciously. When their father passed away, Nolbu took the entire fortune and threw Heungbu and his family out of the house. One day, Heungbu fixed a baby swallow's leg and was rewarded with great wealth, as the swallow brought him a gourd seed that he planted, producing a many great things. Nolbu tried to achieve this too by breaking a swallow's leg, but the result of this was that the gourds brought only misfortune. Eventually he asked Heungbu to forgive him. Heungbu was willing to help, and they lived together happily ever after.

In the early phase, Nolbu takes part in many wicked and cruel acts. He dances at a funeral and forces a man to sit on his stool when he relieves himself. Even more cruelly, he rapes a young woman. Finally, he deliberately fractures a swallow's leg and bandages it, in order to receive material gain. In the middle phase, instigated by the swallow world, he is attacked and deprived of wealth. Furthermore, a large quantity of excrement floods his house, and he feels fearful and helpless. In the final stage of the story, Nolbu seeks Heungbu's forgiveness, and eventually his brother offers Nolbu his support. As in Psy's "Gentleman" and in Ravel's opera, music is the form by which this transformation occurs. Audiences feel ugly because of Nolbu's bad acts. However, they are able to experience the repair of all of this destruction within the music. Again, I would argue that, in their minds, the ugliness is transmuted into beauty.

In both these examples the musical form is similar to Psy's "Gentleman", but within the more extended structures there is also an acknowledgement of damage. This leads to regret. In the short music videos, regret is missing. Without regret, is repair possible? If not, how is the aesthetic experience for the viewer different?

A contemporary example of the importance of violence as a precondition for aesthetic experiences

In these two traditional illustrations in the Western and Eastern arts, we find aggression prior to an aesthetic experience, because these are associated with the process of reparation. Thus, art is always accompanied by aggression. Stokes (1965, p. 24) stated: "A painter, then, to be so, must be capable of perpetrating defacement; though it be defacement in order to add, create, transform, restore, the attack is defacement none the less."

After violence, that which is smashed and shattered is transformed into art. Bacon said that he was only able to paint in an atelier that was messy and dirty, full of dust (Sylvester, 2016). Although Bacon owned beautiful studios, such as the one belonging to John Everett Millais in Cromwell Place, he gave them up because he couldn't be inspired working there. He felt that in beautiful places he lost his imaginative power. Thus, he chose another atelier and didn't clean it for several decades. He gathered dust and debris in his studio, mixed them with oil paint, and then drew. In my opinion, he transformed ruins after destruction into artworks. Segal wrote:

> [A]ll creation is really a re-creation of a once loved and once whole, but now lost and ruined object, a ruined internal world and self. It is

> when the world within us is destroyed, when it is dead and loveless, when our loved ones are in fragments, and we ourselves in helpless despair—it is then that we must re-create our world anew, re-assemble the pieces, infuse life into dead fragments, re-create life
>
> [Segal, 1952, p. 199]

Although Bacon's masterpieces have grotesque, deformed and bizarre contents, perhaps they evoke aesthetic experiences in viewers through an internal process of restoration from the "ugly".

Short but enough—two music videos: Michael Jackson's "Beat It", and Psy's "Gentleman"

Can short music videos that have only several minutes' running time be enough to bring about an aesthetic experience in a viewer? Traditional arts have well-organized structures and narratives lasting a few hours; in comparison with these, it might be said that music videos are too short to have an appropriate format for people to feel beauty. However, as stated above, there seems to be an aesthetic experience between Psy's "Gentleman" and fans all over the world, despite its brevity. Before exploring some factors that may contribute to an aesthetic response in spectators, another music video, Michael Jackson's "Beat It" needs to be discussed.

Michael Jackson's "Beat It": contemporary Western culture

Michael Jackson released "Beat It" in 1983, and it topped charts throughout the world. According to *Rolling Stone* (2011), it was ranked 344th in the list of "The 500 Greatest Songs of All Time" and the music video contributed to the song's success. Its storyline is as follows: Gangsters from different places form two rival mobs. Michael Jackson sings and dances, cross-cutting between himself and the mobsters. The two gangs meet in a storehouse. Starting with the background music of the rock guitar solo played by Eddie Van Halen, two leaders fight with their jackknives as it reaches its climax. However, Jackson intervenes between them, singing the refrain, and begins his dance. Finally, the leaders of the two gangs stop their fight and start to follow his dance. In the refrain, Jackson leads, and all the gangsters dance harmoniously in group.

Michael Jackson's "Beat It" is different from Psy's "Gentleman" in many ways: the location (Western vs. Eastern); era (1980s vs. 2010s); musicians, and storylines. However, they share a common feature—namely, the structure of a group dance with a refrain. With this refrain, aggression is modified.

How can these short music videos with such limited narrative structure evoke an aesthetic response in viewers? There is so little content that doubt, uncertainty, and questions arise in the viewer's mind. In the case of "Gentleman", we might wonder, for example, "Who is that guy in the tuxedo? Why does he tease men and women? Who is that woman?" There are no answers to these questions, leaving viewers with a lot of ambiguity, thereby stimulating their imaginations.

According to Donald Meltzer and Meg Harris Williams (1988a), the roots of aesthetic conflict lie in the infant, who is caught between the "aesthetic impact of the outside of the beautiful mother and the enigmatic inside which must be construed by imagination" (p. 40). I would like to suggest that, like the infant, a viewer is fascinated by the gentleman who wears a tuxedo in a luxurious boutique, but they also feel mystery because they cannot make sense of his behaviour, provoking an aesthetic conflict in their minds. It might be painful for us to stay in vagueness and incertitude; however, if we can remain with the pain, we are able to reach within ourselves to an aesthetic experience (Salomonsson, 2006, p. 4).

Beats and dances that are enormously emphasized in these music videos seem to be associated with aesthetic experiences. In Ravel's opera these are, of course, important components in its structure; however, they are more crucial in the music videos; because they cover almost all the running time. Beat and dances acting as a container seem to allow us to feel an aesthetic experience. Our ability to apprehend beauty can be related to the presence of a container for our pain (Mitrani, 1998, p. 121), and the reason why beats and dances can play a leading role as a container for emotion is that they are associated with an early experience with the mother. The foetus can hear at 24 weeks (Birnholz & Benacerraf, 1983). According to Teie (2016), the foetal acoustic environment, where the mother's heartbeat, respiration, footfall, and voice can be heard in utero, may form the foundation of musical elements. Moreover, this acoustic information is associated with not only the development of the limbic area responsible for our emotions, but also systems adjacent to the brainstem responsible for repetitive movement. These scientific opinions correspond to Meltzer's thought about proto-aesthetic experiences: "Proto-aesthetic experiences can well be imagined to have commenced in utero" (Meltzer, 1988, p. 36).

Beat, rhythm, and dance in music videos act as a container for emotion, and this enables the viewer to endure ambiguity and the uncertainty of the aesthetic conflict, to then apprehend the beauty.

Lastly, in the music videos of both Psy's "Gentleman" and Michael Jackson's "Beat it", the group dance is one of the most critical factors, which helps viewers feel an aesthetic experience when they watch it. It is especially meaningful that rhythms and dances occur in the form of the group. Let's review the changes in the dance routine in the "Gentleman" video. At first, figures, including the gentleman, dance alone or separately, and in the group dance in this early phase the dance is back-to-back. However, in the later part of the video everyone dances rhythmically and harmoniously to the beat of the music.

It could be argued that the group could be the container into which the individual transfers his/her own desires and experiences (Hinshelwood, 2008, p. 286). Bion suggests that the relationship between the container and the contained expands to the group beyond the individual (1970b, pp. 15–16). Jaques states:

> Individuals may put their internal conflicts into persons in the external world, unconsciously follow the course of the conflict by means of projective identification and re-internalize the course and outcome of the externally perceived conflict.
>
> [Jaques, 1955, pp. 496–497]

Therefore, when they watch, spectators move their suspicion and ambiguity into figures who dance en masse in the video; they then relocate those emotions modified in the group into themselves. Through being contained in the group, they can apperceive aesthetic experience.

There are two attractive elements in "Gentleman". One is that the gentleman's most aggressive or perverse behaviours appear just before scenes of the group dance. Viewers who feel disgust and aversion can quickly gain relief by watching the group dance.

Another alluring point is that all the group dances are timed to coincide with the song's chorus. As stated above, this sounds like the obscenity "motherfucker". Although it provokes discomfort and disgust in spectators, it might also be associated with some primitive relation to a maternal object. These entwined emotions could be contained within the harmonized group dance.

In short, music videos' characteristics, such as brevity, beats, and group dances, could contribute to aesthetic experiences in spectators, though their structures do not allow for a narrative arc.

Conclusion

Although Psy's single, "Gentleman", has enjoyed worldwide chart-topping success, it has also provoked debate. Some criticize the song due to its refrain sounding like the profanity "motherfucker", and others renounce its music video for scenes in which the gentleman teases many women with his perverse behaviour. Despite these controversies, the song and video have many fans all over the world. Viewers of the video actively record and upload their response via YouTube; in this way, they are not passive listeners but active re-producers. I consider the song's huge success to be related to the spectator's aesthetic experiences.

To explore this from a psychoanalytic viewpoint, I have used Hanna Segal's theory about aesthetic experience. First, I reviewed the song's lyrics. Because the meaning of the song is vague, I believe that "Gentleman" evokes a preverbal and archaic emotion in the minds of its audience. In addition to the lyrics, I examined the accompanying music video, which consists of three phases. In the early and middle phase, the gentleman exhibits many perverse and aggressive behaviours. As a result of being subjected to this content, viewers experience ugliness. However, after the gentleman is attacked by the woman but is then reconciled with her in their dance, everyone dances together harmoniously in the last phase. Throughout this process, the dances and beats that form the basis of the video can be considered the driving force towards reparation. As the gentleman's solo and indifferent dance is continuously transformed into a balanced and well-coordinated group dance, viewers also feel that the ugliness is transformed into the beautiful by identification with the gentleman.

It could be argued that these aesthetic experiences during reparation are a widespread element in the arts across cultures. In my opinion, two traditional examples, Ravel's opera, *L'Enfant et les sortilèges* and the traditional Korean *Song of Heungbu* illustrate this. In each of these stories, the main character behaves aggressively towards people and things, and as a result of their acts, their victims subject them to retaliatory attacks, leading to their suffering. However, both regret their actions and make an effort to right their wrongdoing. Eventually, all that was destroyed is repaired. As in Psy's "Gentleman", the form of music is an important factor in the reparation.

We find that short music videos like "Gentleman" and "Beat it" can give spectators an aesthetic experience despite their brief running time. Uncertainty and ambiguity originating from insufficient narratives invoke aesthetic conflicts in the viewer's mind. Through enduring pain, and this being contained, people feel aesthetic appreciation. Moreover, the forms—such as beats and group dances—amplify the processes between screen and audience.

It can be concluded that Psy's worldwide hit "Gentleman" might be associated with the audience's aesthetic experiences with reference to Segal's and Meltzer's theory about aesthetics, and I found that this same process could be applied beyond time and place. Perhaps the outstanding question remains as to whether, from a psychoanalytic viewpoint, a true aesthetic experience can come about without some acknowledgment of damage or regret, leading to a deeper feeling of pain than is perhaps experienced in these short videos.

Note

1 The exact words cannot be reproduced here, for copyright reasons, but readers who want to see the words of the refrain can a link to the YouTube clip (https://www.youtube.com/watch?v=Yj4jed7-LJM).

CHAPTER FOURTEEN

Living the dream: a psychoanalytic exploration of the sport of BASE jumping

Gabrielle Smith

BASE jumping is an extreme sport in which participants launch themselves from fixed objects, using a parachute to return safely to the ground. "BASE" is an acronym that stands for the four categories of objects: building, antenna, span (bridge), and earth. Each jump involves a freefall for a number of seconds before the parachute is deployed. In higher jumps, where freefall time is longer, the jumper "tracks" away from the object by holding the body in a horizontal position—horizontal motion, combined with vertical descent, turns falling into flying. With the evolution of the wing suit (a garment with fabric between the limbs and body, creating wings), jumpers have gained an increased range of movement and control and can chart a more deliberate "flight" through the landscape, sometimes lasting a few minutes. In the early years of BASE jumping, the intention was to get as far away from the object as possible; now, with wingsuit and "proximity" flying, the aim can be to get as close as possible to the object—"buzzing the walls" (Holmes, 2007). In contrast to parachuting from a plane, there is little margin for error in BASE jumping: there is no reserve parachute, as there would be no time to deploy it, and there is limited space between the object and the ground. It is an accepted fact that each time you pack your parachute, it contains the seed of your own survival or your own demise.

DOI: 10.4324/9781003564867-19

BASE jumpers unanimously state that the moment after stepping off the object is unlike any other in life:

> When I launch there is complete peace, total release from the rest of life. What has happened has happened, what will happen will happen and there's nothing I can do about either. I exist in that moment, just me and the universe. Clarity, tranquillity, harmony.
>
> [Hurd, 2005]

The death rate is high in BASE jumping, though exact data are difficult to find. On the Wingsuitfly.comwebsite there are the following statistics: "The fatality rate for skydiving is around 1 death per 100,000 jumps. . . . The fatality rate for BASE jumping . . . is . . . a roughly estimated 1 death per 500–1000 jumps."[1] This may happen on a first jump or a thousandth jump. On one of the main BASE jumping websites, the following advice, compelling in its contradiction, reads: "I would never advise someone to get into it (and I have found it to be the most rewarding experience of my life)" (Aiello, 2002). The idea of jumping from an object into space is provocative. It is associated with suicide rather than recreation. And yet to be able to do this and survive also suggests freedom and power. This is not supposed to be possible. It belongs in the realm of fantasy. What might the implications be if a fantasy can be made real: in this instance, the fantasy of flying, via the sport of BASE jumping? If dreams are, as Freud proposed, symbolic representations of wishes that necessitated repression, my interest lies in examining what is happening, in psychoanalytic terms, if one is able to "live the dream".

In his paper "Formulations on the Two Principles of Mental Functioning" (1911b), Freud explains the initial development of mental processes as a necessary function of the appearance of the reality principle. Repeated experiences of disappointment demonstrate to the infant that wish fulfilment by hallucination (his original response to displeasure) is not actually effective. This leads the infantile mind to develop consciousness, to attend to external events, to learn to judge, to act (by means of "motor discharge"), and, ultimately, to restrain action through the process of thinking. However, Freud states that there is a great reluctance in the human mind to renounce sources of pleasure, and so one type of thought process is separated off in the service of what he referred to as the "pleasure principle". Freud called this "phantasying", and it forms the basis of children's play and, later, daydreaming. As a pleasure-oriented activity attached to unconscious processes, it operates with complete disregard to reality and is closely connected with the sexual instincts, while ego development remains in the realm of reality and consciousness. For those who are able to transform their phantasies into actual lived experience, what might be the outcome? The possibility seems to spell danger. Freud's civilization is built on the renunciation of instinct, and phantasy is the mental playpen for repressed desire. If magical thinking becomes a real possibility, is this equivalent to the breaking of a taboo?

No human being is immune to the appeal of flight. Gravity binds us to the earth, and the sky, unbounded and out of reach, intrigues and beckons. One does not have to wish to occupy this space oneself to understand why others might. Eight million people watched Felix Baumgartner fall from space and break the sound barrier (14 October 2012), the largest audience ever for a live-streamed event. Throughout history, Gods and angels have been allowed to have wings, but not mortals. In the Greek myth, Icarus and his father, Daedalus, escape Crete on constructed wings. Icarus flies higher than his father, but the sun's heat melts the wax holding the feathers together. He falls into the sea and drowns. Curiously, however, it is Icarus who acts as a source of inspiration today, and not his father, Daedalus, who reached his destination unharmed. That quiet journey doesn't resonate in the same way as the exhilarating boundary-pushing of his son. Michael Abrams writes in *Birdmen, Batmen and Skyflyers*: "Ballooning, aviation, and bungee-jumping companies have named themselves after the wax winged hero. . . . Icarus Canopies is perhaps the best known parachute manufacturer in the world" (Abrams, 2006, p. 17). Early balloonists were the first to launch themselves into the air and were rapturous in their descriptions of the experience. Julian Barnes captures this feeling in his book *Levels of Life*, with this quotation from the physicist J. A. C. Charles, who participated in the first ascent of a hydrogen balloon in 1783: "When I felt myself escaping from the earth my reaction was not pleasure but happiness. It was a moral feeling. I could hear myself living, so to speak" (Barnes, 2013, p. 12). Wingsuit designer and one of the first wingsuit proximity flyers, Loïc Jean Albert, describes his experience: "The feeling was as good as it can get, I think. I would call it freedom. For a certain moment, for a certain time, I don't feel gravity. You feel that you are flying. . . . And wow you feel pretty powerful" (Loïc Jean Albert, in Schatz, 2012).

In *The Interpretation of Dreams* Freud investigates the typical childhood dream of flying. He is unable to draw a conclusion as to its full significance but suggests that it points to a child's oedipal strivings: a quest for knowledge and truth and a longing to be capable of sexual performance. Children know that adults are able to do something that they are forbidden both to know about, and to do themselves—it is illicit and wonderful, and the child's "violent wish" (Freud, 1900a, p. 392) expresses a desire to do this forbidden thing oneself. He talks about flying dreams in connection with the child's first experiences of exhilaration and terror, associated with physical acts performed in combination with adults. The child is thrown into the air, bounced on a knee, almost dropped but saved. Here excitement and threat are combined to breathless effect; an event occurs that is beyond the child's own motor capacity but not beyond their emotional repertoire. Something is felt but not understood.

Freud suggests that dreams speak to the present from the past. They are communications from the unconscious into the conscious mind, and almost always they express unfulfilled wishes. In the unconscious, and so too in the dream, "No" does not apply, and contradictory ideas as well as time frames can co-exist. Inherent in every BASE jump is this tension of contradictory forces. Jumpers, without exception, state that they feel high levels of fear before leaving the edge, which must be overcome in order to make the leap. As Matt Gerdes says in the film *Birdmen:*

> "I think when you're standing on the edge of a cliff you're faced with two different sides of our mind, first of all humans are naturally afraid of heights, second of all, all humans kind of dream of flying. . . . You're sitting there and it's like 'it's wrong' but at the same time you want to do it. The dream of human flight is overpowering for some of us and it's far more important than the fear of the unknown."
>
> [in Sheridan, 2012]

This tension is resolved at the point of commitment. Fear disappears as the BASE jumper steps off the edge, "in that moment, when pushing off to jump, I never think about what's coming next. The past doesn't exist. The future doesn't exist. There's only now" (Espen Fadnes, in Boisen & Fävremar, 2012). The capacity to act against instinct, to take the leap, gains the individual a freedom that operates not just in a physical sense, but also in leaving behind attachment to life and relationships. The tension in this paradoxical edge moment could be an exacerbated form of the tension inherent in being human; living with the unknown, with the possibility of loss, the fear of moving towards change and the anxieties that accompany this.

In "Creative Writers and Daydreaming", Freud compares the creative writer with "a child at play, in creating a world of phantasy where the motive forces of phantasies are unsatisfied wishes, and every single phantasy is the fulfilment of a wish" (1908e [1907], p. 146) "the past, present, and future are strung together, as it were, on the thread of the wish that runs through them" (p. 148). He writes: "we can immediately recognise His Majesty the ego, the hero alike of every day-dream and every story" (p. 150). In BASE jumping, the phantasy is also the reality. The BASE jumper is his own wish fulfilled: he has created a world in which he can live out his fantastic story wearing his own wings—he does not have to renounce his pursuit of pleasure, his narcissism is permitted, applauded even. Hervé Le Gallou became the first person to jump off the Burj Tower in Dubai, in 2008, and has spoken of the seconds leading up to the launch, "In that moment everything below seemed to belong to us. We felt like kings and this was our kingdom" (Caesar, 2009).

There may be many unconscious wishes underpinning the phantasy to fly: to omnipotently look down from above, to penetrate forbidden space, to fall into the abyss, to act out aggressive sexual wishes, to renounce attachment, to return to the anti-gravity state of the womb, to achieve oneness and oceanic bliss. And in this moment the BASE jumper can actually fulfil (some, or all, of) those unconscious wishes, as he *can* fly.

In BASE jumping the symbolic has become real. Falling or flying off an object is now a concrete act, embodied by a living representative. Its symbolic value was derived in part from its essential impossibility: flying is not an action that one usually performs with one's own body—rather, it is to be dreamt about, "The scene of action of dreams is different from that of waking life" (Freud, 1900a, p. 536). Transforming a symbolic act into a concrete reality lends it the quality of a psychotic dream. Or does this anxiety reside only in the spectator? The jumper does not believe in the likelihood of her own death, and plans even greater feats—she has already replaced that dream with a new dream:

» Steph Davis (climber, BASE jumper and wingsuit flyer) wants to fly "up", proposing that ". . . the real visionary change is going to happen with wingsuit ridge soaring" (in Megroz, 2012*Outdoor Adventure Magazine*, 2012).
» Loïc Jean Albert (helicopter and light aircraft pilot, BASE jumper and wingsuit flyer) says his motivation is "to enlarge our flight envelope, to enlarge the flying capacities of the human body" (Sheridan, 2012).
» Jeb Corliss (BASE jumper and wingsuit flyer) dreams of the day when he can land without a parachute. He refers to this as "The Landing Project" (Laurendeau, 2009, p. 105).

It is perhaps, then, only in the mind of the observer that this dream has become vertiginous, unstable with the weight of a real person. In the next section I explore some of the analogies that link the BASE jumping experience with various stages of human development, from birth through infant play and adolescence to negotiation with death and loss.

Birth

The physical journey of a BASE jump is not unlike the journey of birth. As the jumper leaves the object, there is a moment of weightless suspension and quiet, akin to the experience of a baby in utero. This sensation lasts for just a few seconds before gravity takes hold and the body begins its descent, with no possibility of turning back. There is a great rush of air and a sense of power as the jumper fights and flies downwards through open space. This part of the journey, like the movement of the baby through the birth canal, is perilous, turbulent, and unknown, apart from its inevitable downward trajectory. After sufficient distance has been achieved relative to the object, the (umbilical) ripcord is pulled, and there is a moment of acute uncertainty before the parachute fills out. Then all the skills of mind and body are mobilized to guide the parachute safely to the ground. Freud wrote about the "compulsion to repeat" (Freud, 1914g, p. 150), referring to an individual's need to repeat a traumatic event over and over again in an attempt to retrospectively "master" the original trauma. Might the jumper be trying to master the anxiety, and fear of death, that belong to the traumatic experience of birth?

In his doctoral thesis "Extreme Dude—A Phenomenological Perspective on the Extreme Sport Experience", Eric Brymer explores the testimonies of a variety of participants engaging in extreme sports, all of which have death as a possible outcome. He discovers a consensus of experience: that of a mind–body connection, while moving through a particular physical space, in which the participant "knows what to do without knowing it" (Brymer, 2005, p. 247). Those involved in Brymer's study describe a powerful sense of integration between mind, body, and environment, often explained as a "transcendent" experience within a physical realm. This seems to involve operating at a level of control within an environment of potential non-control, "Accepting that there is a potentially fatal element of randomness that cannot be controlled" (p. 248). This relates to the experience described by Stephen Lyng in his paper "Edgework", "negotiating the boundary between life and death, consciousness and unconsciousness, and sanity and insanity" (Lyng, 1990, p. 855). One must respond at a point where one is a moment away from being entirely overwhelmed. One of Brymer's subjects says "when I'm skiing my very best I feel like I'm on the edge of complete destruction . . ." (Brymer, 2005, p. 247). Surviving this solo journey, in which body and mind are in contact with, and reactive to, the immediate surrounding surface, often in states of great fear, yields a profound sense of personal satisfaction and deep feelings of joy. BASE jumpers experience an indescribable exhilaration upon landing, and a powerful sense of self-belief. And with this self-birth (or gift of life) comes the desire to do it again. Freud's repetition compulsion can involve not only an attempt to master, but also a refusal to renounce a source of pleasure. Certainly, there is a consensus in BASE jumping narratives that once you have had the experience, it is not to be relinquished. Géraldine Fasnacht (BASE jumper, wingsuit flyer) says: "When you do it you wonder how you managed without it for so long, you can't live without it" (Montaz-Rosset, 2012).

In interviews, BASE jumpers frequently articulate an inability to explain the experience using words. This declared inadequacy becomes the fundamental means of describing it. Brymer's subjects stated as much: "there are no words because it's a complete sensation, it's a sensation that's taking in all our senses and then some you didn't know you had" (Brymer, 2005, p. 270). Christopher Bollas, in *The Shadow of the Object* (1987), develops his own terminology to describe a child's pre-verbal memory of the relationship with its primary object. He proposes that from birth the child has an experience of being interacted with (positive, negative, or both) and despite the lack of verbal representation, this is retained somewhere in the psyche as an "unthought known" (p. 107). In a therapeutic setting the analyst may find herself being used in the transference in a particular way that can function to reveal this early relationship, despite it having been originally processed outside the reach of language. The analyst can then help the patient, with words, to understand what they have already known. A pre-verbal memory could also exist from the baby's experience in the womb. The foetus is growing inside another organism; it is, on the one hand, tiny, protected, part of something far bigger than itself, which supports and contains it in all directions. At the same time, it is the very centre of an organism that is perhaps unlimited in its power. Here the "unthought known" combines contradictory experiences. The baby is simultaneously powerful and vulnerable, subject and object. The foetus is growing in a paradoxical environment. This duality becomes part of its DNA and could be the beginning of the original experience of narcissism.

Another legacy of the growing environment of the foetus might be described as a feeling of faith; the residue or imprint of an awareness of having been created by something larger and more powerful than oneself. This interconnectedness or religiosity (without a specific God) is spoken about by Freud in *Civilization and its Discontents* after a discussion with the poet Romain Rolland. Rolland describes it as "a purely subjective fact", this feeling he called "a sense of 'eternity', a feeling of something limitless, unbounded—as it were 'oceanic' " (Freud, 1930a, p. 2). Intriguingly, Freud says he cannot detect even a trace of it in himself. Further on, he writes about another friend, who has experimented with yoga and breathing, leading to states that this friend interprets as "regressions to ancient conditions in the life of the psyche that have long been overlaid. He sees in them a psychological justification, so to speak, for much of the wisdom of mysticism" (p. 12). Others might describe this feeling as belonging to an earlier state of interconnectedness with the natural world. Many BASE jumpers describe feelings that belong to this realm of experience:

> [Y]ou're part of the environment . . . you get an insight into the fact that life and everything is connected and we're all . . . part of this cycle. . . . [Y]ou can stand on the edge of these huge cliffs . . . and put your arms in the air and you're totally vulnerable and totally part of the environment at the same time.
>
> [Brymer, 2005, p. 277]

> As you leap off, you cross over from . . . the world that you know, to the world beyond. And it's a feeling which you cannot describe to anyone unless they have done it.
>
> [Dan Whitford, in Overton, 2006]

> BASE jumping helps you . . . become inordinately humble but inordinately self-possessed and confident at the same time.
>
> [Brymer, 2005, p. 277]

Playing or reality

In post-Freudian psychoanalysis much has been written about play and how it functions for the developing child. Playing is one way for a child to make sense of the world and her experience in it. In her paper "Libidinal Phases, Ego Development and Play" (1954), Lili E. Peller explains how different types of play are used to master the anxieties that accompany each libidinal phase. The child can repeat a situation in play that in reality was felt to be traumatic or beyond assimilation, and so transform a passive experience into an active one. This might involve changing their role in the original event (from victim to aggressor, for example), or changing the ending of their story to a positive outcome, rather than its experienced opposite. Other types of play simply involve the repetition of a pleasurable experience. She quotes Freud's use of the word "*Spielrausch*" (dictionary definition: "gambling fever", "*Rausch*" being the word for drunkenness, a state of euphoria, a high, ecstasy, transport, rapture, thrill), to say that all play brings "wish fulfilment, pleasure, elation, a feeling of euphoria, well-being" (Peller, 1954, p. 80) but adds that this pleasure functions in the service of the previously mentioned compensatory role. Peller's study focuses on the play of children, but she makes clear that the survey does not exclude adult play.

BASE jumping recalls a game Freud observed his grandson playing with a cotton reel. Freud called the game "*Fort, da*". The little boy would throw the reel away and then retrieve it by pulling the string, as he uttered the words "*Fort!*" (away) and "*Da!*" (back again) (Freud, 1920g, p. 15). Freud believed that the child was using his own capabilities to actively explore his awareness and anxieties about his mother's separateness, her ability to leave him and his fears about her return. In the game he was able to change the passive experience of being left into one in which he, instead, had an active role. In BASE jumping the jumper uses his own body to control absences and reappearances in the lives of his primary objects. He does the leaving, always displaying through the element of uncertainty in each flight, that he is master of his own birth or death. If the game is successful, all possible outcomes are realized: full possession of the mother at the point of exit (with the return to anti-gravity bliss and oneness with nature), followed by her displacement in avoiding death and giving birth to himself. The experience is described as "reality in its truest sense; life and death separated only by your own decisions" (Dedijer, 2004).

Peller writes that "play . . . is an attempt to compensate for anxieties and deficiencies, to obtain pleasure at a minimum risk of danger and/ or irreversible consequences. Play is a step towards sublimation" (Peller,1954, p. 180). But BASE jumping is not a game in which unconscious wishes and their associated anxieties can be manifested and transformed through the actions of play, at minimum risk of danger. The threat to the individual is all too real. BASE jumping has been called "the most serious play in the world" (Laurendeau, 2012, p. 109). If play involves a recognition and management of loss as the stages of the oedipal journey are negotiated, in real terms BASE jumpers lose more people than most. The game does not offer a purely psychic experience of absences or separation: theirs are concrete losses. Does the game, instead, deny dependence, separation, and loss? Winnicott believed that it was only in playing that people are entirely their true selves. He saw the creativity within play as facilitating mental growth and therefore health. In his lecture "Play and Reflection in Donald Winnicott's Writings" (2005), André Green defines playing as "a category beyond good and bad" (Green, 2005, p. 16) and refutes Winnicott's claim that play "belongs to health" (1971b, p. 41). He highlights the fact that play is motivated by sexual and destructive drives and expands on Freud's notion that play can develop in many directions—creatively, as in writing, but also in neurosis, through an attachment to an alternative piece of reality, and in psychosis towards delusion. Underpinning all play is loss, and the play in effect becomes a measure of sickness or health, relative perhaps to the dimension of loss or the individual's capacity to process its trauma. According to Green, Winnicott sees the destructiveness in play as a kind of excitement belonging within a healthy love/hate relationship to the primary object. Green suggests that destructiveness can also belong to a type of play that is not about an interchange: "It is a kind of play that is impregnated with destructiveness . . . a sort of play that brought not only enjoyment but was also a way of feeding one's omnipotence" (Green, 2005, p. 12). He refers to Bion's development of the symbols K, representing knowledge, and –K, representing its antithesis (an anti-knowing), to suggest that play is a form of thought and can therefore be used as its inverse, as a way of not thinking.

In BASE jumping pleasure is obtained at maximum risk of danger, and the success of the jump provokes a quite reasonable sense of omnipotence. The play here turns fantasy into lived experience. Fear is conquered in order to continue this particular mode of play, because the reward is great. Freud wrote "the opposite of play is not what is serious but what is real" (Freud 1908e [1907], p. 144). Is the game of BASE jumping a triumph of narcissism, or is it sublimation in the realm of self-discovery? Participants describe a sense of freedom, feelings of truth, an appreciation of one's place in the universe, a mind–body connectedness: "jumping into the space between life and death and that's a pretty good description of it because it's another type . . . you know it's like a different universe" (Brymer, 2005, p. 227). And then there is the sheer physical joy expressed by participants.

Howard M. Katz, in "Escaping Gravity: Movie Magic and Dreams of Flying" (2002), uses an examination of the film *Crouching Tiger Hidden Dragon* to remind the reader of the fundamental importance of mastery in the locomotive sphere for every child's development. He suggests that inadequate attention has been devoted in psychoanalytic literature to this as a primary aim—the desire to sit, stand, crawl, and walk. A child is expected and expects to master this. Achievement in the physical sphere is one of the first ways a child satisfies her own sense of agency and intent. Realization of physical aims is vital to the developing sense of self and ego as the child explores her world and its physical boundaries in the service of reality testing. Marian Tolpin's paper "The Daedalus Experience: A Developmental Vicissitude of the Grandiose Fantasy" (1974) draws on the work of Kohut to elaborate on the idea that an original grandiose phantasy exists within an appropriate phase of primary narcissism and, if realistically integrated into the ego and de-instinctualized, can contribute to the positive development of elevated interests and achievements. She uses the examples of Tolstoy and Churchill, suggesting that their fantasies of flying (both men had childhood accidents in the belief that they could fly) were intrinsic to their striving towards individual feats of the imagination and storytelling, or of oratorical and military power. She writes about this grandiose feeling as a memory from when the child had been held in the mother's arms, able to move at a height and pace that would be impossible on his own. At this stage, unable to differentiate between himself and a mother who is separate, the child has an experience that appears wholly self-generated. Tolpin proposes that any attempt to recapture or retain his unique uplifted feeling will always be beyond his physical scope, but can be the motivation for acquiring skills in the service of achieving real goals and real successes, and the basis of positive feelings of self. In fact, for some individuals, this uplifted feeling will literally be within their physical scope and, as such, the real goal will be to fly.

Douglas Bond was a psychiatrist with a US Air Force regiment stationed in England during the Second World War. In his book, *The Love and Fear of Flying* (1952), he writes about pilots in wartime, addressing the problems of different members of air crews from a psychoanalytic perspective. He echoes Freud in stating that the basis for the human love of flying is the gratification of deep unconscious drives, which are associated with sexual and aggressive phantasies. In BASE jumping aggression and erotic impulse are satisfied by "playing" within the gravitational field, defying its turbulent forces for a short time, and the accompanying bodily sensations that transform a plummeting to earth and possibly death, into a triumphal descent. The jump has all the thrill of combat without an active enemy, like a fighter pilot joyfully negotiating a giant, sleeping dragon. Matt Gerdes talks about the excitement of flying close to the cliff:

> our generation grew up with all these fantastic sci-fi movies in the eighties. I'll never forget the image of the Ewoks speeding through the forest on their speeder bikes or Luke Skywalker diving into canyons on the death star or even just the classic image of Superman flying head first. To me wingsuiting is all those things rolled into one. It's the ultimate dream of flight realised.
>
> [in Sheridan, 2012]

But is there a more direct expression of aggression in pursuing a sport that contains the very real possibility of death in every jump? Is there an element of "anti-thinking" in leaving others to carry the anxiety of potential loss? Chris McDougall writes,

> It's funny, when we go on a big base mission these days, it's like going in to battle. You pretty much know one of you is not going to come back alive. It sounds full-on but it's just a realistic view that has unfortunately been proven over and over again to be true.
>
> [McDougall, 2009, p. 162]

Or is this no different from the separation that is required of every developing individual? By toying with death, beckoning death to come a little closer, does the BASE jumper confront his own mortality, or deny it?

Adolescent retreat

The BASE jumping world is in some ways reminiscent of Peter Pan's "betwixt-and-between" adolescent world of Neverland. This is not just an outsider view—BASE jumpers reference Peter Pan as self-description:

> I used to call him Peter Pan, the boy who can fly and refuses to grow up and is surrounded by lost boys. He would smile in recognition and call me his Wendy. Goodbye Peter Pan, have fun in Never Never Land and keep on flying! [Written by Lesley Assersen, Darcy Zoitsas' girlfriend, on an online remembrance board after his death at Kerjag. 22 July 2005. *Sydney Morning Herald*, 22 July 2005]

Margot Waddell (1998b) writes about adolescence being a period characterized by the impulse to act and get rid of disturbing feelings. This period comes with a new awareness of the self as now physically capable of fulfilling oedipal wishes: the boy is strong enough to hurt his father, the girl is in reality able to have her father's baby. Unconscious guilt around these oedipal wishes, coinciding with real bodily capacities, may give rise to a need to perform destructive acts and be punished, or to act out these aggressive and sexual possibilities in another, "safer" sphere. Boundaries are tested, and children spend a period of time moving away from the parents and returning to this seat of safety as self-definition develops. The BASE jumper does something similar; however the seat of safety in this case is literal, and the acting out of unconscious wishes takes place in an unsafe sphere.

In *Playing and Reality*, Winnicott writes about the unconscious phantasies of adolescence. He explains that growing up is essentially an aggressive act that requires the murder of a parent:

> If the child is to become adult, then this move is achieved over the dead body of an adult. (I must take it for granted that the reader knows that I am referring to unconscious fantasy, the material that underlies playing).
>
> [Winnicott, 1971b, p. 145]

He proposes that adolescence is a time of appropriate and healthy immaturity, which should be protected and allowed for, not rushed through via false maturation. The adolescent can experiment with new ideas, creative thoughts, their own ideals, and the excitement of optimistic solutions, without actually having the real responsibilities of an adult. For some adolescents, however, managing the murderous fantasy and its triumph is a difficult or impossible task and may be turned, instead, into a suicidal impulse. This period is not easy for the parents either, and their role is basically to survive, to remain intact. BASE jumpers are aware that what they have chosen can be very painful for those closest to them—who live with the knowledge that any jump could be their last. Parents live under a shadow of anxiety, neither released from responsibility nor able to exercise authority. Espen Fadnes, in the film *Split of a Second* (Boisen & Fävremar, 2012), explains: "I feel bad because I know that my mum and dad worry that at some point, it will all go wrong. I know a lot of my friends are concerned. It's a choice I've made, making people who care about me worry." Chris McDougall says of his father, "He knows the dangers and accepts the fact that one day he will get the phone call saying that I have gone in" (McDougall, 2009, p. 208).

Margot Waddell talks about the significance of groups during these turbulent adolescent years as the child has to deal with difficult physical developmental realities as well as emotional states—separating from family and not yet ready to make an adult couple. Attempting to integrate different parts of the personality, the group can become an environment for experimentation as well as performing a positive, if temporary, holding function. The relationships are intense, passionate, and significant, although they can change rapidly. Groups can also function in a more negative way, by being used to sanction destructive behaviour and attitudes that cannot be resisted. In the case of BASE jumping, group relationships become the new primary relationships. The temporary holding function becomes a permanent holding pattern. Ellen Brennan says: "The relationships you make in BASE jumping seem to be a lot stronger than any other relationship you have because you're able to share something that's so unique and few other people understand the feelings you get from BASE jumping" (Sheridan, 2012).

In its early days BASE jumping was described by those on the inside as a closed world: "It was very hard to break into. No one ever talked about it. It was like some kind of Mafia" (Boole, 2009). This closed world brings to mind John Steiner's *Psychic Retreats* (1993). He writes about pathological organizations of the personality that serve to protect the individual from overwhelming anxiety. This is achieved through the creation of a delusional world that appears to offer the solution to all problems. However, the freedom from pain comes at the expense of real relating and prevents genuine growth and development. The protective "group" is essentially a complex defence, organized against internal destructiveness and associated anxiety. Steiner credits Herbert Rosenfeld's definitive description of destructive narcissism as being the basis of his development of ideas about pathological organizations (Steiner,1993, p. 45). Rosenfeld writes about the idealization of destructive parts of the self, which are split off and projected outwards as a means of coping with primitive envy and dependent states. In BASE jumping it is a real group, rather than a collection of internal objects, that might be seen to be operating as a pathological organization. Certain truths are evaded, and aspects of reality denied: destructive elements are implicitly idealized via the understanding that death, who waits in the wings, is a negligible price to pay for the experience. The jumper possesses knowledge that the uninitiated, and those outside the "organization", cannot know and therefore cannot contradict. The omnipotence is encapsulated in choosing to perform this counterintuitive act and surviving it, and in generating a physical, sensuous experience of incomparable intensity. This momentary achievement of perfect sensation under one's own mastery is a self-administered dose of pure id pleasure.

Won from the void

To outsiders, BASE jumping may seem perverse, and many jumpers admit that the price is high in terms of the suffering inflicted upon loved ones, but the actualization of this desire is considered more fundamental to the self than any other part of life. As such, relatives and friends are compelled not to inflict a "living death" on the jumper by taking away the very thing that makes them feel most alive. To the observer it can appear as if the cheating of death becomes more important than the living of life. One BASE jumper explains his attitude to life as follows:

> People say we have a death wish and that we are crazy but that couldn't be further from the truth. It's people like us that are really living our lives. They may not be the longest lives, but they are definitely filled with maximum fun and maximum excitement, with real appreciation of what living life to the fullest is truly about. Yes every death makes you step back and have a look at it all and makes you question what you're doing and why you're doing it, but so far the answer is still the same and at this stage I will keep powering on through this amazing journey that has become my life.
>
> [McDougall, 2009, p. 175]

Every BASE jumper knows someone who has died. Often jumpers die in front of their friends, who may continue to jump on the same day as a tribute to the lost friend. Memorial jumps are organized to commemorate a death, and it has happened more than once that on such a jump another friend will die. And another memorial jump is arranged. The denial of death could be seen to be literally enacted by the survival of the memorial group. At this point the idealization of destructive elements of the self is visible, albeit disguised as an appropriate expression of mourning—a tribute performed under full cognizance. In John Steiner's terms, the psychotic structure of the organization remains intact.

As Freud developed his ideas around "repetition compulsion", he struggled to reconcile observations that people frequently repeated negative or destructive experiences. This did not fit within his original theory of the pleasure principle and led him to posit the existence of an alternative motivating force, "something that seems more primitive, more elementary, more instinctual than the pleasure principle which it overrides" (Freud, 1920g, p. 23). He suggested that there might be two instincts at work in an organism: the life instinct (or self-preservative, sexual drive) and, competing with that, the death instinct, which seeks to reduce tension by returning the organism to an inorganic state. He writes:

> It is as though the life of the organism moved with a vacillating rhythm. One group of drives rushes forward so as to reach the final aim of life as swiftly as possible; but when a particular stage in the advance has been reached, the other group jerks back to a certain point to make a fresh start and so prolong the journey.
>
> [pp. 40–41]

Freud retained his concept of a death instinct and used it in later works to explain particular behaviours, but his investigations, in *Beyond The Pleasure Principle*, into the nature and substance of a death drive were never completed and remain speculative. The fact that the BASE jumper travels so close to death invites one to revisit the notion. In so far as Freud was able to conclude: "What we are left with is the fact that the organism wishes to die only in its own fashion" (p. 39).

BASE jumps are, almost always, meticulously planned. Jumpers have a vast technical knowledge of parachuting, the environment, weather conditions, the physics of flying and their own equipment. Many BASE jumpers will have physical fitness levels equivalent to those of elite athletes. The risks are carefully considered and minimized. BASE jumpers are adamant that they do not want to die. A successful jump is one in which everyone lives.

The focus on death can prevent one from appreciating the very real creative and "frontier" aspects of these individual journeys in flight. I wonder if the potential deathliness in BASE jumping is engendering a tendency towards an anxious and reductive view.

Considering BASE jumping in relation to Bion's ideas, he expanded Klein's concept of the depressive position, suggesting that, throughout life, there is a continual movement back and forth between the paranoid–schizoid and the depressive positions, which involves a constant rhythm of breaking up and coming together again. This rhythm is described by Michael Eigen in "Towards Bion's Starting Point: Between Catastrophe and Faith" as follows: "the self is born, evolves and dissolves with a sense of catastrophe" (Eigen, 1985, p. 325). The first signs of thinking are a response to this sense of catastrophe or trauma, and Bion suggests that this rhythm, which persists throughout life, is the basis of all creative acts. He explains that in order to tolerate an ongoing movement between the paranoid/schizoid and depressive states, we need faith. He uses F to denote this: a faith in what he calls O or the "ultimate truth". Bion situates O in opposition to any possessiveness towards understanding: O is the emotional reality or truth of a moment. According to Emanuel (2001, p. 1081), Bion suggests that all truly creative acts or new ideas have to be "won from the void and formless infinite" (Bion, 1970b, p. 88), and this involves tolerating the disintegration and reintegration, or dividing and uniting, that is an essential part of the creative process. Faith is regenerating in the sense that the survival of each catastrophic falling apart then strengthens faith. This rhythm is reflected in the nature of the BASE jump quite literally: each jump "won from the void" involves the breaking up and reconstituting of elements, and the act itself is potentially catastrophic. Jumping could be said to involve a personal "leap of faith", and jumpers refer to "the pull of the void" (Gerdes, 2010, p. 14). Uncertainty must be tolerated throughout the journey. The creative aspect of the jump, obviously different for each individual, is made explicit in these varied testimonies from BASE jumpers:

» Géraldine Fasnacht (extreme snowboarder and wingsuit flyer) says she "paints lines in the sky" to create her flight path (Montaz-Rosset, 2012).
» Geoffrey "Geo" Robson researched balance in human body flight for his PhD at the Institute for Dynamic Systems and Control in Zurich. He said "It's a magical and life changing experience, just stepping off a cliff, spreading your arms and flying like a bird. You really do feel like a bird. That's my research. I'm a very lucky man" (Sheridan, 2012).
» Espen Fadnes (fastest flying human in the World BASE Race 2010) says, "It's that sense of voluntarily putting myself in a potentially life-threatening situation and then getting out of it safely. Solving the problem elegantly is such a tremendous joy. I live off that" (in Boisen & Fävremar, 2012).

> Chris "Douggs" McDougall arranges jumps for groups, teaches a first jump course, and introduces the sport of BASE jumping worldwide. He writes about his unique experiences in nature; to quote just one here: "After running off the waterfall, I entered freefall with the water moving faster than me, but there was one point (even though it was only for a split second, it seemed to last for minutes) that I was travelling at exactly the same speed as the water and everything went still. . . . It was truly magical. After this moment everything sped up again."
>
> [McDougall, 2009, p. 54]

Any individual's journey of self-discovery is not without danger. If this involves pushing physical limits, then the risks are visibly greater. This investigation into what might happen if a phantasy could become a reality has generated more questions than it has answered. At times I felt as if I was unwittingly pinning a butterfly to a cork board. For every possibility, there was an equal and opposite alternative. BASE jumper and wingsuit pilot Matt Gerdes, who has written a thoughtful and comprehensive guide to BASE jumping, asks the question *Why BASE jump in the First Place?* (Gerdes, 2010, p. 24). He has jumped with nurses, doctors, surfers, builders, airline pilots, psychologists, engineers—as he puts it, "all sorts of normal people" (Gerdes, in Sheridan, 2012). He explains that enquiries have been conducted within different disciplines, and psychological theories proposed, but no satisfactory conclusion has yet been drawn. He continues:

> thus, the why remains answered and unanswered. Regardless of why we do jump, we know that we want to and we love it. It makes us happy, and gives us pleasure. It is fulfilling, rewarding and gratifying. It is one of the most positive parts of our lives and for some people the most important part.
>
> [Gerdes, 2010, p. 24]

To those like myself, who do not BASE jump, it remains in the realm of a phantasy or "feat of the imagination". Mine is a different dream from that of the actual BASE jumper, who lives his dream as well as dreaming it. This comes with reward and danger, perhaps in equal measure. It appears that society too, might collectively require people to perform such feats. We want to vicariously experience the pushing of boundaries, the risking of life, and to see people attempt and accomplish the impossible. We are inspired by seeing that dreams do come true. The story of Icarus offers us the option to fall either side of the narcissistic duality that is our birthright. Ideally, in life every individual will find a way to balance the paradoxical sense of power and vulnerability, of omnipotence and humility, that we inherit from the womb. It is the important developmental work of the child's early years, possibly of a lifetime.

To finish with another quote from Espen Fadnes:

> About once a month I dream about flying. I fly upwards and outwards. And in the dream I'm not wearing any gear. But the sensation I have in my dreams is often similar to the way I feel in real life as a BASE jumper. And both experiences are fantastic.
>
> [Fadnes, 2011]

Note

1 http://www.wingsuitfly.com/risk/4572000812

CHAPTER FIFTEEN

The hidden inner world of littering

Leila Taheri

The Welsh Harp (Brent Reservoir) is a Site of Special Scientific Interest (SSSI) and Local Nature Reserve (LNR) in London. It is a 170-acre open mosaic habitat of water, wetland, marshes, woodland, and grasslands. In the 1980s, it was transformed into world-class wetlands—becoming an important breeding site for wetland birds. But its heyday was not to last for long. By the time I encountered it as a teenager in the 1990s, it was already known as being heavily littered and a fly-tipping[1] hotspot. So when, decades later, I moved nearby, I had little interest in exploring it. But then COVID-19 arrived, and everything changed.

Looking locally

Like many people, the COVID-19-imposed lockdowns forced me to explore my immediate surroundings. I took to walking in the Welsh Harp, which, I discovered, was actually quite pleasant despite all the litter. In the summer of 2020, during the reprieve between the lockdowns that began in the Spring, I even organized a clean-up.

But the real turning point came in January 2021. The Canal & River Trust (CRT), which owns the reservoir, lowered the water level by one metre to conduct a flood risk assessment, and in doing so revealed an environmental catastrophe. Entire shores were seemingly made up of nothing but litter. Plastic bottles and aluminium cans were present in

DOI: 10.4324/9781003564867-20

huge quantities, as far as the eye could see. Birds were nesting and feeding among wheelie bins, broken Styrofoam packaging, wet wipes, and tyres. The protected SSSI status of the Welsh Harp was revealed as a sham.

Why so broken?

In addition to plastic pollution, a myriad other problems faced the Welsh Harp: a variety of urban pollutants and contaminants in the water, toxic silt, colonized willow, and invasive plant species, no control of activities detrimental to an SSSI (e.g. fishing), no biodiversity plan, broken bird breeding rafts, . . . What was the explanation?

A new local campaigner cited the "broken windows theory" first introduced by social scientists James Q. Wilson and George L. Kelling (1982). It proposes that people are more likely to break windows, write graffiti, or deface a space if it has already been defaced. In other words, one broken window leads to more broken windows. This is because social signifiers of disorder, such as littering, lead people to think an area is unsafe. The subsequent withdrawal of the community weakens social controls that had previously kept antisocial behaviour in check, which, in turn, leads to further disorder and crime. This certainly seemed to be the case at the Welsh Harp.

Then there was the issue of the owners, of which there are five: CRT, Barnet and Brent Councils, the Environment Agency (EA), and Natural England (NE)—all of whom have statutory responsibilities for various aspects of the SSSI. The blurred physical boundaries and progressive budget cuts seemed to promote a culture of "passing the buck" and a reluctance to collaborate with other stakeholders to come to any meaningful, holistic solutions.

Meanwhile, the Welsh Harp Conservation Group, dedicated to preserving the Welsh Harp as a haven for wildlife, once so active and vibrant and responsible for gaining huge grants and re-profiling the wetlands, had stagnated. Most of its members were now interested exclusively in bird watching—even if it was in a rubbish dump. At one point they even actively opposed litter picking by local grassroots group Friends of the Welsh Harp (FOWH), which I later become involved with.

But despite knowing the "facts"—the broken windows situation, multiple ownership, budget cuts, and defunct conservation group—the question still remained: why would anyone litter and fly-tip? Didn't they care? And why didn't those responsible for this green and blue space do anything about it? Why was it left to volunteers?

We are living in a waste age

This is not a situation unique to the Welsh Harp. Plastic pollution is an environmental crisis requiring urgent action. Much plastic ends up as litter, posing a threat to food chains and blighting landscapes. Since the generation of waste began with the mass production of plastics in 1950, we have created 8.3 billion metric tons of it, of which 80% accumulates in landfills or in the environment, and currently only 15% of all plastics produced is recycled (Simon, 2021). Technology and recent advances in AI might give us the illusory sense that our world is dematerializing, but, in fact, the opposite is true, and we are producing more waste—crucially, plastic waste—than ever before (McGuirk, 2022).

We see litter everywhere because we live in a waste age. And if we don't see it, it is because it has broken down into microplastics—tiny pieces, smaller than 5mm. At this size, plastic waste enters water and soil and consequently the food chain (McGuirk, 2022). Microplastic pollution has now been detected at the summit of Mount Everest (National Geographic, 2020), in the deep ocean (Barrett et al., 2020), in human blood (Carrington, 2022), and in the feces of babies (Zhang, Wang, Trasande, & Kannan, 2021). This year, a new disease caused by plastics was discovered for the first time in sea birds. According to scientists, plasticosis, which scars the digestive tract, probably affects other types of birds, too (Horton, 2023).

Littering vs litter

Here I look specifically at the act of littering and litterers. However, it is important to note that the problem with litter is primarily one of disposability—an inherent quality of most litter. From a psychoanalytic point of view, the existence of litter exposes the "entitled exceptionalism" (Weintrobe, 2021) displayed by profiteering manufacturers and our throwaway culture. In contrast, the act of littering reveals how our unconscious inner lives interact with the outside world—and it is this I explore psychoanalytically. My aim is not to psychologize individuals and thus collude with policymakers who would rather blame people than the systems that facilitate the problem (Hoggett, 2013). Rather, it is about exploring the intersection of individuals, society, and culture to reveal hidden truths about each. This "litter litmus test" can be used to stress test grass-roots strategies and rethink policies and campaigns around littering and plastic pollution. My goal is to understand the litterer, rather than shame, abuse, or belittle them—under the psychoanalytic premise that only through true understanding of ourselves can we expect lasting change.

Beginning with Freud

It is somewhat of a tradition to start a psychoanalytic exposition with a quote from Freud. And while he did not have anything to say on the subject of litter, he does talk about rubbish dumps—and so this is where I begin.

Psychoanalysis is, according to Freud, "accustomed to divine secret and concealed things from despised or unnoticed features, from the rubbish-heap, as it were, of our observations" (Freud, 1914b, p. 222).

By this, he, of course, meant the unconscious. Freud claimed that unconscious processes revealed themselves through slips of the tongue, dreams, and jokes. He also recognized the power of "free association" and actively encouraged his patients to engage in it, understanding that before long, the drivel and "random" musings would lead to a revelation about the suffering individual (Freud, 1900a).

My exploration of why people litter, why litter persists in our environment, and how littering can be minimized all have at their core the idea that humans have an unconscious. This means that people are not rational, consistent, and logical but are, instead, ambivalent, torn, full of contradictions, ruled by powerful narratives, and overwhelmed by emotions such as despair, anxiety, hopelessness, and regret (Hoggett, 2013).

In this chapter I ask and present my arguments to these three key questions: why people litter, why litter persists in the environment (i.e. why most people don't pick it up), and what can be done to reduce it.

Why do some people litter?

Litterers develop rubbish phantasies

People who do not litter find littering difficult to fathom. They ask questions such as, "Why can't litterers throw their rubbish in a bin?", "Why are they behaving so selfishly?", and "Don't they respect anything?"

> **Vignette 1.** *The environmentalist:* I was on a walk with a friend and her son. He handed her his chewed and flavourless bubble gum to dispose of. To my surprise, she tossed it on the ground. She must have registered my reaction, because she said, "it's just a bit of gum, it's not a big deal". My surprise stemmed from the fact that before getting married and starting a family, she had studied environmental science, worked for an NGO, and organized litter picks. She was having marital difficulties at the time.

As this vignette shows, my friend had all the information, experience, and personal conviction not to litter. And yet she did.

For Melanie Klein, unconscious phantasies[2] underlie all dreams, thoughts, and activities (1946). Klein thought that phantasies are shaped by what happens with the infant's body. In this way, she carried forward Freud's body-centred theories of the mind (1923b). Phantasies modify external events, endowing them with significance.

> Infantile feelings and phantasies leave, as it were, their imprints on the mind, imprints that do not fade away but get stored up, remain active, and exert a continuous and powerful influence on the emotional and intellectual life of the individual.
>
> [Klein, 1936, p. 290]

Crucially, phantasies become more and more elaborate as one continues into adult life. Character and personality themselves are related to phantasies that arise from a defence against specific situations in infancy (Isaacs, 1948).

The act of turning rubbish into litter is thus influenced by a range of complicated phantasies that go beyond explanations that centre on selfishness or lack of respect. The out-of-character behaviour exhibited by my friend, a once staunch environmental advocate, underscores this.

So what are the phantasies associated with rubbish and litter? They are, of course, varied, but I present two contenders based on my observations.

The first is phantasies of a toilet–breast mother. Our attitudes towards the external world are rooted in our earliest experiences—that is, the baby's bodily and emotional needs. "The schemas, attitudes and expectations that grow from these basic needs remain unconsciously active throughout life, although they are often obscured or rationalized by later, more sophisticated ways of thinking" (Keene, 2013, pp. 145–146). At first the infant is relentlessly demanding. Gradually, it develops varying levels of a "capacity for concern", becoming aware of the mother as a person with her own needs and moods (Winnicott, 1965). Keene (2013) sees the unconscious obstacles to caring for the planet as being rooted in these experiences with our primary caregiver. He suggests that for those who have not developed this capacity for concern early on, the planet is experienced as a limitless "toilet–mother"—a great dumping ground with an infinite capacity for absorbing our waste products. Like the real mother, mother earth provides our urgent needs and a holding environment—something we take for granted unless it lapses (Winnicott, 1965). She is experienced as "utterly enormous in relation to our individual activities and therefore often believed to be quite immune to our puny demands on her" (Keene, 2013, p. 146). Similarly, littering or fly-tipping is an attack on "mother" earth with polluting objects. The phantasy is that "she can take it" and will absorb the waste. Litterers and fly-tippers are thus operating from an entitled and demanding position, having not learnt to temper demands through a capacity for concern. The infant phantasies of an infinitely bountiful breast–mother on the one hand, and forgiving toilet–mother on the other, combine to form an idealized, indestructible toilet–breast mother, who endlessly provides for us and absorbs all our waste (Keene, 2013). Litterers engaged in this phantasy might unconsciously harbour the idea that their litter will be absorbed by the earth, eaten by animals, biodegraded by plants, removed by the council or by volunteers. Letting go of this idealization infringes upon our sense of narcissistic entitlement and the belief that we can do as we wish. It involves developing a capacity for concern and mourning the loss of living under restrictions.

The second phantasy centres around being back in a womb. Psychoanalysts, psychologists, and sociologists have variously described our culture as "narcissistic, perverse, consumerist, extractive, entitled, arrogant, psychopathic, instrumental, and manically triumphant" (Weintrobe, 2018). In my proposed model, developed to encapsulate the "culture of narcissism" (Lasch, 1979), I argue that in this context the concept of a placenta–womb mother is more relevant than a toilet–breast mother. Rooted in pre-infancy, the placenta–womb mother, like the toilet–breast mother, endlessly provides and automatically absorbs and removes all our waste. But, significantly, operating within our narcissistic culture, this combined object allows us to exist alone and cut off from reality. The placenta–womb mother protects us not only from the "outside world" and its dangers, but also from our own envy and hatred. This placenta–womb phantasy underlies unrestrained littering with the "expectation" that it will be automatically dealt with. I put expectation in quotation marks because in reality, there is no expectation, owing to the automation of the womb environment. This phantasy destroys the other—even (or especially) the mother. One cannot be concerned for someone or some thing that does not exist. This is in line with the core of narcissism—a hatred of the relational, which seeks to destroy any separateness (Symington, 1993). Traditionally, psychoanalysis considers this an interpersonal failure of separateness. However, in line with Searles' emphasis on the nonhuman environment (1960), littering—and, indeed, all environmental crime—is a sign of a failure to relate to the nonhuman environment. Paradoxically, this happens because we destroy the separation that exists between us and nature. Another way to understand this is that animal life or plant life becomes an extension of, and serves, the self. They do not exist for themselves, independent of and separate from us. The litterer does not consider the needs or rights of these nonhuman others, instead resorting to control and abuse—that is, littering—to eliminate the other. In fact, any impingement on the self by the other, such as "do not litter" signs, is hated precisely because it destroys the illusion that there is no other.

Rubbish phantasies propel littering

Phantasies underlie our projections and introjections, which are the ways in which our inner world interacts with the outer world. In projection aspects of one's internal world are projected onto (usually) someone else. It is defensive in that it is used to expel and externalize uncomfortable inner thoughts and feelings. Littering can be thought of as a physical manifestation of projection. This is particularly obvious when considering littering from cars—taking the car to represent the self, the polluting driver the projective mechanism, and litter the uncomfortable inner feeling (projection). When there is a lack of a psychic capacity to hold onto what is uncomfortable (rubbish), it is projected out (as litter).

In this state of mind, there is a splitting of good from bad to protect what is good and keep the bad from spoiling and attacking it. This is Klein's paranoid–schizoid position (1946), in which things and people are perceived in black and white and are one-dimensional: either purely good or bad. Rubbish is transformed from what it was (such as a clean tissue) to something dangerous and bad that must be got rid of immediately (such as a dirty tissue). The person relates to part-objects rather than whole objects, missing the "big picture". The many consequences of littering cannot be thought through. The litterer is *compelled* to project out the bad, since in Klein's view healthy development requires splitting to allow introjection and identification with the good. This reveals the urgent, uncaring, unconscious quality of littering.[3]

Living in a "culture of uncare" exacerbates littering

> **Vignette 2.** *Uncare perpetuated*: BBC London covered the plastic pollution crisis at the Welsh Harp in early 2021. In response, a CRT representative cited "few resources" and said there was a "small on-site team doing what they can". She asked for volunteers to help them. In separate correspondence, the EA and CRT both blamed the public for littering and fly-tipping. Shortly afterwards, Welsh Harp campaigner and musician Ben Watt (2021) asked in a report: "Why should the public respond responsibly when all they see are marshes filled with supermarket trollies and wheelie bins; a shoreline awash with litter; trash traps overflowing; streams awash with urban runoff; woodlands filled with rotting mattresses; reeds and brambles choked with

> invasive weeds and plastic bags; and no clear signage anywhere to even tell them they are entering a SSSI and a Local Nature Reserve, and what that signage might mean, what they might see, and how they might tread carefully, or be inspired?"

Weintrobe (2018) describes how a "culture of uncare"—dominating the period of globalization since the 1980s—works to break links with the caring parts of the self. She argues that it has bolstered the uncaring, selfish, competition-led parts of us (which the current sociocultural narrative touts as "human nature"), at the expense of our caring, nurturing, compassionate parts. Its aim is to "break links with care and encourage spatial distancing of the victims of our uncare in the internal world of the psyche" (p. 412). In this way it keeps us "defended against feeling conflicted and anguished at our collectively damaging way of living" (p. 414).

This can be seen clearly in Vignette 2. At that time, the CRT took a defensive approach. It had clearly, visibly, and unequivocally failed in its statutory duty to manage the wetland habitats. By displacing blame onto the littering public, both the CRT and EA created distance with their victims—the littering and non-littering public. By citing its limited funds and people power, it could break links with its responsibility to care. The fact that CRT is now actively engaged at many levels, from funding wildlife walks to spending over £100k on habitat managements with more investment on the way, shows that their initial response was dominated by a culture of uncare that had been allowed to perpetuate, not by an actual lack of funds or ability to gain funds.

Litterers see signs of uncare and react negatively

Klein said that the absence of the good object is experienced as the presence of the bad object (1975). In a space like the Welsh Harp, good object absences include: broken/graffitied council noticeboards, lack of appropriate signage, no interpretation panels, absence of park wardens/rangers, absence of an ecologist on the council, unmaintained paths, and lack of habitat management. These hated frustrating objects can quickly become persecutory, as they are imagined to want to exact revenge similarly to how they are treated. This establishes a vicious cycle: uncare experienced as persecutory, which is attacked in phantasies and projected out. People who are sensitive to environmental cues and lacking in other good objects in their lives are particularly susceptible to persecution by uncared-for spaces. These individuals are more compelled to project, expel, pollute, and destroy. Littering and fly-tipping become tools with which to combat the persecution. A culture of uncare activates the uncaring parts of the self—and all the underlying phantasies—that say, "it's ok to chuck this can of coke there, the bin men will pick it up, I pay enough council tax!" or "it's only a little piece of chewing gum". These deeply internalized objects let us off the hook (Weintrobe, 2021) as regards littering.

In summary, I argue that powerful unconscious phantasies underlie projections, which is one way our inner world interacts with the outer world. Littering is a defensive projection of aspects of one's internal world onto the external world. It is defensive in that it is used to expel and externalize uncomfortable inner thoughts and feelings. It can suggest a lack of capacity for concern and relating narcissistically. Living in a culture of uncare exacerbates littering. It bolsters our selfish parts at the expense of our caring parts. Such a culture enables us to mentally distance the perpetrators of littering—litterers, but also manufacturers and consumerism—from its victims, thus avoiding having to face the plastic pollution crisis. Certain people are particularly susceptible to uncared-for spaces. These individuals are more likely to experience uncare as attacking and are feel compelled to "fight back" in the form of littering. A culture of uncare activates the uncaring parts of the self in most people.

Why does litter persist in the environment?

Litter stirs up anxiety and defences

Litter is, by definition, matter in the wrong place or out of place, as described by Freud (1908b) and Douglas (1966). Most people don't go near it because "the recognition of anomaly leads to anxiety and from there to suppression and avoidance" (Douglas, 1966, p. 6). Because of its "inbetweenness" and the disorder it represents, many people consider litter dirty.[4]

Psychoanalyst and philosopher Julia Kristeva calls this the "abject". She describes the loss of distinction between subject–object or self–other as threatening meaning, causing a reaction of horror, which she calls "abjection" (Kristeva, 1982). "It is thus not lack of cleanliness or health that causes abjection but what disturbs identity, system, order. What does not respect borders, positions, rules. The in-between, the ambiguous, the composite" (p. 4) Her examples of the abject include corpses, waste, nail clippings, the skim on milk, etc.

Thus a discarded crisp packet leads to abjection in me because it represents the free-floating rejected parts of an identity that is other, but could also be mine—that is, the litterer within me or the rejected parts of me. The abject is also therefore that which has been repressed—what one does not want to see, smell, touch, or experience. Litter stirs horror and anxiety. We deal with this through a variety of defences, including denial.

> **Vignette 3.** *Words matter:* In January 2021 the CRT, which has the guardianship of all of Britain's waterways including the Welsh Harp, downplayed the plastic pollution crisis by describing it as "unsightly rubbish". In February 2023, NE wrote to us to "support the litter removal ... to improve the aesthetic".

We utilize defences when faced with anxiety. Denial—more specifically, negation—is a psychological defence that involves the outright rejection of reality. It is claiming that something that is, is not, in order to defend against feelings of anxiety and loss (Freud, 1925h). In disavowal reality is not denied, but its importance is minimized and devalued (Freud, 1927e). Disavowal is "knowing and not-knowing at the same time" (Weintrobe, 2013, p. 7).

At first glance negation might seem the more problematic defence. But disavowal is the more serious and intractable of the two, because while negation can be a first step toward accepting reality and "says no to the truth", it "does not distort the truth" (p. 7). Disavowal systematically avoids reality by distorting the truth or making it insignificant. This increases unconscious anxiety further (because you both know and don't know something), which leads to even greater disavowal (p. 7). As Vignette 3 shows, disavowal can characterize organizations that presumably are aware of the impact of plastic pollution. Both CRT and NE focused on the aesthetic impact of litter rather than on the harm it causes to wildlife and humans. Acknowledging the latter would, after all, force their hand in acting to resolve the issue. But even when disavowal does not dominate a group's culture, there are other challenges that impact on litter picking.

People dislike those who handle litter

Ironically, the act of cleaning is not, itself, clean. In many cultures, including our own, cleaning and waste management is considered degrading and polluting—though this doesn't apply to cleaning one's own dirt (Spelman, 2016). Indeed, in the US people doing community service often pick litter as part of their punishment.

> **Vignette 4.** *An anecdote about "rubbish girl":* A group of men made derogatory comments in a dialect of my mother tongue while I was picking litter. When I respectfully invited them to join, they were caught off-guard, surprised I could speak their language. They were offended by my suggestion and declined. But they were also apologetic about their comments.

As the vignette shows, litter picking can be considered undesirable and even taboo. If dirt is matter out of place, then those who clean dirt are out of place or without place. By not occupying a place, you do not occupy a space, and therefore do not matter or even exist. A person with an uncertain social status or insecure sense of self cannot be associated with anything out of place, ambiguous, or taboo (unless they are forced to for reasons of survival). One must be confident of one's place in society to be able to risk associating with dangerous and polluting objects.

Shameful anti-litter campaigns are ineffectual

Some anti-littering campaigns tell people off or threaten them (with fines), like a punitive superego. But the current most widely used anti-littering campaign is based on shame. Variations of "Don't Be a Tosser" have been used by leading UK litter charity Keep Britain Tidy as well as many councils around the UK (Keep Britain Tidy, 2022).

Tosser has a double meaning—it is a person or thing that tosses something, and a person who masturbates. The "Don't Be a Tosser" campaign employs the traditionally shameful trope of masturbation in order to embarrass people into stopping littering. It is of interest that no other public campaign in the UK openly uses a term of vulgar abuse directed at a group of people in order to persuade them to change their habits.

Shame is inflicted by the superego, it is a sign of failure to attain the ego ideal (with an associated threat of abandonment and rejection), and it may lie at the centre of the narcissistic patient's pathology (Morrison, 1983). Such campaigns provoke the narcissistic personality as well as reinforcing beliefs about one's shameful status. Morrison says that "working with shame involves recognizing, acknowledging, accepting, and investigating the patient's shame. Only after such empathic investigation can underlying conflictual and genetic derivatives be productively pursued" (1984, p. 503).

Instead of shaming and provoking the narcissistic parts of the self, anti-littering campaigns might focus on the impact of littering and what is being done by a culture of care. This can tie individuals with local spaces more strongly, and contribute to creating what is called a "psychic skin" (Anzieu & Segal, 2018), a concept that is explored later.

To conclude, I argue that litter isn't picked up because it is thought of as "dirty" owing to its "in-betweenness" and the disorder it represents. This anxiety is dealt with by utilizing defences. Disavowal is a defence that allows individuals and organizations to systematically avoid the reality of the plastic pollution crisis—that it kills animals and gets into human food chains—by distorting the truth or making it insignificant (by calling it "unsightly", for example). The anxiety that litter triggers also "pollutes" those who come into contact with it. Those who occupy an uncertain social status, possess low self-esteem, and so on, may find this anxiety more difficult to bear and consequently will not try to remove it from their environments. The most popular anti-littering campaign, which should lead to reduced littering, is ineffectual because it relies on shame, provoking the narcissistic parts of the self, which, in turn, triggers the person to more deeply occupy their existing position in order to protect themselves.

What can be done to reduce littering?

Create a containing culture of care

> **Vignette 5.** *Clean-ups:* My involvement in FOWH geared up in January 2021, when the reservoir water was lowered by one metre to allow for dam repairs. It revealed an environmental catastrophe marked by a phenomenal amount of historic litter. I initiated a daily, solo, COVID-19-friendly clean-up campaign. It was a huge success—by a conservative estimate, volunteers cleared at least 2,000 bags of rubbish in the first three months of 2021 alone, not to mention hundreds of tyres and oddities such as a parking metre from an affluent central London borough, and even a gun.

With an organizing framework in place, provided by FOWH, people's caring parts were activated, and difficult, painful emotions—such as: anger at the authorities that had neglected this area and allowed this to happen; frustration with the slow progress of removing litter; the guilt of being a consumer and contributing to the plastic pollution crisis; ambivalence about whether this work would actually really make a difference "in the grand scheme of things"—were worked through.

While hundreds of volunteers turned out every single day for the entire 4-month period, the CRT continued to lament their lack of resources, and the EA sent a man with a wheelbarrow to clean the trash screen at the River Brent, which feeds into the Welsh Harp. The stakeholders were all caught off-guard by this mounting public outcry and, crucially, *action*. For a culture of care to develop, the culture of uncare must be broken. Friends groups such as FOWH can engender a culture of care and oppose uncare.

"To be caring we need to feel cared for", Weintrobe tells us in her discussion of what a culture of care looks like (2018, p. 417). This caring is of a special kind, according to Wilfred Bion's container–contained theory (1962a). He describes a state of "reverie", whereby the mother displays a capacity to hold her baby's anxieties and to go on thinking, offering her inner resources. In this state, the mother engages, understands, and contains her baby's distress, offering back to it a true version of itself. Gradually, over time, the baby introjects this containing function, building it into its personality. In this way the mother helps the infant to process thoughts and emotional experience (Bion, 1962a). Crucially, the mother does not "mirror" the infant's moods but, rather, has an active role in helping the infant understand its own emotions by transforming meaningless, fragmented, disconnected impulses into meaning.

A culture of care depends on "frameworks of care". Such a culture would have a containing function, repair broken links with care, and forge new ones, "expanding the experience of self and of feeling alive" (Weintrobe, 2018, p. 412). However, this may often be difficult and painful to do, because, first, it requires organizations to display what I call "organizational reverie" by functioning in a containing way, and, second, it requires acknowledging loss. A mature, caring culture faces reality, recognizes the staggering scale of issues, and apologizes for past neglect, rather than engaging in denial, disavowal, idealized thinking (for example, "only if we had £1 million could we save this place"), or omnipotent thinking (for example, "one day plastic-eating bacteria will save us"). Such a culture successfully mourns the fact that the earth is not a toilet–breast mother and has limitations. It recognizes that it must engage in actual care of humans, wildlife, and plant life through thoughtful action and collaboration.

A caring culture sets up frameworks for reparation. This is a defining feature of Klein's depressive position. Reparation, for Klein, is the psychological need to mend and repair relationships, accompanied by guilt over destruction of the other as well as feelings of love (Klein, 1959). A caring culture recognizes that dealing with loss and damage is difficult and can lead to disengagement and a need to protect one's emotions (O'Shaughnessy, 2018). So it facilitates reparation by, for example, supporting friends groups to flourish, as well as fulfilling their own responsibilities. Klein differentiates this genuine reparation from manic reparation, which is a defence mechanism that works to conceal or preserve phantasies of aggression, without any feelings of guilt or admiration for the other (Segal, 1973).

Let love bloom

Searles (1960) and the philosopher Slavoj Žižek (2008) both argue that rather than "merging" or "feeling at one" with nature, we must stand apart from it in order to relate to it. Searles (1960) says that mature persons (or mature organizations) develop a depth and breadth of relationships not only with other humans, but with all life. They grasp the clear relation between self- and nonhuman environment, relate to the environment on an individual basis and creatively, and act as constant, vigilant, caring stewards. In this depressive position (Klein, 1946), we can notice little changes and details, develop loving feelings and attachment, feel loss when our objects are damaged, and develop a desire to repair (e.g. by picking litter).

> **Vignette 6.** *Building relationships:* When I first started organizing litter picks, I was very focused on removing as much litter as possible. Over time, and quite unconsciously, I have come to realize the importance of building relationships. This includes spending more time chatting to volunteers instead of furiously clearing litter, making sure we always have refreshments after our events, and organizing funded nature walks and workshops. The conscious realization came after I reflected on my own experience: during lockdown I walked the Welsh Harp every day, which, in turn, enabled me, for the first time in my life, to deeply and consistently relate to aspects of a natural environment. I knew and charted the development of trees and plants, noticed sounds I'd never heard before, and waited in anticipation for spawning frogs. All this transformed into love of the place, which I shared with others, and effected caring action.

Freud is not known for his romanticism or sentimentality. He barely mentions the word "love" in his writings—so its use in his paper on narcissism is striking and memorable: "We must begin to love or we must fall ill. And we must fall ill if we are unable to love" (1914c, p. 85).

A culture of care requires love. Love, a true recognition of the external reality of "the other"—not projected phantasies or wishful thinking or idealizations—is the antidote to narcissism, according to Freud. In a culture of narcissism, building loving links with others and the nonhuman world is crucial to achieving a culture of care. This can be achieved with frameworks of care that nurture and build consistent, lasting relationships that are both physical and emotional.

Litter pick in groups to grow a common psychic skin

> **Vignette 7.** *From "mashang" to meaning:* Historically, my father has been ambivalent about my volunteer work. For a time, he would jokingly call me "mashang", which is a derogatory Persian word for someone who is naïve, confused, and a bit stupid. Nevertheless, bored at home one day, he decided

to join one of our conservation events. After clearing litter from a secluded woodland, we joined the rest of the group at the roadside. He did so reluctantly, because he didn't want to be spotted by anyone he knows; but, to his credit, he quickly got stuck in. He has since attended every litter pick we have run and recently told me how much he enjoyed them. He was surprised that the volunteers are young and "respectable", have "good jobs", and are educated. He enjoys talking to them and working alongside them, doing what he now describes as important and worthwhile work. On a recent trip to Iran, he WhatsApped me a photo of himself standing in a narrow mountain pass popular with hikers, ankle deep in a cold stream, next to a much younger man, beaming. They are holding three full bags of litter each. I cried.

"The ego is first and foremost a bodily ego", Freud famously said in *The Ego and the Id* (1923b), continuing, "it is not merely a surface entity, but *is itself the projection of a surface*" (p. 26). The statement is followed by a footnote:

> I.e. the *ego is ultimately derived from bodily sensations*, chiefly from those *springing from the surface of the body*. It may thus be regarded as a *mental projection of the surface of the body*, besides . . . representing the superficies of the mental apparatus.
>
> [Freud, 1923, p. 26; italics added]

This statement about the ego—that part of the human personality that is experienced as the "self" or "I" and is in contact with the external world through perception—implies a non-dualism and body–mind centredness that was developed by the French psychoanalyst Didier Anzieu (Anzieu & Segal, 2018).

Anzieu saw the psychological significance of the skin and psychic envelopes as "wrappings" for our feelings and thoughts. In the same way as the skin is the body's protective envelope, Anzieu thought that the skin-ego acted like a psychic envelope—containing, delimiting, structuring, and protecting the psyche. For Anzieu, the ego is first and foremost a skin-ego, the projection in the psyche of the body's skin (Anzieu & Segal, 2018). His idea is that the psyche is built on the body in interaction with the environment—a powerful notion for environmental movements and something I experienced as I built a relationship with my local space, as outlined in Vignette 6.

In short, the skin-ego's function is to distinguish what belongs to the self and what does not; to differentiate between one's own thoughts and feelings and those of other people; to demarcate inner reality from one's body and the outer world (Centre for Sensory Studies, 2023).

Therefore, someone with a "leaky" skin-ego, which develops as a result of inadequate holding and handling by the caregiver, could be more prone to projective littering. It also means that *continuing* inadequate containment could compound the leakiness.

Litter picking thus requires strong containment—particularly as the psyche is required to deal with undesirable, rejected, unwanted, contaminated matter. The skin and skin-ego protect against the outside world and its contaminations. So just as when one's skin is cut and is liable to infection from outside contaminants, so a leaky skin-ego is particularly prone to rubbish and all its unconscious associations. Where the skin-ego has formed and a boundaried thinking ego has also developed, the "otherness" and contamination of rubbish does not threaten. The inside and outside is clearly defined and understood, and picking up litter then becomes possible.

The skin-ego concept can help us to understand that operating in groups can create a psychic envelope that contains groups of individuals with varying levels of leaky skin-egos. Anzieu said that "there is no group without a common skin, a containing envelope, which makes it possible for its members to experience the existence of a group self" (1990, p. 97). We can think of the group as giving a "borrowed psychic skin" in which to operate and feel contained for a time. This is clearly demonstrated in Vignette 7, where my father is only happy to pick up litter with others—surrounded by people he can identify with. Even during our solo litter-picking campaign in early 2021, a collective psychic skin was created by the organized presence of a campaign under the umbrella of an established group.

In Vignette 6 I detail the social side of our conservation events. This is a space for people to talk about their worries and fears about plastic pollution, climate change, and a variety of other environmental topics. Anzieu believed that words symbolize, replace, and re-create touch (Anzieu & Segal, 2018). Thus, psychoanalysis, otherwise known as the "talking cure", can contribute to healing deficiencies and injuries to the skin-ego. In a similar way, exchanges between volunteers can work through emotions in a mutually understanding environment where people who have shared cares gather together to act.

Move away from a skin ego and towards an eco skin

Mohammadpour-Yazdi builds on the idea of the skin ego and discusses the notion of an "eco skin"—a psychic skin that "has the potential to allow us to more fully experience our human skin as shared with the skin of nature" (Mohammadpour-Yazdi & Lafrance, 2023, p. 582). He explains that in societies and cultures characterized by ecological alienation (by a lack of emotional connection to and affective engagement with ecology), the eco skin is often underdeveloped, exacerbated by our "culture of narcissism" (Lasch, 1979). "Not surprisingly, those who make up these societies and cultures tend not to have forged secure attachments to nature by means of a common skin phantasy with it" (Mohammadpour-Yazdi & Lafrance, 2023, p. 582).

Developing an eco skin—through "sensory inputs from the ecological body"—is therefore absolutely vital in order to "bring into being a renewed commitment to care for, protect, and connect with a natural world that is now under siege as never before" (Mohammadpour-Yazdi & Lafrance, 2023, p. 582).

In summary, to prevent and reduce littering, I argue that organizations must create a containing culture of care by facing reality, recognizing the staggering scale of issues, and apologizing for past neglects. Engaging in denial, disavowal, idealized thinking, and or omnipotent thinking should be avoided. They should facilitate reparation by supporting friends groups to flourish, as well as fulfilling their own responsibilities. Love, a true recognition of the external reality of "the other" (not projected phantasies, wishful thinking, or idealizations), is the antidote to a narcissistic culture. Building loving attachments with the nonhuman world is crucial to achieving a culture of care. This can be achieved with frameworks of care that nurture and build consistent, lasting relationships. Developing an eco skin—through "sensory inputs from the ecological body"—is absolutely vital in order to remediate the ecological alienation many of us grow up with. Forging secure attachments with nature can be brought about by engaging with one's local green and blue spaces, facilitated by friends groups and local authorities.

Conclusion

Feeling unloved, excluded, and disrespected all contribute to littering and a lack of care for the environment. Littering is a kind of revenge on society and the world. Shaming and denouncing litterers' attitudes do not work. Rather than a blaming, moralistic attitude towards them, we might do better adopting a more thoughtful and understanding stance. A "hello and how are you" is far more effective than a "you tosser, pick that up". Sometimes telling people off can make them worse.

Through increasing understanding of the psychoanalytic underpinnings of littering, I hope this chapter can relieve some of the intense anger and frustration felt when confronted by litter and engender compassion towards litterers. Friends groups such as FOWH may prefer to see themselves as performing a continuous, caring role in helping to manage people's littering, thus focusing on people as well as the environment. They have a more important function than "just" dealing with plastic pollution: developing and strengthening a community's psychic skin in relation to environmental issues must be the goal of any group.

My conservation work and writing this dissertation have helped me to reflect on the growth of my own eco skin and experientially understand the importance of strengthening one's human and nonhuman relationships. If we want to have litter-free spaces and, more broadly, surmount the climate crisis we are facing, we must mobilize love of our natural spaces, their wildlife, and the people who frequent them—whether they are behaving as we wish or not.

Acknowledgements

Thank you to my father, Seyed Ahmed Reza Taheri, for giving his consent to be included in this chapter, but more importantly, for coming on this journey with me. Thank you also to my fellow campaigners, particularly Daniella Levene, Livia Forte, Leo Batten, and Ben Watt, as well as the volunteers, without whom none of this would be possible. I am grateful to my supervisor, Professor Michael Rustin, for his wisdom and support. Last but not least, my heartfelt thanks go to Dr Ahmad-Reza Mohammadpour-Yazdi—*merci baraye hame chiz*.

Notes

1 Although sometimes used interchangeably, there are, in fact, differences between the terms "rubbish", "waste", "litter", and "fly-tipping". Rubbish, or waste, is any unwanted or unusable substance. Litter is rubbish that has been discarded incorrectly, without consent, at an unsuitable location. It is usually less than a black-bin-bag's worth. Fly-tipping is the illegal depositing of more than a black-bin-bag's worth of waste onto land that does not have a licence to accept it. It is dumped illegally to avoid disposal costs.

2 "Phantasy is the imaginative activity that underlies all thought and feeling. . . . Conscious mental activity is accompanied, supported, maintained, enlivened, and effected by unconscious phantasy, which begins in childhood, is primarily (originally) concerned with biological processes and relations, and undergoes symbolic elaboration" (Rycroft, 1995).

3 By contrast, in a sufficiently developed ego, the bad can be integrated, and ambivalence and conflict can be tolerated (Klein, 1946). A person in

the depressive position can wait until reaching home to dispose appropriately of a late-night McDonald's. The ego is able to hold together the good and bad object, and therefore able to see things and people more for what they are (whole object relations).

4 "Dirt is us. There is no such thing as dirt or cleanliness in nature. Dirt is a distinction we make and impose on our environment. There is no reality of dirt, independent of humans. It is relative to us and lives on our fantasies." (Schiller, 2008). While dirt *can* be grounded in a reality of biological contamination, it is not necessarily so. It is, instead, a complex system of unconscious phantasies (Kubie, 1937) that some have exploited to gain societal control and power (Douglas, 1966).

CHAPTER SIXTEEN

Beyond competence in social work: where are we now?

Clare Parkinson

Twenty or so years ago, and not long after I had completed my Masters in Psychoanalytic Studies at the Tavistock, I wrote a paper based on my dissertation about approaches to social work learning and teaching. In this chapter I revisit the themes that were my focus then (Parkinson, 2000). Then, as now, I was writing about social work through the lens of Wilfred Bion's work.

Here, I consider changes over the last three decades in the arrangements for how social workers learn to practice. Looking at the current context, I ask about the space available for social workers to learn from experience. What are the implications for social work and those we work with if contemporary structures do, or do not, enable this? I indicate recent developments that seem, at least at first glance, to offer practitioners the opportunity both to face the tough realities of social work and achieve some satisfaction and success.

After a decade in practice, I was at the start of the "social work academic" phase of my career. My main preoccupation was with ideas about learning inspired by reading Bion, which I first encountered through the theory teaching on the Psychoanalytic Studies course. I was particularly affected by Bion's (1962b) paper, "A Theory of Thinking": the wonderful clarity in the statement that thinking is preceded by thoughts rather than the other way around; that first there is a thought, and in response to the thought we develop an apparatus for thinking; that once there are

DOI: 10.4324/9781003564867-21

thoughts, these can come to be used in a process called thinking and that problems can arise in both the development of the thought and in the development of the apparatus for thinking them. From reading Bion, one can see the significance of our very first thoughts, for all aspects of development and future social relationships, and for the increasingly complex thinking processes we engage in from the start. In "A Theory of Thinking", Bion's example is of a baby. The baby is in the temporary absence of the breast or food source. At this moment, the baby either is or is not able to think. Whether or not the baby can think, Bion suggests, is determined by their capacity or incapacity to tolerate frustration. If the baby can tolerate frustration, then the gap between the absent "breast" and the previously experienced available breast can be bridged. This gap is bridged by the baby's thought of the breast, and, through that thought, frustration can then be faced and modified. So, that which bridges the gap may be regarded as the baby's first thought—a prototype, Bion suggests, from which all subsequent thoughts and thinking spring. Importantly, toleration of frustration is also, according to Bion (1967b, p. 114), what "initiates procedures necessary to learning by experience".

In this chapter, I consider the value of Bion's theory to be not just for understanding infant development. One can apply this theory of thinking to wider contexts too—for example, what happened in the social work profession following the death of two children known to the social work service can, perhaps, helpfully be understood through the lens of Bion's ideas about when conditions are or are not conducive to learning from experience.

Bion proposes important variations on the theme of thinking. He describes what may happen if frustration cannot—or can only partially—be tolerated. He is clear that a baby's capacity to tolerate frustration is born of the baby having been sufficiently responded to on enough previous occasions by a primary carer, someone who is themselves able to think and can, often enough, lend their mind to the experiences and communications of the baby. The emotional state for the infant and the interaction between these emotions and those of the containing parent are the basis for the mental life of the individual. I suggest that we can therefore ask: do professional bodies help practitioners to think? If yes, might the opposite also hold true, might those leading a profession at any one time falter and so produce the opposite effect?

A section of Bion's "A Theory of Thinking" paper that resonated for me then (and now) as relevant to difficulties in thinking that we as social workers may face concerns the place of what Bion termed *omniscience*. Omniscience is one of the variants that occurs if frustration is somewhat tolerated, but not sufficiently tolerated to enable thinking. Omniscience, according to Bion, is employed as a substitute for thinking. He proposed that omniscience arises when the reality principle (as described by Freud) is not securely in place. Instead of a state of mind that is open to reality, an all-knowing, quite rigid state of mind comes to the fore. In this state of mind, Bion suggests, one is unable to differentiate between truth and non-truth. In the omniscient state we cannot tolerate the anxiety associated with not-knowing, and so we pre-judge situations in a search for certainty.

One of the strongest aspects of social work education that has had a significant impact on the work of students and qualified practitioners over the last three decades is what has been variously referred to as equal opportunities, anti-discriminatory practice, anti-oppressive practice, diversity and inclusion, and, more recently, intersectionality (Ahmed, 2012; Lowe, 2014; Dominelli, 2018; Stephenson, 2020). This ethical strand has been central to the professional values and identity of individual social workers and for the profession (Reid, 2020). In a multidisciplinary team, or a group event, it is quite likely that it will be the social workers who pick up and respond to instances of injustice that occur along the axes of ethnicity, gender, disability, and, though perhaps less often, class and sexuality. Student social workers on their qualifying courses are keen to learn about anti-oppressive approaches. They listen attentively when these topics are explored. Without much prompting—although we do prompt through assessment rubrics and course materials—students include anti-oppressive perspectives in their essays, dissertations, theses, and in practice portfolios from placement. Students on placement are alert to expressions of prejudice as encountered by themselves, their colleagues, and their service users. Social workers are strong advocates for the oppressed party in such situations. The professional body consistently commits to encouraging this aspect of professional practice.

Since the death of George Floyd in 2020 in America and the increasing prominence of Black Lives Matter, social work commentators have been energized and articulate about ways in which we might refresh the social work curriculum and the very many strands of social work practice. What has been given less attention during this period of heightened consciousness, particularly concerning racism, is the difficulty for social workers to consider our own conscious and unconscious racism, or what Davids (2011) has termed "internal racism". I know in myself the ease with which I can identify the needs of others compared with the difficulty sometimes of acknowledging my own needs and frailties. We are drawn to assist others and can readily identify anyone who requires assistance (Parkinson, 2017). It seems likely that the same is true for recognizing prejudice. It is often easier to see prejudice in others than to face it in ourselves. It may be helpful to view this as a problem specific to those in the helping profession, and as a pertinent example perhaps of what Bion calls an omniscient state of mind. Can we, as social workers, take heed of the need not to rush too quickly into all-knowing positions to avoid the pain of facing prejudice in our midst? Bion (1967b, p. 114) suggests that the omniscient state of mind involves a "dictatorial affirmation that one thing is morally right and the other wrong". In order to work out what communications and actions may best achieve changes in ourselves and the wider milieu in which we work, it is as important as ever to think and to reflect through bearing such frustrations as we encounter *en route*.

Was the process of learning obscured when competences held sway?

In 2000, when I asked the question about how social workers learn and are taught, my critique was of the social work education paradigm that held sway at the time. This paradigm was strongly underpinned by the notion of competence. The model, as I examined it, was based on a kind of further education system: the National Vocational Qualifications. The social work training body had picked this up and run with it (CCETSW, 1989). One characteristic of this approach is that all that must be learned by the professional is set out, in advance, in discreet statements of competence. The learning programme then entails presenting the individual learner with the opportunity to demonstrate, to a trained assessor, that they do/do not yet/are unlikely ever to evidence these competences. It seemed to me that depth of understanding, engagement with complexity, capacity for reflectiveness, and reflexivity are all skimmed over in this model. I argued that little or no consideration of the process of learning was likely when the intention was only the achievement of competence. The social work profession wanted to be seen as knowing what it was doing, but at the cost of covering up the uncertainties and anxieties involved in any learning process.

Learning from experience certainly did not appear in the early iterations of the qualifying award, the Diploma in Social Work. Yet it is interesting to note that the educational regulators came to add the requirement of "reflective practice" to their prescriptions for social work educational providers just a few years later (CCETSW, 1995). It was as if they could see, even while committing to the competence-driven approach, that something crucial, which we might think of as learning from experience, was missing. This addition of "reflective practice" brought many rich opportunities in its wake.

Changes to social work education prompted by the sad fact of children's deaths

Children's deaths at the hands of their carers continue to loom large in contemporary life. As I write, Nurse Lucy Letby has just been convicted of the murder of seven babies in her care and the attempted murder of six others. How are we, as a society, to begin to understand the horror and devastation that this represents at the heart of a beloved yet besieged National Health Service? How was it that the thoughts and worries raised by clinicians were denied and silenced?

In the year 2000, 8-year-old Victoria Climbié was killed by her great aunt and her boyfriend. Victoria's death was swiftly followed by big changes to social work education. There was an increase in the base-line length and level of the qualifying training for social workers, which was at last increased in England and Wales from a two-year diploma to a three-year degree course. Another aspect, in 2004, was the first iteration of a government plan—"Every Child Matters"—setting out key outcomes for children and young people. This was given legal force by the amendments to the Children Act 1989 in the same year.

The murder of Peter Connelly (Baby P) by his family in 2008 brought further changes, though in a different, more ambivalent, and sometimes hostile mood. The Government initiated what was referred to as a deep-dive investigation into social work practice and education. A task force (Social Work Task Force, 2009) was established to conduct this and to propose wide-scale reform of the child protection system. The task force issued calls for evidence and outlined priorities in a first interim report, which found, in the arrangements for social work practice: "weak leadership, lack of a national voice, poor IT support, and excessive bureaucracy". The Reform Board (Social Work Reform Board, 2010), introduced by the task force, called for the establishment of an independent College of Social Work; this was set up in 2012.

Two inquiries were invited to examine the state of child protection in England and Wales. Lord Laming led one of these and reported in 2003 that children's social workers suffer from "low staff morale, poor supervision, high caseloads, and under-resourcing". Social work academic Eileen Munro led the other. In her 2011 report Munro emphasized the need to cut the levels of bureaucracy that hampered social work practice and place more trust in the professional judgement of individual social workers. The Government had nominally accepted all recommendations from both reports despite the fact that when Lord Laming had reviewed the situation in 2009 the progress was, he said, dismal.

Many things have changed for social work education since Peter Connelly's death. But some of these seemed eventually to have a more destructive side to them, as described by Ray Jones (Jones, 2014). There followed two changes of social work regulator. The College of Social Work, which was tasked with approving each qualifying course alongside the then regulator the Health and Care Professions Council, had developed a Professional Capabilities Framework (PCF). Note the change in terminology from "competence" to "capability". This framework was described as a holistic model for social work training: a rainbow fan from pre-qualification stage to the most experienced and advanced levels of post-qualifying practice. But in 2014 the Government unceremoniously disbanded the College from which the PCF originated. The abolition of the College and the sacking, on live TV, of the Director of Social Services for the team working with Peter Connelly and his family, showed a hateful and unthinking reaction from the Government in collusion with the bullying press of that time.

The Professional Capabilities Framework (PCF) has endured and is mostly protected by the British Association of Social Workers (BASW, 2018), although the College of Social Work, as the originator of the model, has been airbrushed out of the more recent edition. Also gone is the commitment of resources for continuing professional development. What had been a rich and imaginative array of post-qualifying courses has been largely reduced to short-course in-house employer-led provision and the occasional sponsorship of doctoral studies. It is evident that the disbanding of the College and the Post-Qualifying framework coincided with the beginning of the Coalition and then Conservative Governments' era of austerity. It seems that these were not conditions conducive to collective learning from experience.

Recent high-profile deaths of children known to social workers, including Arthur Labinjo-Hughes, Star Hobson, and Hakeem Hussein, have led to another round of government scrutiny producing official reports such as the independent Review of Children Social Care (MacAlister, 2022) and the report into these deaths by the Child Safeguarding Practice Review Panel (CSRP, 2022). Social work researchers continue the quest to make sense of the factors contributing both to the children's deaths and to society's response. A 2023 research paper by Ciaran Murphy asks: what can be learnt about the current system from researching the lived experience of child protection social workers? Harry Ferguson comments: "Support for social workers is the missing piece of the Star and Arthur review" (2022).

The turn to relationship-based practice

Bion (1967b, p. 111) suggests that the process of thinking, where it goes well, results in the creation of a concept. A concept, he suggests, is a named thought. In social work education one can perhaps describe the relationship-based approach as the named thought that, for at least a decade, has increasingly been accepted as central to what we do and how we think and learn. This shift has, of course, resulted from the considerable struggle between contesting forces within both the profession and the state. Here is some of the story of how it was achieved.

Imagine a group of social work academics informed by and committed to psycho-dynamic approaches to learning and teaching gathering in advance of the introduction of the three-year degree programme. How might we influence/interpret the new curriculum? What could we include? It was clear that focussing on both the content and the process of learning on social work qualifying courses might strengthen reflective and relational aspects alongside teaching about legal and policy contexts. We would add baby and young child observation underpinned by developmental theory (Briggs, 1992; Le Riche & Tanner, 1998; Trowell & Miles, 1991), provide different versions of reflective practice groups (Rustin & Bradley, 2008), and emphasize experiential learning, including the use of self (Ruch, Turney, & Ward, 2010) and the relevance of the organizational context (Hinshelwood & Skogstad, 2002).

Some influential fringe groups have continued to promote a psychodynamic approach to the work. *The Journal of Social Work Practice* (owned by the Group for the Advancement of Psychodynamics and Psychotherapy in Social Work [GAPS]) is committed to doing just that. Other groups involved with policy, practice, and research, as well as collaborations of practitioners and educators, have valued and developed relationship-based approaches to social work. There have been some key texts produced too. Before the turn of the century, some texts specifically focused on reflective practice were Yelloly and Henkel's (1995), *Learning and Teaching in Social Work: Towards Reflective Practice*, similarly, Gould and Taylor's *Reflective Learning for Social Work* (1996), and Marion Bower's *Psychoanalytic Theory for Social Work Practice* (2005), incorporating in her subtitle Bion's fantastically useful phrase, *Thinking under Fire*. In the same year Cooper and Lousada's *Borderline Welfare* arrived, with, again, a memorable subtitle, *Feeling and the Fear of Feeling in Modern Welfare*. This hints at a central theme of the book, which explores the defences that are viewed as characteristic of social workers and the situations faced in practice that give rise to these. Wilson, Ruch, Lymbery, and Cooper (2008) offered a substantial introduction to what were termed relationship-based and reflective approaches.

In 2010, and emerging out of what became the Centre for Social Work Practice (recently wound up), Ruch, Turney, and Ward edited a text entitled: *Relationship-Based Social Work: Getting to the Heart of Practice*, now in its second edition. Three substantial texts were then published within a short interval. First came Hingley-Jones, Parkinson, and Allain's (2017) *Observation in Health and Social Care*, followed by Bower and Solomon (2018), *What Social Workers Need to Know: A Psychoanalytic Approach*. This edited text includes chapters such as Narenda Kavel's "Exploring Racist States of Mind" and Joanne Stubley's "Working with Traumatised Refugees". The third of this series of psychoanalytically informed texts for social workers was Andrew Cooper's 2018 collection of many of his seminal papers. This volume, *Conjunctions: Social Work, Psychoanalysis, and Society*, includes papers intended to orient social workers with reference to practice, politics, organizations, and research.

A reflective space scenario

In a weekly workshop for family therapy clinicians, an update of ongoing work was presented. The clinicians, both psychotherapists and social workers, spoke of the confusion and loneliness of a mother of now young-adult children. The focus of her current confusion was her tax situation. Her ex-husband has refused to help her sort it out. The clinicians described how, stepping out of their usual roles as therapists, they had signposted her towards reliable financial advisors. In the workshop, two reflections were offered. First, how is it that the clinicians had resorted to what we all agreed is more usually a social work response? Second, how might the confusion over taxation be understood? Perhaps it is the case that this person no longer knows what she owes to whom? She struggles over having been exploited (overtaxed) by those closest to her. She feels depleted, perhaps because of a tendency to project her difficulties into her three daughters and former husband. But she wants to find the balance and to set the record straight. It seems likely here that the practical reaching out of the therapists, prepared to be temporarily pushed off their usual stance, communicated preparedness of the service to get alongside family members to connect to their difficulties as they were verbalized. The reflections and analyses of the workshop were also experienced as an essential part of staying on track with the family work, including restoring its more recognisably therapeutic frame.

This is an example of one of the different faces of contemporary social work. It has felt like a fruitful period for thinking and learning in social work.####

How did we fare when teaching and learning remotely through the pandemic?

For social work educators, teaching and learning during the Covid pandemic was on-line only for the two-year period between 2020 and 2022. What did that mean for our relationships with our students, and for theirs with service users, given that many frontline social workers continued to visit families at home during this time? What, if anything, was lost through working remotely?

As teachers and learners, we suffered in the absence of face-to-face contact and, especially, of valued informal friendships and incidental contact, such as meetings that occur on stairways, corridors, and in foyers and cafés. Some students had Covid 19-related illness and deaths in their families. Others reported facing severe economic hardship. There was more movement in the student group, which is typically very stable. Some students deferred. Some left their courses. The cameras of some remained firmly switched off, perhaps in part suggesting the need for more privacy in their intimate and familial spaces. Some individuals avoided sessions or topics that they anticipated would be too distressing.

Both student and staff groups worked with new challenges, changes, and the need to adapt, regroup, and reassign resources. How to continue to make and retain connections with each other? Black Lives Matter asked for our urgent attention and action. It was imperative to address this through messaging and other demonstrations of solidarity. We persisted with integrating intersectional learning materials, written and experiential. We made space to acknowledge and process the feelings in the learning group in the face of the pandemic and the sudden centrality of death and the fear of dying suddenly touching us all.

Following up on student absences during this time seemed to be more appreciated than resented. This was part of keeping the structure and culture of the courses in place, as was anticipating and exploring the impact of breaks before and after they occurred. We were emphatically aware of the need to hold the learning frame. We met even more regularly as staff.

It is true that we managed to keep going. We continued to be immersed in the learning and teaching tasks and relationships. Where possible, we acknowledged the losses from teaching and learning remotely. We were open to the possibilities of our current shared reality—for a time it was the only one we had and, for incoming students, the only one they had known. In some respects, as teachers and students we were drawn closer together than ever.

The idea of the organization-in-the-mind (Armstrong, 2005) had a new pertinence. What is an organization beyond the physical building that had housed us before? We acknowledged the team around the course in an explicitly interdependent way, recognizing our need for each person's role: as course administrator, technical assistant, librarian, section manager. We filled out the organization-in-the-mind with our own thoughts, feelings, and lively interaction. We continued to create the shape, purpose, and culture of the teaching/learning organization, even from our individual, separated-out rooms and settings.

Following Winnicott (1971b), perhaps, we articulated the aim of "good-enough" on-line teaching that continued to allow for the student contributions and resourcefulness to flourish.

Revisiting some key questions

These were the questions that I explored in my first iteration of this theme (Parkinson, 2000). Now it is possible to pose them again, but in the context of the current time.

Is there current capacity for reverie in social work education structures?

Bion theorized that the baby needs the mind of the mother to help them to process and make sense of their experiences for the baby to come to know itself as well as the world around them. Bion (1967b, p. 116) refers to the capacity of the mother to provide this help as reverie. If reverie is not available, Bion suggests that the baby must make stronger and more frequent contact with the mother, projecting ever more forcefully in an effort to be heard. But if the mother is still unavailable, Bion states, perhaps the baby is increasingly met by what he calls "a wilfully misunderstanding object". Instead of a feeling of being understood, what the baby suffers then is "a nameless dread" (Bion, 1967b, p. 116).

At the time of writing my earlier paper, I was preoccupied with what felt like a competition between a competence framework for social work education and a more observation-based and reflective model of learning. The former was characterized by what appeared to be an over-emphasis on omniscient, assessment-driven learning, particularly of the tick-box variety, with an absence of interest in thinking and the process of learning. Concerns of social workers at the time were that there was little in the way of reverie or containment offered to them by supervisors or educators, despite this being expected of them in their work with clients. In the 1990s, the climate was one of attacks on social workers by the media and the government, with charges of "political correctness" levied at those who challenged injustices and inequalities. It was evident then, as now, that if a containing space is not available for practitioners to process the difficult projections the work exposes us to, then a more defensive state of mind might be resorted to. As Bion asserted, if conditions are not conducive to it, thinking cannot occur.

The fight over the form that social work education should take has only partly been won in favour of providing thinking spaces. As discussed above, the relationship-based approach to practice is still in the ascendency. Nevertheless, the insistence by the government that it controls the nature of social work practice also continues. The legislation that produced the current regulator, Social Work England, originally also contained a clause to make it possible for child protection services to be run by private companies generating profit. The professional association and pressure groups intervened in time to prevent this aspect of the Social Work and Communities bill going through. For now.

Quite different in form and intention from the College of Social Work's Professional Capabilities Framework (PCF), as discussed above, is the checklist against which the newly qualified social worker is still assessed in their first year of practice. Rather than the PCF framework, which invites development according to degrees of experience, we have a competence-based document. This is a set of assertions of what the newly qualified practitioner must evidence—the Chief Social Workers': Knowledge and Skills Statements (KSS). One of these is written by the Chief Social Worker for Children and Families and one by the Adults Chief Social Worker. Both individuals are government appointees. On the Children and Families side, the KSS represents a tiny part of a much larger aspiration for control and testing included and endorsed in the 2022 report from the Independent Review of Children's Social Care (MacAlister, 2022). This development arguably takes responsibility and control of the social work curricula and learning process out of the hands of social work educators and places them firmly into the hands of government officials.

It can be seen that the Chief Social Worker's intention of assessing and approving the children and family practitioners, even after they are fully qualified and including when they may move into leadership roles, retains many characteristics of a competence paradigm. It does not appear to be one that offers space for observation, containment, and imaginative thinking, advanced by Bion as the most creative kind of learning. Nevertheless, as when the competence model was first introduced into social work qualifying training, an unexpected development parallel to this was the training body's requirement that their courses also made space for reflection. Perhaps something similar is happening now. Two interesting and hopeful developments are evident in our current times. One of these flowed directly out of the Knowledge and Skills Statement for Practice Supervisors. A consortium, the Practice Supervisors Development Programme, included a research-into-practice agency and participants from different universities and a teaching centre. It came together to create a training scheme and set of resources for those who supervise front-line social workers. It would seem from all accounts that this offered a valuable space in which supervisors could think deeply about their approach to supervising staff. The resources developed by the consortium continue to be freely available for all to use, and it appears that the value of this initiative could be widespread and lasting.

Another strand of considerable importance in this current time has been a product of the Black Lives Matter movement. The professional body BASW and many others have been galvanized into action. The phrase "decolonizing the curriculum" is taken seriously by social work education providers and their students. Course lists and experiential learning activities are scrutinized and refreshed to create and take account of the myriad relevant materials for social workers to breathe fresh air into practice. These materials support anti-racist and intersectional approaches. They include texts that specialise in challenging white supremacy and white fragility. They offer black perspectives on the range of practice specialisms in which social workers find themselves. The corrosive impact of racism in contemporary life is indeed an obstacle to thinking and learning. It seems likely that it is only if we continue to be alert to the existence and effects of racism and other forms of oppression that we can benefit from the increasingly available spaces for reflection and development.

What are the consequences for social work of the current structures of learning?

In my original paper, I included this portrayal of social work from psychotherapist Margot Waddell:

> A central characteristic of work in the public sphere is the immense pressure it entails: the practical burdens, the sheer quantity to be done—and with wholly inadequate resources—quite apart from the specific nature of the stress and anxiety involved. On one level, and in quite a contradictory way, the function of working that intensely is effectively to eliminate space for thinking and digesting experience.
>
> [Waddell, 1989, p. 14]

This still rings true as a description of what social work practitioners so often face. Doctoral research, for example by Charlotte Noyes (2017), bears this out. Noyes' study presents an examination of the traumatic impact of direct work on practitioners in the field of statutory child protection, often still experienced many years after a practitioner has worked with a specific case.

Another psychoanalytic exploration of the impact on social workers of an organization that does not provide space to think was undertaken by Amina Adan (2020). Adan researched child protection social workers and found that the paradigms within their setting were so constricting that the choices of response open to them were either to become machine-like in what Adan termed a "compliant-techno-rational" practice pattern, or else to disconnect in one of two possible ways, which Adan labelled as "idealistic-disconnected pattern" or "anxious/avoidant intuitive" pattern. The healthier, more hopeful pattern this author refers to is what she calls the "holistic reflective" pattern. Sadly, Adan's ethnographic field research in a children's service did not find any participants to include in this healthier practice pattern. It was clear from her findings that those in the dysfunctional patterns found it difficult to relate constructively not only to their organization but also to their service users. it was the lack of containment in their setting that seems to have prevented this from being possible.

Bion (1962a) asserted that the consequence of the failure of a containing connection (between parent and child) is "a severe disorder of the impulse to be curious, on which all learning depends" (p. 77). Social workers engage with people who are suffering. They may be dependent, often disenfranchised, possibly damaged, bewildered, sometimes violent and abusive, sometimes mentally ill and in need of hospital care. As Adan's research into a child protection setting shows, in the absence of containment, not only does the direct contact with the client become impoverished, but the structure for offering this contact will be increasingly weakened and ineffective.

Conclusion

I was on my way to becoming a social work academic when I signed up for the Psychoanalytic Studies MA. The infant observation and theory sessions and their applications inspired me. I gained confidence in the approach and applied it to my leadership of a new course for mental health social workers. When I started to teach and supervise students, I designed courses that offered infant, young child, and organizational observation. I felt, from reading especially Bion, Klein, and Winnicott and from the lasting impact of the MA course, that I understood something about how I wanted to approach my work.

It seems likely in this post-pandemic world that there will be many other, possibly unimagined forms of impingement on social workers' and their teachers' capacities to think. The emergence of Artificial Intelligence and machine learning is very much to the fore, with consequences that are yet unknown for how we persist with learning to help those who are suffering. There are urgent concerns, not least about the environment, high levels of debt, and extremes of poverty. One of the last budgetary statements of the previous government contained not a word about funds for the social care sector, the parlous state of which has become abundantly clear in recent times.

Social Work has another new regulator. Can we begin, though, to have any more confidence in them showing commitment to sound relational learning and practice? There are reasons to be hopeful, given that psychoanalytically informed social work research is becoming well established and productive. Studies based on researching below the surface continue to shed light on the possible defences, not just of research participants, but also of the researcher, incorporating greater emotional connectedness and reflexivity into social work practice at all levels. Courses and curricula are increasingly adopting an intersectional stance to working with aspects of ethnicity, gender, sexuality, class, and disability. And yes, we are at last decolonizing our curriculum and refreshing content to highlight the cultural history and context of social work students and those with whom we work (Barnard & Harris, 2016; Reid, 2020; Tedam, 2020).

How might Bion have viewed the educational models discussed in this chapter? In "A Theory of Thinking" Bion proposed (1967b, p. 118) that the tendency towards abstraction in the formulation of scientific communication is in order to diminish feelings of persecution that communication can evoke in the group. What is also possible, instead, through communication, is what he terms "correlation". Correlation can lead to what Bion calls a "commonsense view" of truth (p. 119). My hope after scanning developments in social work over the three previous decades is that understanding gained from such reflections may help us to maintain a more harmonious and truthful approach in our work, so that practice and teaching retains and sustains those qualities we have found, individually and as a community, to be conducive to thinking and learning from experience.

Afterword

Margaret Lush

I am delighted that this project, conceived jointly with Kate Robertson several years ago, has finally been realized, and the book has taken its place in the Tavistock Clinic Series. Along the way, we had many setbacks—the book's gestation spanned a period when pressures on the NHS led to turbulence and reorganization within the services we work (or worked) in—a situation that resulted in considerably increased demands on our time. However, when we could, we also found time to have many interesting discussions, as we tried to work out which of the many excellent essays and dissertations that came out of the course stood out as being particularly distinctive, original, and suitable for inclusion.

During this period Kate took on the prestigious and high-profile role of Chair of the Association of Child Psychotherapists, and she was in this role when the 2020 Covid 19 pandemic struck. Again we found ourselves with significant additional demands, as we were both in roles where we needed to reconfigure courses, teaching, clinical work, and, in Kate's case, support to the child psychotherapy profession, to make these available in a meaningful way online. Work on the book slowed, although we continued to mull it over as we met frequently during the pandemic to walk the green spaces of North London.

In the early period of preparation, Kate showed her particular talent for developing the contributions where needed, and I was always impressed how, by adding a new idea or taking something one step further

DOI: 10.4324/9781003564867-22

theoretically, sometimes suggesting quite small changes, she added depth and a greater sense of completeness.

Very sadly, in the summer of 2022 Kate became ill, and in the autumn she was diagnosed with pancreatic cancer. She stepped down from her role at the Association of Child Psychotherapists in January 2023 and anticipated that this would allow her time to work on the book. We had hoped that she would be able to co–write the Introduction, the introductions to each part, and the Appendix, but despite her wish to do this, she found that it was not possible. Kate died in October 2023.

Nearly all the contributors had known Kate as Course Lead when they were students, and, following her death, many sent me heartfelt messages expressing what she meant to them and how they remembered her. One wrote, "I first met Kate when she interviewed me for the Psychoanalytic Studies course and was immediately struck by her kindness, warmth, and sincerity." Another said, "Kate was such a dear mentor, and from the moment she interviewed me for the course she played such a big role in my learning through her consistent support and belief in me."

In all her professional roles she was widely respected for her many qualities: her passion, depth of understanding, clarity of thought, kindness, sense of justice, and sense of humour, as well as her dedication to the profession. One of her child psychotherapy trainees wrote: "Kate was incredibly thoughtful, went further than she needed to in terms of her support and caring of staff and patients. People really felt held in mind in a truthful and deep sort of way."

The experience of "feeling held in mind in a truthful way", a feeling I recognized from being with her myself, is echoed in the many comments I received from former students. A member of the course staff commented, "Kate will always be remembered for her huge contribution to the Psychoanalytic Studies course and her generous support and containment of the students and teachers."

It is important to acknowledge that two of the chapters are also being published posthumously. Jenny Abbott died in 2021, and I would like to thank Jenny's family for allowing us to include her chapter, "Sam: Observations and Reflections on the First Eighteen Months". I am also grateful to Michael Rustin and Iain MacRury, who prepared Diana Webster Thomas' chapter, "Identity, Identification, and Narcissistic Phantasy in the Novels of Kazuo Ishiguro", following her death in 2022. Diana had agreed to them editing an article from her PhD thesis and was pleased that this would be published.

During Kate's illness, by which time we had agreed the book's structure and the chapters were being developed, I continued to work on the book, including writing the introductory sections and additional material. It had become clear that what had started as a joint endeavour had, by that time, become a solo project. Nevertheless, as well as having the continued support of the Series Editors and the contributors, I benefited from Kate's continuing interest in and hopes for the book, and her pleasure in the knowledge that it would indeed come to fruition. I had always been determined to get the book to the point of publication, but after Kate's death I persisted even more resolutely. She was my good friend as well as my co-editor, and I felt it was vital to see this through to the end—for her. The book, which I hope reflects her creativity and passion, is dedicated to Kate.

APPENDIX

Fundamental psychoanalytic concepts

1. The inner world and the good object

Melanie Klein laid out her final explanation of her view of the inner world and internal objects in her 1959 paper, "Our Adult World and Its Roots in Infancy". The concept links with Klein's emphasis on the unconscious mind as something that is constantly present and active. The inner, or internal, world could be described as the dynamic, living theatre of an individual's mind, which is built up from earliest infancy onwards through the unconscious processes of projection (expelling) and introjection (taking in), working on and in conjunction with innate factors and constitution. The makeup of the internal world is determined by complex interactive processes between nature and nurture—the quality of experiences on offer to the infant and young child is important, but so, too, is the infant's capacity to make use of those experiences. Sometimes constitutional factors such as excessive envy or destructiveness mean that good experience cannot be taken in, and this would impede the development of an internal good object. These processes of projection and introjection are rooted in the infant's relationships with his caregivers, the environment, and his physical reality, but they colour the individual's view of external reality throughout life so that an inner world is only ever partly a reflection of the external one. It affects a person's relationship with others and his view of external situations, so that no interaction is ever free from interpretation coloured by the individual's internal world.

The central feature of Klein's formulation of the internal world is unconscious phantasy, which, following Isaacs (1948), she sees as accompanying all psychic life. The spelling "phantasy" denotes *unconscious* phantasy, as distinct from "fantasy", which is usually understood as a conscious phenomenon. As Klein's work developed, she increasingly emphasized the importance of the introjected good object in the development of the self. The good object gives strength to the ego and lays the foundation for a whole phantasy world that forms the basis of the mind and enriches it, but her view of the good object needs to be balanced by her emphasis on a lifelong conflict between love and hate, life and death. In this way, development is about an increasing ability to contain hate and envy.

2. Paranoid–schizoid and depressive positions

Klein described two levels of mental development, one more primitive, the other more developed.

The paranoid–schizoid position is the more primitive state, characterized by splitting, denial, idealization, and its opposite, denigration (Klein, 1946). Klein saw it as an early stage in the infant's psychological development, where, partly because of the young infant's limited conceptual capacities, he can only experience the mother as separate parts, such as the breast that feeds and the hands that hold. These parts are experienced as unrelated to each other. The infant's early experiences are felt to be either wholly good or wholly bad. A satisfying feed leads to feelings of love in the baby; the discomfort of hunger is likely to give rise to feelings of hate and persecution. Splitting is developmentally necessary for the infant to feel that he can hold onto something good inside without being overwhelmed by badness. At this early stage, the frustration and deprivation caused by the absence of a "good" object are experienced by the infant as if they are caused by the presence of a "bad" object. Persecutory anxiety, which is a fear for the self, predominates in the paranoid–schizoid position. With every physical development comes a psychological development, and as the infant is increasingly able to recognize their mother fully, the way is paved for a more complex state of mind, where conflictual feelings are struggled with. Klein called this the depressive position.

Klein's formulation of the depressive position describes a more integrated state of mind, where, over time, in ordinary good circumstances the infant develops the capacity to experience the mother as a whole person who is both loved and hated (Klein, 1935). A capacity in the infant to sustain these conflictual feelings is central to the achievements of the depressive position. Because of this greater integration, the infant recognizes that his hostile feelings and his destructive unconscious phantasies might have harmed or destroyed the loved mother. This gives rise to feelings of concern for the mother and anxiety that his hostile feelings might be more powerful than his good feelings and also leads to guilt for damage felt to have been done. The predominant anxiety of the depressive position is depressive anxiety, characterized by a fear for the survival of the loved object rather than the self.

Klein used the term "position" to emphasize that these are not developmental stages but "a constellation of anxieties, defences, object relations and impulses" (Hinshelwood, 1989, p. 393). She recognized that everyone fluctuates between these states of mind throughout life. Later theorists developed the idea that movement from the depressive position to the paranoid–schizoid position, as well as the other way round, is to be seen as part of a normal process of development. Bion (1970a) and Britton (1998a) emphasized the fluidity and iterative nature of movement between the two positions, introducing the idea of a "post-depressive paranoid–schizoid position".

3. *Projective identification*

Projective identification refers to the phantasy, far removed from conscious awareness, of entering the object—for example, the maternal object—with the whole or part of the self. This may lead to an altered perception of the self and object in relation to one another or a merging of the two in an attempt to avoid awareness of separation.

The mechanism was first defined by Klein in 1946 in her work on the emotional life of early infancy and is understood as active from the beginning of life. The term can be confusing, as there is variation in the way it is understood by theorists, and there are different underlying drivers.

Bion (1959, 1962a) identified two categories of projective identification—normal and abnormal—where the difference lies in the degree of violence with which the mechanism is executed. He described the abnormal use as the violent evacuation of a painful state of mind forcibly into an object, in phantasy, with the aim of gaining immediate relief and often with the aim of controlling the object.

A more normal use is to introduce a state of mind into the object as a means of communicating a particular mental or feeling state. This communicative use of projective identification can only be achieved if there is a sufficiently available container, usually the mother, who can take in the infant's projection and withstand its impact, including its aggressive elements, while maintaining her adult capacities and without being unduly disturbed. This is the foundation of ordinary psychic development. If a container is not available in this way, the projection is returned to the infant with increased toxicity, as it is now also infused with mother's anxiety. Bion described the infant's experience of this as "nameless dread". In this situation the infant will increasingly resort to evacuatory projective identification, leading to a depletion and disturbance in the developing personality.

As described in the Introduction to Part III, the extent to which an individual makes use of projective identification has an important impact on their psychological development. It is a question of how much of the self is in the self. Transient processes of projective identification during the development of identity are ordinary; more stuck processes, where much of the self is elsewhere (lodged in others), cause distortion in the development of the personality and the individual's sense of their own identity.

Many post-Kleinians have worked to further understand projective identification, including, notably, Rosenfeld (1965) and Meltzer (1967).

4. Containment

The concept of containment has become central in the British Object Relations school of psychoanalysis. It originates in Bion's model of "container–contained" (1962a) and draws on Klein's understanding of the mechanism of projective identification (1946). In this model the mother is seen as a container for the infant's projected feelings, such as distress caused by early primitive anxieties or unsatisfied needs. The containing function is provided by the mother through an unconscious capacity Bion called "reverie". This implies a particular state of mind in which the mother is open to receiving what the baby projects, can take it in and psychically digest it. Through this process she conveys to the baby that his anxieties and communications are bearable, have meaning, and can be understood.

Over time the baby will internalize this process, identifying with the mother's containing function, and this enables the baby to be open to the impact of new experience without being unduly disrupted by it. The baby himself becomes a container. This is the beginning of the capacity to learn in the genuine sense, which is to learn from experience.

The therapeutic relationship is seen as a containing relationship where, within a setting based on regularity and predictability, the psychoanalyst or psychotherapist brings his reverie and capacity for reflective thinking to the communications of the patient.

5. *The Oedipus complex*

Freud's formulation of the Oedipus complex arose out of the self-analysis he undertook following the death of his father and is first mentioned in a letter to his friend Fliess in 1897 (Masson, 1985, p. 272). The complex is seen in psychoanalysis as universal, and, as Freud saw it, it centres on the child's unconscious wish to have sole possession of the parent of the opposite sex and exclude or eliminate the parent of the same sex. This is the complex in its original formulation and its most florid state, but what we see in infant observation and in work with young children is the infant wanting to possess each parent and exclude the other.

Freud named the complex after the mythical Oedipus who killed his father and married his mother without being aware that they were his parents. In Freudian theory the complex was thought to emerge between the ages of 3 and 5, and working through of the complex, resulting in the child achieving identification with the parent of the same sex, was thought to bring about its resolution. However it is arguable whether the Oedipus complex is ever fully resolved.

Klein places the emergence of the complex considerably earlier, as the infant begins to have a sense that he is not the only one, and there is "another", felt to be an intrusive third, in reality and in mother's mind. As a feed comes to an end, the infant's mind turns to who has got mother now.

At this stage any other figure can represent this intrusive third. In line with the infant's need to keep things separate in the paranoid–schizoid position, these figures are kept separate in time or in the infant's mind to avoid the experience of a triangular configuration. In the infant's experience, when he is having a good experience with a good object, he is in full possession of it, both internally and externally (Hinshelwood, 1989).

Through the development of his cognitive and emotional capacities over time, the infant becomes increasingly able to bring objects together as he moves towards the depressive position, and this culminates in him being able to witness the possession of two objects by each other and to be "on the outside" of this couple, rather than himself being in "in possession of" the object. He can be a witness, not a participant.

Britton (1989) emphasized the importance for psychological development of the achievement of the capacity to experience oneself as the third, the one excluded from the parental couple or "on the outside". This involves feeling left out, and the capacity to bear this feeling of exclusion is to experience fully the pain of the oedipal situation. Not only has the infant become increasingly aware that his parents have a relationship with each other from which he is excluded in external reality, he has also achieved an internal situation in which he can observe and reflect on himself from an internal "third" position.

The move away from Freud's original formulation, which focuses on the traditional family constellation of mother, father, and baby, towards the contemporary emphasis on the importance of "the third", maintains the relevance of the Oedipus complex for infants and children growing up within any family structure today. There will always be "another" of some sort in the primary carer's mind, whether that be an external or an internal figure.

6. *Narcissism*

Narcissism is a difficult concept to define succinctly, as the term is used in different ways. Freud (1914c) described "primary narcissism", which he saw as a universal stage in early infancy, before there is recognition by the infant of an object and where the infant takes himself as the object of his own libidinal love.

Klein (1952b) disagreed with this formulation, as she saw the infant as object-related from birth. She put forward the idea of narcissistic *states* that are moved in and out of, rather than Freud's more static idea of the narcissistic *stage*.

In the narcissistic state the focus is on the self and the needs of the self, and the individual and his object are felt to be "of one mind". A vivid description of the narcissistic state appears in the novel *Middlemarch*, where George Eliot describes a state of mind in which we believe that everything in the world exists for our benefit—in other words, we see ". . . the world as an udder to feed our supreme selves" (Eliot, 1872, quoted in Waddell, 1998, p. 7).

Klein described states of mind that fluctuate throughout life between those that are predominantly self-serving (paranoid–schizoid position or more narcissistic) and those where capacities for generosity and concern for the other predominate (depressive position). The achievement of the depressive position depends on the capacity to introject good experiences, which allows the development of an independent self built on what has been taken in from others. The building of this independent self relies on an ordinary capacity to allow dependence on another. (See the Introduction to Part III for a more detailed exploration of Rosenfeld's thinking about pathological narcissism and narcissistic character structures, where the avoidance of any dependent relationship severely hinders psychic development.)

7. Transference and countertransference

These two concepts belong in the realm of clinical psychoanalysis, as they describe aspects of the relationship between patient and analyst. As there is no patient in applied psychoanalysis, these concepts are mentioned infrequently in this book but are included in the Appendix to give a broader context.

"Transference" refers to the way the patient experiences the analyst. The phenomenon has been known since the beginning of psychoanalysis but has been understood differently over time. Transference came to Freud's attention particularly sharply in the treatment of one of his patients, Dora (Freud, 1905e [1901), and this case proved to be an important but painful learning experience for him. Freud had previously experienced patients having unnaturally positive feelings towards him, but Dora broke off her analysis suddenly, with much ill feeling towards him. After the breakdown, Freud came to understand this as an enactment of Dora's feelings towards Herr K, who had made sexual advances towards her, here played out in Dora's relationship with her analyst. The dynamic was active in the moment, and she was always expecting Freud to act in the same way as Herr K. Thus Freud understood it as an enactment in the present of something from Dora's past and a demonstration of how the transference is something that needs to be worked on in the analysis to guard against detrimental acting out.

Kleinian theory brought a development in the understanding and use of the transference relationship. At the core of Kleinian theory is the concept of unconscious phantasy, which is active in the mind constantly and underlies all psychic life. What is played out in the transference relationship came to be understood as an enactment of current phantasy experience in the here and now of the clinical setting. Patients come to analysis bringing with them unconsciously everything that has ever happened to them, and this inevitably leads to unconscious expectations of the analyst. These expectations are influenced by, but don't correspond directly to, their experience of previous relationships; conversely, the way the patient experiences the analyst will never reflect external reality wholly, as their perception is always coloured by their own phantasy life.

One of the expectations of psychoanalysis is that, over time, distortions in the patient's view of reality can be modified by being worked through in the transference.

Psychoanalytic thinking about "countertransference" changed significantly in the second half or the twentieth century as a result of Heimann's work (Heimann, 1950). In the early days of psychoanalysis, there were some who thought that the analyst should put aside his own feelings altogether and present as a blank slate for the patient; others recognized that analysts would inevitably have feelings, but these were seen as inconvenient interference. Heimann revolutionized these ways of thinking and introduced the idea that feelings evoked in the analyst during work with a particular patient could be understood as giving potentially helpful information about the patient's own state of mind and feelings.

The blank-slate approach implies that analysts were not open to their patients' emotional communications but were, perhaps, making interpretations about the patient's verbally expressed stories predominantly on a cognitive level. However, understanding was increasing about the need for a mind to have another mind to make use of in order for psychic change to take place, and thinking about projective identification was taking more of a central place. The concepts of countertransference and projective identification belong together, as it came to be understood that some of the feelings or feeling states that analysts were picking up and experiencing were being communicated by their patients through projective identification. However, making sense of the countertransference is not an easy task—the analyst has feelings, just as the patient does, and has the very complex task of sorting out what belongs to him and what might be being communicated by the patient. The patient makes use of and may intrude into the analyst's mind in all sorts of ways, and the countertransference has become an important instrument for understanding the transference.

8. Mourning

In his paper, "Mourning and Melancholia", Freud is compelling in explaining how anger that would consciously be directed at someone else is unconsciously shifted onto the person's own ego through identification with the object. In this way the object need not be relinquished, but the price is the "countless separate struggles" of melancholia (Freud, 1917e [1915], p. 256). By comparison, mourning seems to be a simpler process of accepting the loss of an object attachment. Freud says that "reality-testing" slowly persuades the person to accept the truth of their loss, and the ego "is persuaded by the sum of the narcissistic satisfactions it derives from being alive to sever its attachment to the object that has been abolished" (p. 255). Yet why mourning is so painful and slow and how, if it is simply a process of letting go, mourning could psychologically enrich a person remain unanswered questions (Freud, 1916a; Spillius et al., 2011a).

Klein addresses these questions by situating Freud's observations on identification and object choice within her theory of early human development. Klein explains that an actual loss later in life revives the mourning of the infant depressive position, which is fundamental to human development (Klein, 1940). The depressive position arises when the infant has begun to recognize its mother/primary carer as a whole person. This very achievement sparks mourning for the lost good—though part-object—breast (and all the security and goodness it has represented) of the earlier paranoid–schizoid position, when the infant had dealt with anxiety by phantasies of splitting, projection, and introjection of good and bad feelings (Klein, 1940). Both the ego and the objects were split, kept tolerably, but insecurely, apart. Klein argues that this way of relating is never given up and can be regressed to in times of stress, such as mourning. As previously mentioned, Bion (Meltzer, 1978) and Britton (1998a) build on this to show explicitly how oscillation between positions exists throughout life and is part of development.

Moving to the depressive-position acceptance that good and bad, love and hate, can co-exist means that absence of the good need not mean presence of the bad, as it does in the paranoid–schizoid position. Insecurity can be more tolerated. In the depressive position, anxiety brings forward concern by the ego both for itself and for its good objects.

Profound losses in later life revive these infantile fears of loss of one's inner good objects: the person feels their inner world threatened as, along with the actual external object loss, their internalized and unconscious good objects are "felt to have gone under, to be destroyed" (Klein, 1940, p. 353). Klein agrees with Freud that adult mourning is slow because it involves "reality-testing", but for her this means that the person's early internal objects and internal world have to be reintegrated and rebuilt. It is this combination that is challenging, painful, and slow. If the loss can be accepted and the mourner can feel that the "lost loved object can be preserved inside", this can support the ego and stimulate sublimations that explain the flowering of life that is often observed after loss:

> painful experiences of all kinds can sometimes stimulate sublimations, or even bring out quite new gifts in some people. . . . Others become more productive in a different way—more capable of appreciating people and things, more tolerant . . . they become wiser.
>
> [Klein, 1940, p. 360]

REFERENCES

Abrams, M. (2006). *Birdmen, Batmen and Skyflyers*. New York: Three Rivers Press.

Adan, A. (2020). "Thinking Outside the Technocratic Box": Understanding Emotional Communication in Child Protection Work. Unpublished doctoral dissertation, Tavistock/UEL, London.

Adorno, T. W. (1955). Cultural criticism and society. In: *Prisms* (pp. 17–34), trans. S. Weber & S. Weber. Cambridge, MA: MIT Press, 1981.

Adorno, T. W. (1961). Trying to understand *Endgame*. In: *Notes to Literature*, trans. S. Weber Nicholsen. New York: Columbia University Press, 2019.

Ahmed, S. (2012). On Being Included: Racism and Diversity in Institutional Life. Durham, NC: Duke University Press.

Aiello, T. (2002). *Getting into Base*. dropzone.com. Available at: https://www.dropzone.com/articles/disciplines/getting-into-base-r49

Alvarez, A. (1992). *Beckett*. London: Fontana.

Alvarez, A. (2003). Foreword. In: H. Canham & C. Satyamurti (Eds.), *Acquainted with the Night: Psychoanalysis and the Poetic Imagination*. London: Karnac.

Anderson, S. (2011). *National Poetry Month Poem-a-Week: Jo Shapcott's "Of Mutability"*. Available at: https://scottedwardanderson.blog/2011/04

Anzieu, D. (1990). A Skin for Thought: Interviews with Gilbert Tarrab on Psychology and Psychoanalysis. London: Routledge.

Anzieu, D., & Segal, N. (2018). *The Skin-Ego: A New Translation by Naomi Segal*. London: Routledge.

Arendt, H. (1994). Eichmann in Jerusalem: A Report on the Banality of Evil. New York: Penguin.

Armstrong, D. (2005). Organization in the Mind: Psychoanalysis, Group Relations, and Organizational Consultancy. London: Karnac.

Auden, W. S. (1949). *Selected Poems*. London: Macmillan.

Auden, W. S. (1966). *Collected Shorter Poems*. London: Faber & Faber.

Badiou, A. (2003). *On Beckett*, trans. A. Toscano & N. Power. Manchester: Clinamen Press.

Badiou. A. (2005). *Being and Event*, trans. O. Feltham. New York: Continuum.

Badiou, A., & Troung, N. (2012). *In Praise of Love*. London: Serpent's Tail.

Bainbridge, C., & Yates, C. (2021). Series Editors preface. In: N. Giffney, *The Culture-Breast in Psychoanalysis: Cultural Experiences and the Clinic*. London: Routledge.

Bardenstein, C. B. (1997). Raped brides and steadfast mothers: Appropriations of Palestinian motherhood. In: *The Politics of Motherhood: Activist Voices from Left to Right* (pp. 170–181). Hanover, NE: University Press of New England.

Barnard, C., & Harris, P. (2016). Safeguarding Black Children: Good Practice in Child Protection. London: Jessica Kingsley.

Barnes, J. (2013). *Levels of Life*. London: Jonathon Cape.

Barrett, J., Chase, Z., Zhang, J., Banaszak Holl, M. M., Willis, K., et al. (2020). Microplastic pollution in deep-sea sediments from the Great Australian Bight. *Frontiers in Marine Science*, *7*: 576170. Available at: https://www.frontiersin.org/journals/marine-science/articles/10.3389/fmars.2020.576170/full

BASW (2018). *Professional Capabilities Framework for Social Work in England: Guidance on Using the 2018 Refreshed PCF*. Available at: https://basw.co.uk/policy-and-practice/resources/professional-capabilities-framework-social-work-england

Bataille, G. (1951). Molloy's silence. In: *Samuel Beckett's Molloy, Malone Dies, The Unnamable*, ed. H. Bloom. New York: Chelsea House, 1988.

Baudry, F. (1984). An essay on method in applied psychoanalysis. *Psychoanalytic Quarterly*, *53* (4): 551–581.

BBC (2012). *Gangnam Style Becomes YouTube's Most Viewed Video*. Available at: http://www.bbc.co.uk/news/technology-20483087

Beckett, S. (1938). *Murphy*. New York: Grove Press.

Beckett, S. (1951a). Malone Dies. In: Three Novels: Molloy, Malone Dies, The Unnamable. New York: Grove Press, 2009.

Beckett, S. (1951b). *Molloy*. In: *Three Novels: Molloy, Malone Dies, The Unnamable*. New York: Grove Press, 2009.
Beckett, S. (1952a). Happy Days. In: Samuel Beckett: The Complete Dramatic Work: London: Faber & Faber, 1986.
Beckett, S. (1952b). Waiting for Godot. In: Samuel Beckett: The Complete Dramatic Work. London: Faber & Faber, 1986.
Beckett, S. (1953). The Unnamable. In: Three Novels: Molloy, Malone Dies, The Unnamable. New York: Grove Press, 2009.
Beckett, S. (1957). *Endgame*. In: *Samuel Beckett: The Complete Dramatic Work*. London: Faber & Faber, 1986.
Beckett, S. (1969). *Breath*. In: *Samuel Beckett: The Complete Dramatic Work*. London: Faber & Faber, 1986.
Beckett, S. (1972). *Not I*. In: *Samuel Beckett: The Complete Dramatic Work*. London: Faber & Faber, 1986.
Beckett, S. (1980). *Rockaby*. In: *Samuel Beckett: The Complete Dramatic Work*. London: Faber & Faber, 1986.
Beckett, S., & Duthuit, G. (1949). Three dialogues. In: *Transition Forty-Nine*, No. 5, pp. 97–103.
Bell, D. (2009). Is truth an illusion? Psychoanalysis and postmodernism. *International Journal of Psychoanalysis, 90*: 331–345.
Berryman, J. (1964). *The Dream Songs*. New York: Farrar Strauss & Giroux.
Bick, E. (1964). Notes on infant observation in psycho-analytic training. *International Journal of Psychoanalysis, 45*: 558–566.
Bick, E. (1968). The experience of the skin in early object relations. *International Journal of Psychoanalysis, 49:* 484–486.
Binswanger, L. (1958). The existential analysis school of thought [trans. E. Angel]. In: R. May, E. Angel, & H. F. Ellenberger (Eds.), *Existence: A New Dimension in Psychiatry and Psychology* (pp. 191–213). New York: Simon & Schuster.
Bion, W. R. (1953). Notes on the theory of schizophrenia. In: *Second Thoughts: Selected Papers on Psychoanalysis* (pp. 23–35). London: Heinemann, 1967.
Bion, W. R. (1957). Differentiation of the psychotic from the non-psychotic. In: *Second Thoughts: Selected Papers on Psychoanalysis* (pp. 43–64). London: Heinemann, 1967.
Bion, W. R. (1959). Attacks on linking. *International Journal of Psychoanalysis, 40* (2): 308–315.
Bion, W. R. (1962a). *Learning from Experience*. London: Karnac, 1984.
Bion, W. R. (1962b). A theory of thinking. In: *Second Thoughts*. London: Heinemann, 1967.
Bion, W. R. (1967a). Notes on memory and desire. In: E. Bott Spillius (Ed.), *Melanie Klein Today, Vol. 2: Mainly Practice* (pp. 17–21). London: Routledge, 1988.

Bion, W. R. (1967b). *Second Thoughts*. London: Karnac, 1984.
Bion, W. R. (1970a). Container and contained transformed. In: *Attention and Interpretation* (pp. 117–124). London: Karnac, 1984.
Bion, W. R. (1970b). Reality sensuous and psychic. In: *Attention and Interpretation*. London: Karnac.
Bion, W. R. (1990). *Cogitations*. London: Karnac.
Birnholz, J. C., & Benacerraf, B. R. (1983). The development of human fetal hearing. *Science, 222*: 516–518.
Bishop, E. (1952). Arrival at Santos. In: *The Complete Poems*. London: Chatto & Windus.
Blanchot, M. (1953). Where now? Who now? In: *The Book to Come*, trans. C. Mandell. Stanford, CA: Stanford University Press, 2002.
Bloom, H. (2000). *How to Read and Why*. New York: Touchstone Press.
Blum, L. D. (2013). Music, memory, and relatedness. *International journal of Applied Psychoanalytic Studies, 10* (2): 121–131.
Boisen, J., & Fävremar, B. [Dirs.] (2011). *Split of a Second* [Film]. Gothenburg: Goovinn.
Bollas, C. (1987). The Shadow of the Object: Psychoanalysis of the Unthought Known. London: Free Association Books.
Bollas, C. (1992). Being a Character: Psychoanalysis and Self Experience. London: Routledge.
Bond, D. (1952). *The Love and Fear of Flying*. New York: International Universities Press.
Boole, J. (2009). Staring death in the face: The truth behind BASE jumping. *Daily Mail*, 5 January. Available at: https://www.dailymail.co.uk/home/moslive/article-1103214/Staring-death-face-The-truth-BASE-jumping.html
Boulter, J. (2008). *Beckett: A Guide for the Perplexed*. London: Bloomsbury.
Bower, M. (Ed.) (2005). Psychoanalytic Theory for Social Work Practice. London: Routledge.
Bower, M., & Solomon, R. (Eds.) (2018). What Social Workers Need to Know: A Psychoanalytic Approach. London: Routledge.
Brazelton, T. B., & Cramer, B. G. (1991). The Earliest Relationship: Parents, Infants, and the Drama of Early Attachment. London: Karnac.
Briggs, S. (1992). Child observation and social work training. *Journal of Social Work Practice, 6* (1): 49–61.
Britton, R. (1989). The missing link: Parental sexuality in the Oedipus complex. *The Oedipus Complex Today: Clinical Implications* (pp. 83–101). London: Karnac.
Britton, R. (1992). The Oedipus situation and the depressive position. In: *Clinical Lectures on Klein and Bion* (pp. 34–45). London: Routledge.

Britton, R. (1998a). Before and after the depressive position. In: *Belief and Imagination*. London: Routledge.
Britton, R. (1998b). Milton's destructive narcissist or Blake's true self. In: *Belief and Imagination*. London: Routledge.
Britton, R. (2003). Sex, Death, and the Superego: Experiences in Psychoanalysis. London: Karnac.
Britzman, D. (2003). After-Education: Anna Freud, Melanie Klein, and Psychoanalytic Histories of Learning. New York: State University of New York Press.
Brophy, B. (1988). *Mozart the Dramatist* (Revised edition). London: Faber & Faber.
Brymer, G. E. (2005). *Extreme Dude! A Phenomenological Perspective on the Extreme Sport Experience*. Doctoral dissertation, Faculties of Education and Psychology, University of Wollongong.
Caesar, E. (2009). The men who fall to earth. *Sunday Times*, 8 March. Available at: https://edcaesar.co.uk/2009/03/08/men-fall-earth-sunday-times
Cancer Research UK (2024). *Cancer Survival for Common Cancers*. Available at: https://www.cancerresearchuk.org/health-professional/cancer-statistics/survival#heading-One
Carotenuto, A. (1980). A Secret Symmetry: Sabina Spielrein between Jung and Freud. New York: Pantheon Books.
Carrington, D. (2022). Microplastics found in human blood for the first time. *The Guardian*, 24 March. Available at: https://www.theguardian.com/environment/2022/mar/24/microplastics-found-in-human-blood-for-first-time
CCETSW (1989). *Rules and Requirements for the Diploma in Social Work: Paper 30*. London: Central Council of Education and Training in Social Work.
CCETSW (1995). *Rules and Requirements for the Diploma in Social Work: Paper 30*. London: Central Council of Education and Training in Social Work.
Centre for Sensory Studies (2023). *From the Skin Ego to the Psychic Envelope: An Introduction to the Work of Didier Anzieu*. Available at: http://centreforsensorystudies.org/occasional-papers/chapter-one-from-the-skin-ego-to-the-psychic-envelope-an-introduction-to-the-work-of-didier-anzieu
Coltart, N. (1998). Slouching towards Buddhism: In conversation with Anthony Molino. In: A. Molino (Ed.), *The Couch and the Tree* (pp. 176–193). New York: North Point Press.
Conrad, P. (1948). A Song of Love and Death: The Meaning of Opera. London: Chatto & Windus.
Cooper, A. (2018). Conjunctions: Social Work, Psychoanalysis, and Society. London: Karnac.

Cooper, A., & Lousada, L. (2005). Borderline Welfare: Feeling and the Fear of Feeling in Modern Welfare. London: Karnac.

Copley, B. (1993). "A Plague on all our Houses": A discussion of Shakespeare's play *Romeo and Juliet*. In: *The World of Adolescence: Literature, Society and Psychoanalytic Psychotherapy*. London: Free Association Books.

Crichton-Smith, I. (2011). *New Collected Poems*. Manchester: Carcanet Press.

Crown, S. (2010). *Jo Shapcott: I'm Not Someone Chasing Her Own Ambulance. The Guardian*, 24 July. Available at: https://www.theguardian.com/books/2010/jul/24/jo-shapcott-poet-interview?view=mobile

CSRP (2022). *Child Protection in England: National Review into the Murders of Arthur Labinjo-Hughes and Star Hobson*. London: Child Safeguarding Practice Review Panel. Available at: https://assets.publishing.service.gov.uk/government/uploads/system/uploads/attachment_data/file/1078488/ALH_SH_National_Review_26-5-22.pdf

Darwish, M. (2002). A love story between an Arab poet and his land. An interview with Mahmud Darwish. *Journal of Palestine Studies, 31* (3): 67–78.

Darwish, M. (2005). *The Butterfly's Burden*, trans. F. Joudah. Port Townsend, WA: Copper Canyon Press.

Davids, M. F. (2011). Internal Racism: A Psychoanalytic Approach to Race and Difference. London: Palgrave Macmillan.

Davids, Z., Miles, G., Paton, A., & Trowell, J. (1999). Issues for seminar leaders in infant and young child observation: A comparative study. *International Journal of Infant Observation and Its Applications, 2* (3): pp. 16–29.

Dedijer, J. (2004). *BASE 66: A Story of Fear, Fun and Freefall*. New York: iUniverse.

Dominelli, L. (2018). *Anti-Racist Social Work* (4th edition). London: Macmillan.

Douglas, M. (1966). *Purity and Danger*. London: Routledge Classics.

Eagleton, T. (1983). *Literary Theory: An Introduction*. Oxford: Blackwell, 1995.

Eagleton, T. (2013). *How to Read Literature*. New Haven, CT: Yale University Press.

Edward, T., Als, H., Adamson, L. Wise, S., & Brazelton, T. B. (1978). The infant's response to entrapment between contradictory messages in face-to-face interaction. *Journal of the American Academy of Child Psychiatry, 17* (1): 1–13.

Edwards, J. (1994). Towards solid ground. *Journal of Child Psychotherapy 20* (1): 57–83.

Edwards, J. (2003). The elusive pursuit of insight. In: H. Canham & C. Satyamurti (Eds.), *Acquainted with the Night: Psychoanalysis and the Poetry Imagination* (pp. 167–189). London: Karnac. Reprinted in: *Love the Wild Swan: The Selected Works of Judith Edwards* (chapter 13). London: Routledge, 2016.

Edwards, J., Arnold, K., Hanson, C., Ngah, Z., Oclander-Goldie, S., & Segal, B. (2006). Making connections: Teaching observation skills to non-clinical students on an MA course in Psychoanalytical Studies. *International Journal of Infant Observation and Its Applications, 9* (3): 221–232.

Eigen, M. (1985). Toward Bion's starting point: Between catastrophe and faith. *International Journal of Psychoanalysis, 66*: 321–330.

Eliot, G. (1872). *Middlemarch*. Edinburgh: William Blackwood.

Eliot, T. S. (1933). *The Use of Poetry and the Use of Criticism*. London: Faber & Faber.

Eliot, T. S. (1983). *Four Quartets*. London: Faber.

Ellis, L. (1997). The meaning of difference: Race, culture and context in infant observation, In: S. Reid (Ed.), *Developments in Infant Observation: The Tavistock Model* (1st edition, pp. 56–80). London: Routledge.

Emanuel, R. (2001). A-void—an exploration of defences against sensing nothingness. *International Journal of Psychoanalysis, 82*: 1069–1084.

Empson, W. (1977). *Seven Types of Ambiguity*. Harmondsworth: Penguin.

Esslin, M. (1960.) The theatre of the absurd. *The Tulane Drama Review, 4* (4).

Evans, D. (1996). An Introductory Dictionary of Lacanian Psychoanalysis. London: Routledge.

Fadnes, E. (2011). *Sense of Flying* [Film]. Goteborg: Goovinn.

Fenichel, O. (1935). A critique of the death instinct. In: *Collected Papers*, New York: Norton, 1953.

Ferguson, H. (2022). Support for social workers is the missing piece of the Star and Arthur review. *The Guardian*, 27 May. Available at: https://www.theguardian.com/commentisfree/2022/may/27/social-workers-star-arthur-review-children-abusers

Finlay, L. (2014). Engaging phenomenological analysis. *Qualitative Research in Psychology, 11* (2): 121–141.

Fisher, J. B. (1999). The Winter's Tale: Marriage and re-marriage. In: *The Uninvited Guest: Emerging from Narcissism towards Marriage*. London: Karnac.

Fraiberg, S., Adelson, E., & Shapiro, V. (1975). Ghosts in the nursery: A psychoanalytic approach to the problems of impaired infant–mother relationships. *Journal of American Academy of Child Psychiatry, 14* (3): 387–421.

Fraiberg, S. H., & Fraiberg, L. (1980). *Clinical Studies in Infant Mental Health: The First Year of Life*. London: Tavistock Publications.

Frank, A. W. (1995). *The Wounded Storyteller*. Chicago, IL: University of Chicago Press.

Frank, A. W. (2004). *The Renewal of Generosity: Illness, Medicine and How to Live*. Chicago, IL: University of Chicago Press.

Freeman Sharpe, E. (1950). Papers on literary interpretation. In: *Collected Papers on Psychoanalysis* (pp. 203—-266). London: Hogarth Press.

Freud, S. (1900a). The Interpretation of Dreams. Standard Edition, 4/5.
Freud, S. (1905e [1901]). Fragment of an analysis of a case of hysteria. *Standard Edition, 7*: 3.
Freud, S. (1908b). Character and anal eroticism. *Standard Edition, 9.*
Freud, S. (1908e [1907]). Creative writers and daydreaming. *Standard Edition, 9.*
Freud, S. (1910c). Leonardo da Vinci and a memory of his childhood. *Standard Edition, 11.*
Freud, S. (1911b). Formulations on the two principles of mental functioning. *Standard Edition, 12.*
Freud, S. (1914b). The Moses of Michelangelo. *Standard Edition, 13.*
Freud, S. (1914c). On narcissism. *Standard Edition, 14.*
Freud, S. (1914g). Remembering, repeating and working through (Further recommendations on the technique of psycho-analysis, II). *Standard Edition, 12.*
Freud, S. (1916a). On transience. *Standard Edition, 14.*
Freud, S. (1916d). Some character-types met with in psycho-analytic work. *Standard Edition, 14.*
Freud, S. (1917e [1915]). Mourning and melancholia. *Standard Edition, 14.*
Freud, S. (1920g). Beyond the Pleasure Principle. Standard Edition, 18.
Freud, S. (1923b). The Ego and the Id. Standard Edition, 19.
Freud, S. (1925h). Negation. *Standard Edition, 19.*
Freud, S. (1927e). Fetishism. *Standard Edition, 21.*
Freud, S. (1930a). Civilization and Its Discontents. Standard Edition, 21.
Fricker, M. (2007). *Epistemic Injustice: Power and the Ethics of Knowing*. Oxford: Oxford University Press.
Froggett, L. (2008). Artistic output as intersubjective third. In: *Object Relations and Social Relations: The Implications of the Relational Turn in Psychoanalysis* (pp. 87–111). London: Karnac.
Fromm-Reichmann, F. (1959). Loneliness. *Psychiatry, 22* (1): 1–15.
Frost, R. (2013). *The Poetry of Robert Frost: The Collected Poems,* ed. E. Conney Latham. London: Random House.
Gardner, M. R. (1994). *On Trying to Teach*. London: Analytic Press.
Gerdes, M. (2010). *The Great Book of BASE*. Hong Kong: Birdbrain Publishing.
Giffney, N. (2021). The Culture-Breast in Psychoanalysis: Cultural Experiences and the Clinic. London: Routledge.
Glover, N. (2009). Psychoanalytic Aesthetics: An Introduction to the British School. London: Harris Meltzer Trust, 2018.
Gould, N., & Taylor, I. (Eds.) (1996). *Reflective Learning for Social Work*. Aldershot: Arena.
Green, A. (2005). Play and Reflection in Donald Winnicott's Writings. London: Karnac.
Greenfield, H. (1980). *Puccini: A Biography*. London: Robert Hale.

Groes, S. (2011). The new seriousness: Kazuo Ishiguro in conversation with Sebastian Groes. In: S. Groes & B. Lewis (Eds.), *Kazuo Ishiguro: New Critical Visions of the Novels*. Basingstoke: Palgrave Macmillan.

Grotstein, J. S. (2013). Dreaming as a "curtain of illusion": Revisiting the "Royal Road" with Bion as our guide. In H. B. Levine & L. J. Brown (Eds.), *Growth and Turbulence in the Container/Contained: Bion's Continuing Legacy* (pp. 107–128). London: Routledge.

Halifax, Edward, Lord (1957). *Fullness of Days*. New York: Dodd, Mead and Company.

Harari, Y. N. (2015). *Sapiens: A Brief History of Humankind*. New York: Harper.

Harari, Y. N. (2018). *21 Lessons for the 21st Century*. New York: Spiegel & Grau.

Harlow, B. (1987). *Resistance Literature*. New York: Methuen Press.

Harris Williams, M., & Waddell, M. (1991). Shakespeare: A local habitation and a name. In: *The Chamber of Maiden Thought*. London: Routledge.

Healthtalk.org (2012). *Living with Breast Cancer*. Available at: https://healthtalk.org/experiences/breast-cancer-women/living-breast-cancer

Heimann, P. (1950). On countertransference. *International Journal of Psychoanalysis, 31*: 81—84.

Herbert, Z. (1985). *Selected Poems*. New York: Ecco Press.

Hindle, D. (2000). L'Enfant et les sortilèges revisited. *International Journal of Psychoanalysis, 81* (6): 1185–1196.

Hindle, D., & Godsil, S. (2006). The song of the siren: Some thoughts on idealization and creativity in Martinu's Julietta. *International Journal of Psychoanalysis, 87* (4): 1087–1102.

Hingley-Jones, H., Parkinson, C., & Allain, L. (Eds.) (2017). Observation in Health and Social Care: Applications for Learning, Research and Practice with Children and Adults. London: Jessica Kingsley.

Hinshelwood, R. (1989). *A Dictionary of Kleinian Thought*. London: Free Association Books.

Hinshelwood, R. D. (2008). Group therapy as psychic containing. *International Journal of Group Psychotherapy, 58* (3): 283–303.

Hinshelwood, R. D., & Skogstad, W. (Eds.) (2002). *Observing Organisations: Anxiety, Defence and Culture in Health Care*. London: Routledge.

Hoggett, P. (2013). Climate change denial in a perverse culture. In: S. Weintrobe (Ed.), *Engaging with Climate Change: Psychoanalytic and Interdisciplinary Perspectives*. London: Routledge.

Holmes, J. T. (2007). Wingsuit flying in Norway. In: *Seven Sunny Days* [Film]. Crested Butte, CO: Matchstick Productions. Available at: https://www.youtube.com/watch?v=S9FUl9x9XYo

Holt-Lunstad, J. (2017). The potential public health relevance of social isolation and loneliness: Prevalence, epidemiology, and risk factors, *Public Policy & Aging Report, 27* (4): 127–130.

Hornstein, G. (2012). Agnes's Jacket: A Psychologist's Search for the Meanings of Madness. Ross-on-Wye: PCCS Books.

Horton, H. (2023). New disease caused by plastics discovered in seabirds. *The Guardian*, 3 March. Available at: https://www.theguardian.com/environment/2023/mar/03/plasticosis-new-disease-caused-by-plastics-discovered-in-seabirds?ref=refind

Hughes, T. (1967). *Selected Translations*, ed. D. Weissbort. London: Faber & Faber.

Hurd, M. (2005). What BASE jumping does to me. In: *What Is Base Jumping*? UkProBASE. Available at: http://web.archive.org/web/20090614001750/http://www.ukprobase.com:80/whatisbase.htm#expand

Hurston, Z. N. (1942). *Dust Tracks on a Road: An Autobiography*. London: Hutchinson.

Husserl, E. (1973). *Cartesian Meditations*. The Hague: Martinus Nijhoff.

Ionesco, E. (1957). Dans les armes de la ville. Cahiers de la Compagnie Madeleine Renaud-Jean-Louis Barrault, Paris, 20 (October).

Isaacs, S. (1948). The nature and function of phantasy. *International Journal of Psychoanalysis, 24* (2): 73–97.

Ishiguro, K. (1982). *A Pale View of the Hills*. London: Faber & Faber.

Ishiguro, K. (1986). *Artist of the Floating World*. London: Faber & Faber.

Ishiguro, K. (1989). *The Remains of the Day*. London: Faber & Faber.

Ishiguro, K. (1995). *The Unconsoled*. London: Faber & Faber.

Ishiguro, K. (2005). *Never Let Me Go*. London: Faber & Faber.

Janaway, C. (Ed.) (1999). *The Cambridge Companion to Schopenhauer*. Cambridge: Cambridge University Press.

Jaques, E. (1955). Social systems as a defence against persecutory and depressive anxiety. In M. Klein, P. Heimann, & R. Money-Kyrle (Eds.), *New Directions in Psychoanalysis*. London: Tavistock.

Jones, E. (1949). *Hamlet and Oedipus*. New York: Norton.

Jones, E. (1961). *The Life and Work of Sigmund Freud*. New York: Basic Books.

Jones, R. (2014). The Story of Baby P: Setting the Record Straight. Bristol: Polity Press.

Joseph, B. (1982). Addiction to near death. *International Journal of Psychoanalysis, 63*: 449–456.

Joseph, B. (1988). Projective identification: Clinical aspects. In: J. Sandler, *Projection, Identification, Projective Identification* (pp. 65–76). London: Karnac.

Jounah, F. (2013). Foreword. In: M. Darwish. *Unfortunately, It Was Paradise*. Oakland, CA: University of California Press.

Judd, D. (1995). Give Sorrow Words: Working with a Dying Child. London: Whurr.

Kahr, B. (2017). *Coffee with Freud*. London: Karnac.

Kanafani, G. (1968). *Poetry of Resistance in Occupied Palestine*, trans. S. Hijjawi. Baghdad: Ministry of Culture, 2009.

Katz, H. M. (2002). Escaping gravity: Movie magic and dreams of flying. *Psychoanalytic Study of the Child, 57*: 294–304.

Keene, J. (2013). Unconscious obstacles to caring for the planet: Facing up to human nature. In: S. Weintrobe (Ed.), *Engaging with Climate Change: Psychoanalytic and Interdisciplinary Perspectives* (pp. 144–159). London: Routledge.

Keep Britain Tidy (2022). *We Warn Car Owners, "Don't Be a Tosser"*. Available at: https://www.keepbritaintidy.org/news/we-warn-car-owners-dont-be-tosser

Kim, R. (2010). Women and Ireland as Beckett's Lost Others: Beyond Mourning and Melancholia. London: Palgrave Macmillan.

Klein, M. (1929). Infantile anxiety-situations reflected in a work of art and in the creative impulse. In: *Love, Guilt and Reparation and Other Works 1921–1945*. London: Hogarth Press, 1975.

Klein, M. (1930). The importance of symbol formation in the development of the ego. In: *Love, Guilt and Reparation and Other Works 1921–1945*. London: Hogarth Press, 1975.

Klein, M. (1932). *The Psycho-Analysis of Children*. London: Hogarth Press, 1975.

Klein, M. (1935). A contribution to the psychogenesis of manic-depressive states. In: *Love, Guilt and Reparation and Other Works 1921–1945*. London: Hogarth Press, 1975.

Klein, M. (1936). Weaning. In: *Love, Guilt and Reparation and Other Works 1921–1945*. London: Hogarth Press, 1975.

Klein, M. (1940). Mourning and its relation to manic depressive states. In: *Love, Guilt and Reparation and Other Works 1921–1945*. London: Hogarth Press, 1975.

Klein, M. (1946). Notes on some schizoid mechanisms. In: *Envy and Gratitude and Other Works 1946–1963*. London: Hogarth Press, 1975.

Klein, M. (1952a). On observing the behaviour of young infants. In: *Envy and Gratitude and Other Works, 1946–1963*. London: Vintage, 1997.

Klein, M. (1952b). The origins of transference. In: *Envy and Gratitude and Other Works 1946–1963*. London: Hogarth Press, 1975.

Klein, M. (1952c). Some theoretical conclusions regarding the emotional life of the infant. In: *Envy and Gratitude and Other Works, 1946–1963*. London: Vintage, 1997.

Klein, M. (1959). Our adult world and its roots in infancy. In: *Envy and Gratitude and Other Works 1946–1963*. London: Hogarth Press, 1975.

Klein, M. (1963). On the sense of loneliness. In: *Envy and Gratitude and Other Works 1946–1963*. London: Hogarth Press, 1975.

Klein, M. (1975). Envy and Gratitude and Other Works 1946–1963. London: Hogarth Press.

Kleinman, A. (1988). The Illness Narratives: Suffering, Healing and the Human Condition. New York: Basic Books.

Knowlson, J. (1996). *Damned to Fame: The Life of Samuel Beckett*. London: Bloomsbury.

Kohut, H. (1950). On the enjoyment of music. *Psychoanalytic Quarterly, 19*: 64–87.

Komesaroff, P. A. (1995). From bioethics to microethics: Ethical debates and clinical medicine. In: P. A. Komesaroff (Ed.), *Troubled Bodies: Clinical Perspectives on Postmodernism, Medical Ethics, and the Body*. Durham, NC: Duke University Press.

Kott, J. (1967). *Shakespeare, Our Contemporary*. London: Methuen.

Krider, D. (1998). Rooted in a small space: An interview with Kazuo Ishiguro. *Kenyon Review New Series, 20* (2). Reprinted in: B. W. Shaffer & C. F. Wong (Eds.), *Conversations with Kazuo Ishiguro* (pp. 125–134). Jackson, MS: University Press of Mississippi, 2008.

Kristeva, J. (1982). *Powers of Horror: An Essay on Abjection*. New York: Columbia University Press.

Kubie, L. S. (1937). The fantasy of dirt. *Psychoanalytic Quarterly, 6*: 388–425.

Lacan, J. (1938). *Family Complexes in the Formation of the Individual*. Unpublished translation by Cormac Gallagher. Available at: http://www.lacaninireland.com/web/wp-content/uploads/2010/06/FAMILY-COMPLEXES-IN-THE-FORMATION-OF-THE-INDIVIDUAL2.pdf.

Lacan, J. (1960a). Position of the unconscious. In: *Écrits: The First Complete Edition in English* (pp. 719–720), trans. B. Frink. New York: Norton, 2006.

Lacan, J. (1960b). The subversion of the subject and the dialectic of desire in the Freudian unconscious. In *Écrits: The First Complete Edition in English* (pp. 671–702), trans. B. Frink. New York: Norton, 2006.

Lacan, J. (1977). *The Four Fundamental Concepts of Psycho-Analysis* (1st edition), ed. J. A. Miller. London: Routledge, 2004.

Laming, W. H. (2003). The Victoria Climbié inquiry: Report of an Inquiry by Lord Laming. London: Stationery Office

Laming, Lord (2009). The Protection of Children in England: A Progress Report. London: Stationery Office.

Larkin, P. (1992). *Selected Letters of Philip Larkin 1940–85*. London: Faber & Faber.

Lasch, C. (1979). The Culture of Narcissism: American Life in an Age of Diminishing Expectations. New York: Norton.

Laurendeau, J. (2012). *BASE Jumping, The Ultimate Guide*. Santa Barbara, CA: Greenwood.

Lechevalier-Haim, B. (2001). From freezing to thawing: Working towards the depressive position in long-term therapy with autistic patients. In: J. Edwards (Ed.), *Being Alive* (pp. 89–102). London: Taylor & Francis.

Le Riche, P., & Tanner, K. (Eds.) (1998). *Observation and Its Application in Social Work: Rather Like Breathing*. London: Jessica Kingsley.

Lewandowsky, S., Ecker, U. K. H., & Cook, J. (2017). Beyond misinformation: Understanding and coping with the "post-truth" era. *Journal of Applied Research in Memory and Cognition, 6* (4): 353–369.

Likierman, M. (1988). Maternal love and positive projective identification. *Journal of Child Psychotherapy, 14* (2): 29–46.

Linebarger, M. (1974). *John Berryman*. New York: Twayne.

Li Qingzhao (Chinese: 李清照, 1084–1155). In: *Song Dynasty*. Available at: http://blog.sina.com.cn/s/blog_6252b0bb0100ro16.html

Llewellyn-Beardsley, J., Rennick-Egglestone, S., Callard, F., Crawford, P., Farkas, M., Hui, A., et al. (2019). Characteristics of mental health recovery narratives: Systematic review and narrative synthesis. *PloS One, 14* (3): e0214678.

Lorde, A. (1997). Today is not the day. In: *The Collected Poems of Audre Lorde*. New York: Norton.

Lorde, A. (2017). Poetry is not a luxury. In: *The Masters Tools Will Never Dismantle the Master's House*. London: Penguin/Random House.

Lowe, F. (Ed.) (2014). Thinking Space: The Model Promoting Thinking about Race, Culture, and Diversity in Psychotherapy and Beyond. London: Karnac.

Lyng, S. (1990). Edgework: A social psychological analysis of voluntary risk taking. *American Journal of Sociology, 95* (4): 851–886.

MacAlister, J. (2022). Independent Review of Children's Social Care: Final Report. London: Department of Education.

Malloch, S., & Trevarthen, C. (2009). *Communicative Musicality: Exploring the Basis of Human Companionship*. London: Oxford University Press.

Mason, G. (1986). An interview with Kazuo Ishiguro. *Contemporary Literature, 30* (No. 3, 1989): 334–347. Reprinted in: B. W. Shaffer & C. F. Wong (Eds.), *Conversations with Kazuo Ishiguro*. Jackson, MS: University Press of Mississippi, 2008.

Masson, J. M. (Ed.) (1985). *The Complete Letters of Sigmund Freud to Wilhelm Fliess, 1887–1904*. Cambridge, MA: Harvard University Press.

Matsumoto, D., & Juang, L. (2013). *Culture and Psychology* (5th edition). Belmont, CA: Wadsworth.

McDougall, C. (2009). Confessions of an Idiot: The Colourful Tale of a Life in Freefall. BASE Dreams.

McDougall, J. (1986). *Theatres of the Mind*. London: Free Association Books.

McGuirk, J. (2022). *The Waste Age*. London: Design Museum. Available at: https://aeon.co/essays/ours-is-the-waste-age-thats-the-key-to-tranforming-the-future

Megroz, G. (2012). The 10 greatest adventure stories of the next century. *Outside Adventure Magazine*. Available at: https://www.outsideonline.com/outdoor-adventure/exploration-survival/10-greatest-adventure-stories-next-century

Meltzer, D. (1967). *The Psycho-Analytical Process*. Strathtay: Clunie Press, 1990.

Meltzer, D. (1978). The Kleinian Development Part III: The Clinical Significance of the Work of Bion. Strathtay: Clunie Press, 1985.

Meltzer, D. (1987). On aesthetic reciprocity. *Journal of Child Psychotherapy, 13* (2): 3–14.

Meltzer, D., & Harris Williams, M. (1988a). The Apprehension of Beauty: The Role of Aesthetic Conflict in Development, Art, and Violence. London: Karnac, 2008.

Meltzer, D., & Harris Williams, M. (1988b). The undiscovered country: The shape of the aesthetic conflict in *Hamlet*. In: *The Apprehension of Beauty: The Role of Aesthetic Conflict in Development, Art, and Violence* (pp. 84–133). London: Karnac, 2008.

Mercier, V. (1956). The uneventful event. *The Irish Times*, 18 February, p. 6.

Mill, J. S. (1865). *Crisis in My Mental History*. New York: Harvard Classics, 1909.

Miller, A. (1949). *Death of a Salesman*. New York: Viking.

Miller, I. (2013). Beckett and Bion: The (Im)Patient Voice in Psychotherapy and Literature. London: Karnac.

Milosz, C. (1968). Ars Poetica. In: *New and Collected Poems*. London: Penguin.

Mitrani, J. L. (1998). Unbearable ecstasy, reverence and awe, and the perpetuation of an "aesthetic conflict". *Psychoanalytic Quarterly, 67* (1): 102–127.

Mohammadpour-Yazdi, A., & Lafrance, M. E. (2023). The eco skin: From an egocentric approach to an ecocentric world view. In: C. Schmidt-Hellerau & M. Erlich-Ginor (Eds.), *Mind in the Line of Fire: Psychoanalytic Voices to the Challenges of Our Times* [Mente en la Línea de Fuego: Voces psicoanalíticas ante los retos de nuestro tiempo] (pp. 580–584). London: IPA.

Mollon, P. (2002). Shame and Jealousy: The Hidden Turmoils. London: Karnac.

Montaz-Rosset, S. (Dir.) (2012). *One Step Beyond: The True Story of Géraldine Fasnacht* [Film]. Montaz-Rosset Studio.

Moore, M. (1935). Poetry. In: *Others: Anthology of New Verse*, ed. A. Kreymbourg. New York: Bartleby Books.

Morin, E. (2017). *Beckett's Political Imagination*. Cambridge: Cambridge University Press.

Morrison, A. P. (1983). Shame, ideal self, and narcissism. *Contemporary Psychoanalysis, 19*: 295–318.
Morrison, A. P. (1984). Working with shame in psychoanalytic treatment. *Journal of the American Psychoanalytic Association, 32*: 479–509.
Munro, E. (2011). The Munro Review of Child Protection. Final Report: A Child-Centred System. London: Stationery Office.
Munwha.com, (2013). '젠틀맨' 웃자고한얘기죽자고달려드네 ["Gentleman", It was just a joke, but you're taking it way too seriously]. Available at: http://www.munhwa.com/news/view.html?no=20130419MW083126847686
Murphy, C. (2023). How learning from the lived experience of child protection social workers can help us understand the factors underpinning workforce instability within the English child protection system. *Journal of Social Work Practice, 37* (2): 263–276.
Music, G. (2017). Nurturing Natures: Attachment and Children's Emotional, Sociocultural and Brain Development (2nd edition). London: Routledge.
Nagel, J. J. (2010). Melodies in my mind: The polyphony of mental life. *Journal of the American Psychoanalytic Association, 58* (4): 649–662.
National Geographic (2020). *Microplastics Found Near Everest's Peak, Highest Ever Detected in the World*. Available at: https://www.nationalgeographic.com/environment/article/microplastics-found-near-everests-peak-highest-ever-detected-world-perpetual-planet
Neumann, E. (1963). *The Great Mother* (2nd edition), trans. R. Manheim. Princeton, NJ: Princeton University Press, 1974.
Nietzsche, F. (1882). *The Gay Science*, ed. B. Williams. Cambridge: Cambridge University Press, 2001.
Noy, P. (2009). *Art and Emotions*. Unpublished manuscript.
Noyes, A. (1952). When Daddy Fell into the Pond and Other Poems for Children. New York: Sheed and Ward.
Noyes, C. (2017). Live Work: The Impact of Direct Encounters in Statutory Child and Family Social Work. Unpublished doctoral dissertation, Tavistock/UEL, London.
Ogden, T. H. (1999). The music of what happens in poetry and psychoanalysis. *International Journal of Psychoanalysis, 80* (5): 979–994.
Ogden, T. H. (2001). A question of voice. In: *Conversations at the Frontiers of Dreaming*. Northvale, NJ: Jason Aronson.
Ogden, T. H. (2006). On teaching psychoanalysis. *International Journal of Psychoanalysis, 87*: 1069–1085.
Oonaka, M., & Sato, Y. (1960). いぬのおまわりさん ["The Police Dog"], trans. L. Greg. Available at: https://www.youtube.com/watch?v=OzD59YsLqXA
Orwell, G. (1949). *Nineteen Eighty-Four*. London: Decker & Warburg.

O'Shaughnessy, E. (1981). A commemorative essay on W. R. Bion's theory of thinking. *Journal of Child Psychotherapy, 7* (2): 181–192.

O'Shaughnessy, E. (2018). Reparation: Waiting for a concept. In: P. Garvey & K. Long (Eds.), *The Klein Tradition: Lines of Development—Evolution of Theory and Practice over the Decades* (pp. 199–203). London: Routledge.

O'Toole, F. (2015). Fintan O'Toole: The truth according to Brian Friel. *The Irish Times,* 2 October. Available at: https://www.irishtimes.com/culture/brian-friel/fintan-o-toole-the-truth-according-to-brian-friel-1.2375988

Overton, P. (2006). No fear. Base jump. *60 Minutes,* 22 May. Available at: https://www.youtube.com/watch?v=PaslcutuVDU

Parkinson, C. (2000). *Beyond Competence in Social Work Training: How Are We Learning?* Psychoanalytic Studies Monograph Series No 1. London: Department of Human Relations, University of East London.

Parkinson, C. (2017). How does it feel? Best interests assessors observe adult group care. In: H. Hingley-Jones, C. Parkinson, & L. Allain (Eds.), *Observation in Health and Social Care: Applications for Learning, Research and Practice with Children and Adults*. London: Jessica Kingsley.

Parmenter, B. (2004). *Giving Voice to Stones*. Austin, TX: University of Texas Press.

Pascal, J., & Sagan, O. (2018). Cocreation or collusion: The dark side of consumer narrative in qualitative health research. *Illness, Crisis & Loss, 26* (4): 251–269.

Peller, L. E. (1954). Libidinal phases, ego development and play. *Psychoanalytic Study of the Child, 9*: 178–198.

Phillips, A. (1999). *The Beast in the Nursery*. London: Faber & Faber.

Pinter, H. (1960a). *The Birthday Party*. London: Methuen.

Pinter, H. (1960b). *The Caretaker*. London: Methuen.

Pinter, H. (1965). *The Homecoming*. London: Methuen.

Pitt, A., & Britzman, D. (2003). Speculation on qualities of difficult knowledge in teaching and learning: An experiment in psychoanalytic research. *International Journal of Qualitative Studies in Education, 16*: 755–776.

Plato (380 BC). *The Republic*. London: Penguin Classics, 2007.

Puccini, G. (1926). *Turandot* [Full score, English edition]. London: Universal Music Publishing Ricordi, 2000.

Quandt, J. (2012). *Robert Bresson (Revised)*. New York: Barnes & Noble.

Quinodoz, J.-M. (2008). Listening to Hanna Segal: Her Contribution to Psychoanalysis. London: Routledge.

Rank, O. (1924). *Trauma of Birth*. New York: Dover, 1993.

Raphael-Leff, J. (1991). *Psychological Processes of Childbearing* (revised edition). London: Chapman & Hall, 2001.

Reid, S. (1997). Introduction: Psychoanalytic infant observation. In: *Developments of Infant Observation: The Tavistock Model* (pp. 1–18). London: Routledge.

Reid, W. (2020). Black Lives Matter: Social work must respond with action—not platitudes. *Community Care,* 12 June.

Reik, T. (1941). *Masochism in Modern Man*. New York: Farrar, Strauss.

Reiner, A. (2012). Bion and Being: Passion and the Creative Mind. London: Karnac.

Rhode, M. (2013). The physicality of words: Some implications of Donald Meltzer's writings on language. *Journal of Infant Observation, 16*: 270–285.

Richards, B. (1994). Disciplines of Delight: The Psychoanalysis of Popular Culture. London: Free Association Books.

Richards, I. A. (1924). Communication and the artist. In: *Principles of Literary Criticism* (pp. 25–33). London: Kegan Paul, Trench, Trubner and Co., 1938.

Roberts, G. A. (2000). Narrative and severe mental illness: What place do stories have in an evidence-based world? *Advances in Psychiatric Treatment, 6*: 432–441.

RollingStone(2011).*500GreatestSongsofAllTime*.Availableat:https://www.rollingstone.com/music/music-lists/500-greatest-songs-of-all-time-151127/jimmy-cliff-the-harder-they-come-35805

Rosenfeld, H. (1964). On the psychopathology of narcissism: A clinical approach. In: *Psychotic States: A Psychoanalytic Approach* (pp. 169–179. New York: International Universities Press.

Rosenfeld, H. (1965). Psychotic States: A Psychoanalytic Approach. London: Hogarth Press.

Rosenfeld, H. (1971). A clinical approach to the psychoanalytic theory of the life and death instincts: An investigation into the aggressive aspects of narcissism. *International Journal of Psychoanalysis, 52*: 169–178. Reprinted in E. B. Spillius (Ed.), *Melanie Klein Today, Volume 1*. London: Routledge, 1988.

Rosenfeld, H. (1987). *Impasse and Interpretation*. London: Tavistock.

Ruch, G., Turney, D., & Ward, A. (Eds.) (2010). *Relationship-Based Social Work: Getting to the Heart of Practice* (2nd edition). London: Jessica Kingsley, 2018.

Rusbridger, R. (2008). The internal world of Don Giovanni. *International Journal of Psychanalysis, 89*: 181–194.

Rushdie, S. (1989). What the butler didn't see [Book review]. *The Observer,* 21 May, p. 53.

Rustin, M. E. (2011). Passion in the classroom. In: *Engaging with Complexity*. London: Karnac.

Rustin, M. E., & Rustin, M. J. (1987). Narratives of Love and Loss: Studies in Modern Children's Fiction. London: Karnac, 2001.

Rustin, M. E., & Rustin, M. J. (2002a). Mirror to Nature: Drama, Psychoanalysis, and Society. London: Karnac.

Rustin, M. E., & Rustin, M. J. (2002b). Shakespeare's *Macbeth*: A matrimonial tragedy. In: *Mirror to Nature: Drama, Psychoanalysis, and Society* (pp. 69–94). London: Karnac.

Rustin, M. E., & Rustin, M. J. (2006). *The Enchanted and the Human: Psychoanalytic Reflections on Handel's Operas*. Paper given at the Centre for the Advancement of Psychoanalytic Studies, Institute of Psychoanalysis, London.

Rustin, M. J. (1989). Observing infants: Reflections on methods. In: L. Miller, M. E. Rustin, M. J. Rustin, & J. Shuttleworth (Eds.), *Closely Observed Infants* (pp. 52–75). London: Duckworth.

Rustin, M. J. (1991). Thinking in Romeo and Juliet. In: *The Good Society and the Inner World*. London: Karnac, 2002.

Rustin, M. J. (2001). "Give me a consulting room . . ." The generation of psychoanalytic knowledge. In: *Reason and Unreason: Psychoanalysis, Science, Politics*. London: Continuum.

Rustin, M. J. (2007). How do psychoanalysts know what they know? In: L. Braddock & M. Lacewing (Eds.), *The Academic Face of Psychoanalysis* (pp. 172–195). London: Routledge.

Rustin, M. J. (2019a). The consulting room as the psychoanalytic laboratory. In: *Researching the Unconscious*. London: Routledge.

Rustin, M. J. (2019b). Psychoanalytic cultural methods. In: *Researching the Unconscious*. London: Routledge.

Rustin, M. J. (2019c). *Researching the Unconscious*. London: Routledge.

Rustin, M. J., & Bradley J. (Eds.) (2008). Work Discussion: Learning from Reflective Practice in Work with Children and Families. London: Karnac.

Rycroft, C. (1995). *Clinical Dictionary of Psychoanalysis*. London: Penguin.

Sagan, O. (2000). *Teaching Psychiatric Patients: A Psychoanalytic Exploration*. Unpublished MA dissertation, Tavistock/UEL, London.

Sagan, O. (2002). Teaching psychiatric patients: A psychoanalytic study. *Psychoanalytic Psychotherapy, 16* (1): 58–73.

Sagan, O. (2003). Not held by words: The refugee child in a new environment. *Early Childhood Practice, 5* (1): 11–18.

Sagan, O. (2008a). Getting It Down on Paper: Mentally Ill Adults' Use of Community-Based Expressive Literacy Provision. Unpublished doctoral dissertation, University of London.

Sagan, O. (2008b). The loneliness of the long-anxious learner: Mental illness, narrative biography and learning to write, *Psychodynamic Practice, 14* (1): 43–58.

Sagan, O. (2011a). Interminable knots: Hostages to toxic stories. *Pedagogy, Culture & Society, 19* (1): 97–118.

Sagan, O. (2011b). Love in a cold climate: Mental illness and learning to write "I love you". In: S. Jackson (Ed.), *Lifelong Learning and Social Justice: Communities, Work and Identities in a Globalised World*. London: NIACE.

Sagan, O. (2011c). Thou art: The multiple gaze of audio-visual, community-based participatory research. *Journal of Applied Arts & Health*, *2*: 125–136.

Sagan, O. (2014). Narratives of Arts Practice and Mental Wellbeing: Connection and Reparation. London: Routledge.

Sagan, O. (2020). The lonely legacy: Loss and testimonial injustice in the narratives of people diagnosed with personality disorder. *Mental Health and Social Inclusion*, *24* (4): 241–255.

Sagan, O. (2022). The loneliness epidemic. *Therapy Today* (December). Available at: https://www.bacp.co.uk/bacp-journals/therapy-today/2022/december-2022/articles/the-loneliness-epidemic

Sagan, O. (2024). The quiet place. *Therapy Today*, *35* (7): 46–48.

Sagan, O., & Miller, E. D. (Eds.) (2018). Narratives of Loneliness: Multidisciplinary Perspectives from the 21st Century. London: Routledge.

Sagan, O., & Sochos, A. (2015). Group attachment through art practice: A phenomenological analysis of being seen and showing. *Therapeutic Communities: The International Journal of Therapeutic Communities*, *37*: 45–56.

Salomonsson, B. (2006). The aesthetic dimension of the psychoanalytic process. *Scandinavian Psychoanalytic Review*, *29* (1): 2–12.

Sartre, J. P. (1943). *Being and Nothingness*. Washington, DC: Washington Square Press, 1993.

Schatz, B. (2012). A life in flight: Wingsuit pioneer Loïc Jean-Albert, "The Flying Dude". *Adventure Sports Journal*, 2 April.

Schiller, B. M. (2008). Saying yes to dirt, desire and difference: *Yes (2004)*. *International Journal of Psychoanalysis*, *89* (6): 1225–1235.

Schore, A. (1994). *Affect Regulation and the Origin of Self*. New York: Psychology Press.

Schore, A. (2001). Neurobiology, developmental psychology and psychoanalysis. In: J. Edwards (Ed.), *Being Alive: Building on the Work of Anne Alvarez* (pp. 57–71). London: Brunner-Routledge.

Searles, H. (1960). The Nonhuman Environment in Normal Development and in Schizophrenia. New York: International Universities Press.

Segal, H. (1952). A psycho-analytical approach to aesthetics. *International Journal of Psychoanalysis*, *33*: 196–207.

Segal, H. (1973). *Introduction to the Work of Melanie Klein*. London: Hogarth Press.

Segal, H. (1983). Some clinical implications in Melanie Klein's work. *International Journal of Psychoanalysis*, *62*: 269–276. Reprinted in: R. Hinshelwood, *A Dictionary of Kleinian Thought* (p. 358). London: Free Association Books, 1991

Segal, H. (1990). The Work of Hanna Segal: A Kleinian Approach to Clinical Practice. Northvale, NJ: Jason Aronson.

Segal, H. (1991). *Dream, Phantasy and Art*. London: Routledge.

Segal, H., & Bell, D. (1991). The theory of narcissism in the work of Freud and Klein. In: *Contemporary Freud Turning Point & Critical Issues. Freud's "On Narcissism: An Introduction"* (pp. 149–174). New Haven, CT: Yale University Press.

Seigneurie, K. (2011). *Standing by the Ruins: Elegiac Humanism in Wartime and Postwar Lebanon*. New York: Fordham University Press.

Shapcott, J. (2010). *Of Mutability*. London: Faber & Faber.

Shenfield, T., Trehub, S. E., & Nakata, T. (2003). Maternal singing modulates infant arousal. *Psychology of Music, 31* (4): 365–375.

Sheridan, M. (Dir.) (2012). *Birdmen—The Original Dream of Flight* [Film]. Proximity Productions.

Simon, B. (1988). Tragic Drama and the Family: Psychoanalytic Studies from Aeschylus to Beckett. New Haven, CT: Yale University Press.

Simon, N., Raubenheimer, K., Urho, N., Unger, S., Azoulay, D., et al. (2021). A binding global agreement to address the life cycle of plastics. *Science, 373* (6550): 43–47.

Social Work Reform Board (2010). *Building a Safe and Confident Future: One Year On—Progress Report*. London: Department of Education.

Social Work Task Force (2009). *Facing Up to the Task: The Interim Report*. London: Department of Health & Department for Schools, Children and Families.

Sodré, I. (2004). Who's who? Notes on pathological identifications. In: E. Hargreaves & A. Varchevker (Eds.), *In Pursuit of Psychic Change: The Betty Joseph Workshop* (pp. 53–68). Hove: Brunner-Rutledge.

Sodré, I. (2014). Even now, now, very now: On envy and the hatred of love (on *Othello*). In: *Imaginary Existences* (pp. 200–215). London: Routledge.

Sontag, S. (1990). *AIDS and Its Metaphors*. London: Penguin.

Spelman, E. V. (2016). *Trash Talks: Revelations in the Rubbish*. New York: Oxford University Press.

Spielberg, S. (Dir.) (2021). *West Side Story* [Film). 20th Century Studios.

Spielrein, S. (1912). Destruction as a cause of coming into being. *Journal of Analytical Psychology, 39* (No. 2, 1994): 155–186.

Spillius, E. B., Milton, J., Garvey, P., Couve, C., & Steiner, D. (2011a). *The New Dictionary of Kleinian Thought*. London: Routledge.

Spillius, E. B., Milton, J., Garvey, P., Couve, C., & Steiner, D. (2011b). Projective identification. In: *The New Dictionary of Kleinian Thought* (pp. 126–146). London: Routledge.

Stanley, L. (1992). *The Auto/Biographical I*. Manchester: Manchester University Press.

Steiner, J. (1993). Psychic Retreats: Pathological Organizations in Psychotic, Neurotic and Borderline Patients. London: Routledge.

Stephenson, S. (2020). A racist attack managing complex relationships with traumatised service users—a psychodynamic approach. *Journal of Social Work Practice, 34* (3): 225–235.

Sterba, R. F. (1965). Psychoanalysis and music. *American Imago, 22*: 96–111.

Stern, D. N. (1977). The First Relationship: Infant and Mother (The Developing Child). Cambridge, MA: Harvard University Press.

Stern, D. N. (1998). The Interpersonal World of the Infant: A View from Psychoanalysis and Developmental Psychology. London: Karnac.

Sternberg, J. (2005). Introduction: Infant Observation at the Heart of Training. London: Karnac.

Stokes, A. (1965). *The Invitation in Art*. London: Tavistock Publications. Reprinted London: Routledge, 2001.

Stone, L. (1977). The Family and Marriage in England 1500–1800. New York: Harper & Row.

Stonebridge, L. (1998). The Destructive Element: British Psychoanalysis and Modernism. Basingstoke: Macmillan.

Stonebridge, L. (2007). The Writing of Anxiety: Imagining Wartime in Mid-Century British Culture. Basingstoke: Palgrave Macmillan.

Sylvester, D. (2016). Interviews with Francis Bacon: The Brutality of Fact. London: Thames & Hudson.

Symington, N. (1993). *Narcissism: A New Theory*. London: Karnac.

Tedam, P. (2020). *Anti-Oppressive Social Work Practice*. Exeter: Learning Matters.

Teie, D. (2016). A comparative analysis of the universal elements of music and the fetal environment. *Frontiers in Psychology, 7*: 1158.

Tempest, K. (2014). Kate Tempest: Rapping changed my life. *The Guardian*, 4 October. Available at: https://www.theguardian.com/books/2014/oct/04/kate-tempest-rapping-changed-my-life?CMP=share_btn_url

Tempest, K. (2016). Interview. *The Guardian*, 26 November. Available at: https://www.theguardian.com/lifeandstyle/2016/nov/26/phoebe-waller-bridge-kate-tempest-conversation-fleabag

The Poetry Exchange (2019). *Of Mutability by Jo Shapcott—A Friend To Hannah* [Podcast, 25 April]. Available at: https://podcasts.apple.com/gb/podcast/of-mutability-by-jo-shapcott-poem-as-friend-to-hannah/id1062530220?i=1000436520108

The Tate (2008). *Interview. Cathy Wilkes: Turner Prize Nominee*. Available at: https://www.tate.org.uk/art/artists/cathy-wilkes-12144/cathy-wilkes-turner-prize-nominee-2008

Thomas, D. A. W. (2012). *Identity, Identification and Narcissistic Phantasy in the Novels of Kazuo Ishiguro*. Doctoral dissertation, University of East

London/Tavistock. Available at: https://repository.uel.ac.uk/download/c0dd6450abe1651f33f410bc577411c44384be377ea987018bc0ae-9647ab2c39/1356766/2013_PhD_Webster_Thomas.pdf

Thompson, P. (2001). The classroom and the crucible: Considerations arising from the emergence of unconscious anxiety in teaching and professional learning. *Psychoanalytic Studies, 3* (1): 23–41.

Tolpin, M. (1974). The Daedalus experience: A developmental vicissitude of the grandiose fantasy. *Annual of Psychoanalysis, 2*: 213–228

Trehub, S. E., Ghazban, & Corbeil, M. (2015). Musical affect regulation in infancy. In: *Annals of the New York Academy of Sciences, 1337* (2): 186–192.

Trilling, L. (1951). Freud and literature. In: *The Liberal Imagination* (pp. 34–57). London: Mercury Books.

Trowell, J., & Miles, G. (Eds.) (1991). The contribution of observation training to professional development in social work. *Journal of Social Work Practice, 5* (1): 51–60.

Tuckett, D. (1994). The conceptualisation and communication of clinical facts in psychoanalysis. *International Journal of Psychoanalysis, 75*: 865–870.

Waddell, M. (1989). Living in two worlds: Psychodynamic theory and social work practice. *Free Associations, 15*: 11–35.

Waddell, M. (1998a). Appendix. In: *Inside Lives: Psychoanalysis and the Growth of the Personality* (pp. 213–217). London: Duckworth.

Waddell, M. (1998b). *Inside Lives*. London: Duckworth.

Waddell, M. (2018). *On Adolescence*. London: Routledge.

Watermeyer, B. (2013). Towards a Contextual Psychology of Disablism. London: Routledge.

Watt, B. (2021). *The Slow Death of Welsh Harp—Crisis Update*. Available at: https://benwatt.com/play/article/the-slow-death-of-welsh-harp-crisis-update

Weintrobe, S. (Ed.) (2013). Engaging with Climate Change: Psychoanalytic and Interdisciplinary Perspectives. London: Routledge.

Weintrobe, S. (2018). Communicating psychoanalytic ideas about climate change: A case study. In: P. Garvey & K. Long (Eds.), *The Klein Tradition: Lines of Development—Evolution of Theory and Practice over the Decades* (pp. 411–426). London: Routledge.

Weintrobe, S. (2021). Psychological Roots of the Climate Crisis: Neoliberal Exceptionalism and the Culture of Uncare. New York: Bloomsbury Academic.

Williams, R. (1963). Recent English drama. In: B. Ford (Ed.), *The Modern Age. Pelican Guide to English Literature, Vol. 7* (2nd edition, pp. 531–545). Harmondsworth: Penguin.

Williams, R. (1968). *Drama from Ibsen to Brecht*. London: Penguin.

Williams, R. (1977). *Marxism and Literature*. London: Oxford University Press.

Wilson, J. Q., & Kelling, G. L. (1982). Broken windows: The police and neighborhood safety. *The Atlantic*, March. Available at: https://www.theatlantic.com/magazine/archive/1982/03/broken-windows/304465

Wilson, K., Ruch., Lymbery, M., & Cooper, A. (Eds.) (2008). *Social Work: An Introduction to Contemporary Practice* (2nd edition). London: Pearson, 2011.

Winnicott, D. W. (1953). Transitional objects and transitional phenomena: A study of the first not-me possession. *International Journal of Psychoanalysis, 34*: 89–97.

Winnicott, D. W. (1960). The relationship of a mother to her baby. In: *The Family and Individual Development*. London: Routledge, 2006.

Winnicott, D. W. (1963a). The capacity for concern. In: The Maturational Processes and the Facilitating Environment: Studies in the Theory of Emotional Development. London: Karnac, 1990.

Winnicott, D. W. (1963b). Communicating and not communicating leading to a study of certain opposites. In: *The Maturational Processes and the Facilitating Environment: Studies in the Theory of Emotional Development*. London: Hogarth Press, 1965.

Winnicott, D. W. (1965). The Maturational Processes and the Facilitating Environment: Studies in the Theory of Emotional Development. London: Hogarth Press.

Winnicott, D. W. (1967). Mirror-role of mother and family in child development. In: *Playing and Reality* (pp. 111–118). London: Routledge, 1971.

Winnicott, D. W. (1971a). The location of cultural experience. In: *Playing and Reality* (pp. 95–103). London: Routledge.

Winnicott, D. W. (1971b). *Playing and Reality*. London: Routledge.

Wodehouse, P. G. (1916). *Leave It To Jeeves*. London: Simon & Schuster.

Wood, D. (Ed.) (1992). On Paul Ricoeur: Narrative and Interpretation. London: Routledge.

Woolf, W. (2009). On being ill. In: *Selected Essays*, ed. D. Bradshaw. London: Oxford University Press.

Wordsworth, W. (1799). The Prelude or, Growth of a Poet's Mind: An Autobiographical Poem. Oxford: Clarendon Press, 1926.

Wright, K. (2009). Mirroring and Attunement: Self-Realization in Psychoanalysis and Art. London: Routledge.

Yang, T.-S. (2008). *The Miserable Nolbu and the Blessed Heungbu*. Seoul: Tree of Thought.

Yeats, W. B. (1924). *Essays*. London: MacMillan.

Yeats, W. B. (1994). The Collected Works of W.B. Yeats. Vol. 5: Late Essays. New York: Simon & Schuster.

Yelloly, M., & Henkel, M. (Eds.) (1995). *Learning and Teaching in Social Work: Towards Reflective Practice*. London: Jessica Kingsley.

Yeshurun, H. (2012). Exile is so strong within me, I may bring it to the land. A landmark 1996 interview with Mahmoud Darwish. *Journal of Palestine Studies, 42* (1): 46–70.

Yousef, T. (2011). Mahmoud Darwish and the quest for identity. *Dirasat, 38* (2): 674–687.

YouTube (2011). *L'enfant et les Sortilèges—Theatro Municipal de São Paulo—outubro de 2011*. Available at: http://www.youtube.com/watch?v=IXKCTIQInfk

YouTube (2013). *Psy—Gentleman M/V*. Available at: http://www.youtube.com/watch?v=ASO_zypdnsQ

Zeman, A., Milton, F., Smith, A., & Rylance, R. (2013). By heart: A study of brain activation by poetry and prose. *Journal of Consciousness Studies, 20* (9–10): 132–158.

Zhang, J., Wang, L., Trasande, L. & Kannan, K. (2021). Occurrence of polyethylene terephthalate and polycarbonate microplastics in infant and adult feces. *Environmental Science & Technology Letters, 8* (11): 989–994.

Žižek, S. (2008). *Examined Life: Philosophy Is in the Streets*. Available at: https://www.youtube.com/watch?v=j_K_79O21hk&t=64s&ab_channel=TOP Documentary

CREDITS

The editors also gratefully acknowledge the permission given to reprint the following materials.

"The Police Dog" by Megumi Oonaka and Yoshimi Sato reproduced by permission of the copyright holder

Edwards, J. "This is not for tears: thinking – poetry and psychoanalysis in orbit" first published in *British Journal of Psychotherapy*, 34, 2 (2018) and reproduced by kind permission of John Wiley and Sons Ltd. Copyright © 2018 John Wiley & Sons Ltd. and the British Psychotherapy Foundation. All rights reserved. No part of this publication may be reproduced, stored or transmitted in any form or by any means without the prior permission in writing from the copyright holder.

"Of Mutability" copyright © Jo Shapcott, 2010 from *Of Mutability* by Jo Shapcott reprinted by permission of Faber and Faber

Mahmoud Darwish, "In Her Absence I Created her Image" from *The Butterfly's Burden*, translated by Fady Joudah. Copyright © 2007 by Mahmoud Darwish. Translation copyright © 2007 by Fady Joudah. Reprinted with the permission of The Permissions Company, LLC on behalf of Copper Canyon Press, coppercanyonpress.org.

Excerpts from *The Remains of the Day* copyright © Kazuo Ishiguro 1989 reprinted by permission of Faber and Faber Ltd.

INDEX